Helio's

MW00454501

Web: www.he

orders@helioslondon.com

Email: info@helioslondon.com

8 New Row
Covent gardens
London, WC2N4LJ
020 - 7379 - 7454

APPLYING BACH FLOWER THERAPY TO THE HEALING PROFESSION OF HOMEOPATHY

PSYCHOLOGY, PSYCHIATRY, PSYCHOSOMATIC MEDICINE

By

Dr. Cornelia Richardson-Boedler,

N.M.D., H.M.D., M.A., BCFM, MFCC

B. Jain Publishers (P) Ltd.
New Delhi

First Complete and Enlarged Printed Edition: 1997 by B. Jain.
Revised Second Edition : 2002

APPLYING BACH FLOWER THERAPY TO THE HEALING PROFESSION OF HOMEOPATHY

Reprint edition 2005

Price. Rs. 229.00

Published by:
Kuldeep Jain
for
B. Jain Publishers (P) Ltd.
1921, Street No. 10, Chuna Mandi,
Paharganj, New Delhi 110 055 (INDIA)
Ph: 2358 0800, 2358 1100, 2358 1300, 2358 3100
Fax: 011-2358 0471; Email: bjain@vsnl.com
Website: www.bjainbooks.com

Printed in India by:
Unisons Techno Financial Consultants (P) Ltd.
522, FIE, Patpar Ganj, Delhi - 110 092

ISBN : 81-7021-786-5
BOOK CODE : BC-5220

```
DEDICATED
TO THOSE
IN SEARCH OF
GENTLE CURE
```

The phoenix Foundation for Spiritual Growth and
The World Health Foundation for Peace

Welcome

Cornelia Richardson, M.F.C.C.

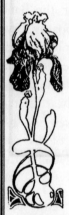

Bach Flower Remedies
for Transformation

Friday, September 23
7.30 p.m.
University Christian Church
2401 Leconte (Entrance on Scenic)
Berkeley
$ 10 Donation

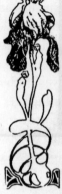

*Cornelia Richardson, M.F.C.C., is a lay homeopath and Bach
Flower practitioner who combines the physical healing powers
of homeopathy with the mental, psychic, and emotional
transformation of Bach Flower remedies. Cornelia will
discuss the many aspects of these vibrational remedies
and their amazing healing properties. All are welcome.*

**The above talk was given by the author on September 23,
1988, in Berkeley, California. The contents of the talk were
based on her experience as psychotherapist and practicing specialist of Bach Flower Remedies and conveyed her
first insights, gained during her early homeopathic training, regarding the combined method of homeopathy and
Bach Flower Therapy.**

PREFACE

he following two books aim at showing the unique use of Bach Flower Therapy in those professions that endeavor to heal human beings from diseases and discomfort in mind/emotions and body. In particular, the Bach Remedies are being applied to the fields of homeopathy, psychology, psychiatry, and psychosomatic medicine. These fields of knowledge consider mind/emotions as causative factors in the development of illness, and, therefore, they lend themselves to the application of the Bach Remedies. Edward Bach, the founder of the Bach Flowers' healing system, saw the imbalances in the personality as the core elements of disease; thus, the disease works from the inner life of the psyche to the outward manifestations of physical illness.

The Bach Remedies, applied to those current treatment methods that include the consideration of mind/emotions, offer a unique and gentle way of cure. The field of homeopathy, profound in its approach to the cure of mind and body, is addressed in book 1. From close observation of patient cases, a unique catalytic effect of Bach Remedies in homeopathic treatment could be determined, with the effect of rendering homeopathic cure more deepened and permanent. For a broader understanding, the historical discovery and systematic analysis of both methods of healing, homeopathy and Bach Flower Therapy, is given, plus a description of their unique differences, and their cooperative healing power.

In addition to the thorough presentation of the Bach Flowers' healing system in book 1, each remedy will be examined further in its dynamics in book 2 and offered as healing medicine in respect of specified conditions and indications. The remedies' psychological dynamics span the field of psychology, shedding light on the diversified nuances of man's consciousness, exploring the various shades of feelings and of cognitive disturbances or hindrances; Bach Remedies are also applied to all major categories of mental illness, as classified in the American Psychiatric Association's *Diagnostic and Statistical Manual of Mental Illness*. In psychosomatic medicine, the physical concomitants of psychological disturbance have been observed; major tendencies of psychosomatic dynamics can be outlined and the Bach Remedies applied accordingly.

In reference to the natural and biological aspects of the plants, and by application of the Doctrine of Signatures, the remedies are further explored in their deeper meaning; the use of imagery and symbolism enhances the integration of the knowledge and opens the mind to the joy and wisdom found in nature.

The remedies are nature's gift to us all, lay persons and professionals alike, and they lend their healing graces to all living and animated creation.

The book is written in such a way as to appeal to all minds that are in search of a deeper understanding of the healing remedies and of healing dynamics in general. It guides lay person and professional alike from the beginnings of homeopathy and Bach Flower Therapy to the exact therapeutic use of the Bach Remedies in the diseases and mental disturbances of our time.

Cornelia Richardson-Boedler,
Westwood Hills,   N.M.D., M.A.
Kansas, 1996.

ACKNOWLEDGMENTS

*T*his work represents years of experience of working with the combined effects of Bach Remedies and homeopathic remedies. Close observation of cases taught me the astounding catalytic power of Bach Remedies in eliciting a clear homeopathic remedy picture and leading to accelerated and more deepened cure. These insights were also formulated for the British Institute of Homoeopathy in my doctoral dissertation of 1993, on which this work is based. The following text, with only minimal revisions and excluding chapters 1 and 8, is also represented in my *Richardson-Boedler Bach Repertory* and offered as computer software since 1993.

I extend my gratitude to Louis DelValle, physicist, for reviewing the original manuscript.

Much of my learning and observation took place within the Homeopathic Study Group of the Eastbay (Berkeley, California), attended by the medical doctor Ellen Gunther, M.D. I am grateful for the introductory words she wrote in regard to this written work:

Sometimes a new way of looking at old principles brings about an important change in the whole order of things. We all recognize that emotions play a large part in the production of disease, and different emotions tend to produce certain kinds of disease.

Now, Cornelia Richardson-Boedler has developed ideas of how this principle can be used in the practical world of therapy. She deals with the emotional components of illness by using the Bach Flower Remedies that were potentized by either direct sunlight or by boiling. The Bach Remedies help relieve the person's original stress. Once the person is more balanced emotionally, he is then ready to be more receptive to the energetic force of homeopathic medicines. It is as if impediments to recovery are put aside and the person's vital force is able to heal at deeper levels and with increased speed.

Cornelia Richardson-Boedler, through her insights as a trained psychotherapist, worked by combining the Bach Remedies within the homeopathic study group which was then under my consultation and medical supervision. Her work is innovative and deserves to be considered by every practicing homeopath. She is to be complimented for teaching Bach Remedies in a new way. I hope you will enjoy this text and learn as much as I did.

Ellen Gunther, M.D.
Berkeley, California, 1992.

viii

CONTENTS

BOOK ONE

BACH FLOWER REMEDIES — CATALYSTS
IN HOMEOPATHIC CURE

Chapter – 1

Chapter – 2

ix

Chapter – 5

Chapter – 6

Chapter – 7

Chapter – 8

BOOK TWO

THE PSYCHOLOGICAL/CONSTITUTIONAL ESSENCES
OF THE BACK GLOWER REMEDIES

BOOK ONE

BACH FLOWER REMEDIES -- CATALYSTS IN HOMEOPATHIC CURE

Includes the Historical Discovery and Systematic Analysis of Homeopathy and Bach Flower Therapy

Bach Flowers

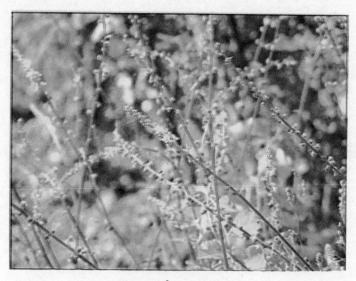

Agrimony

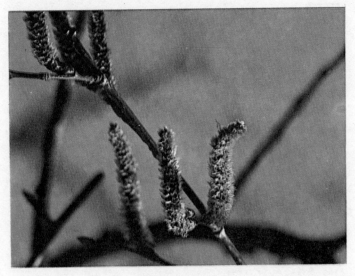

Aspen

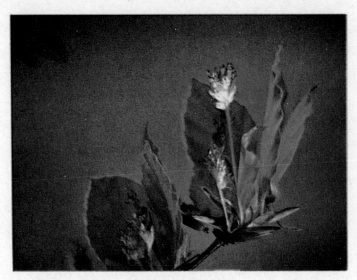

Beech

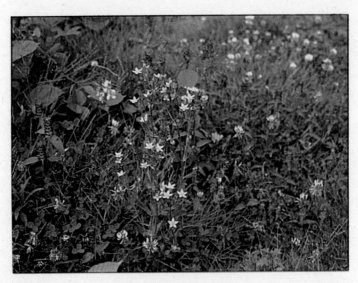

Centaury

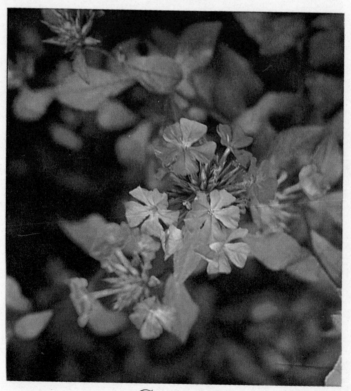

Cerato

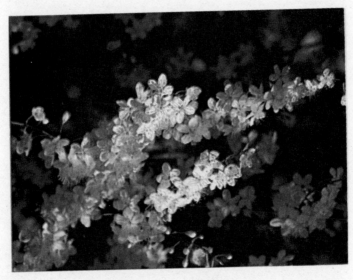

Cherry Plum

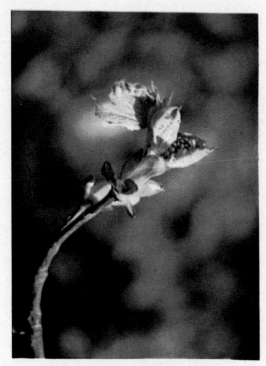

Chestnut Bud

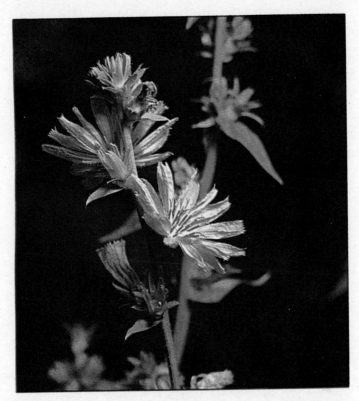

Chicory

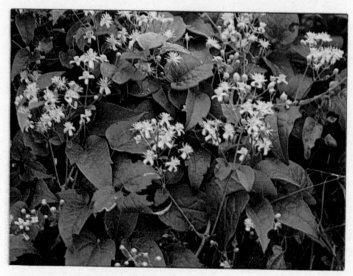

Clematis

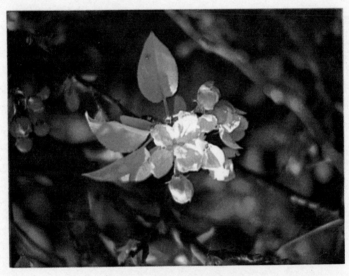

Crab Apple

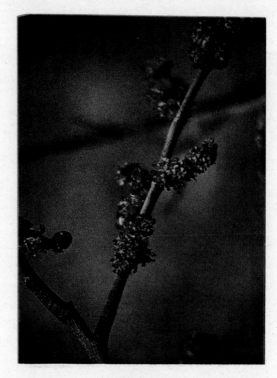

Elm

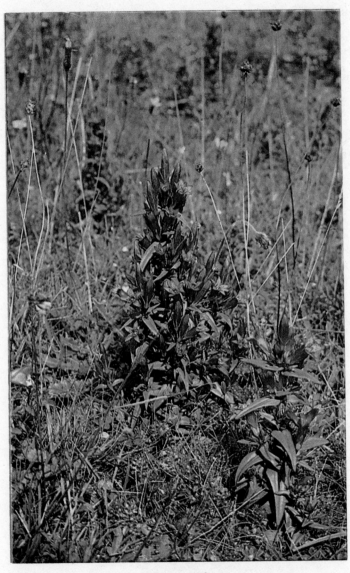

Gentian

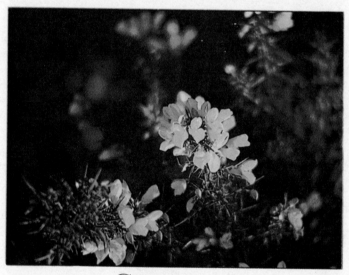

Gorse

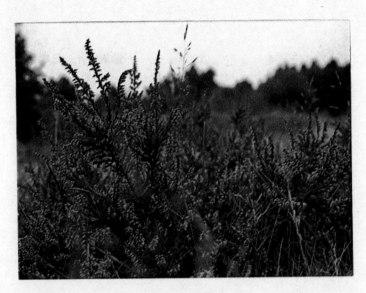

Heather

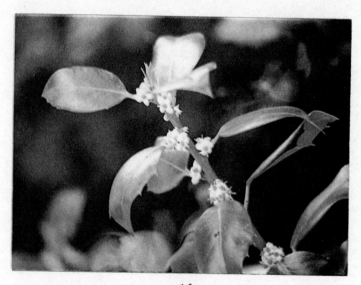

Holly

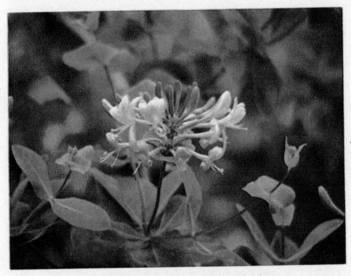

Honey Suckle

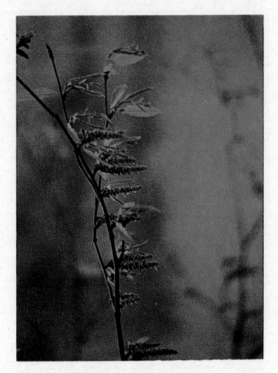

Horn Beam

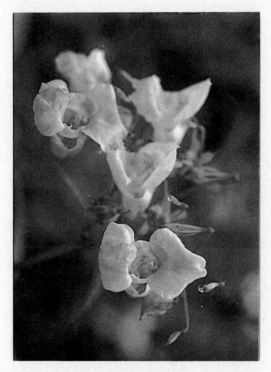

Impatiens

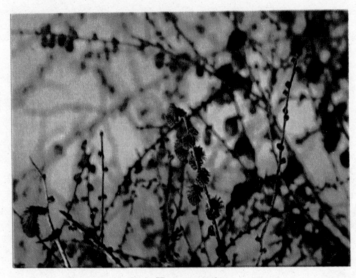

Larch

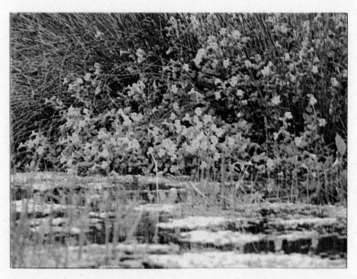

Mimulus

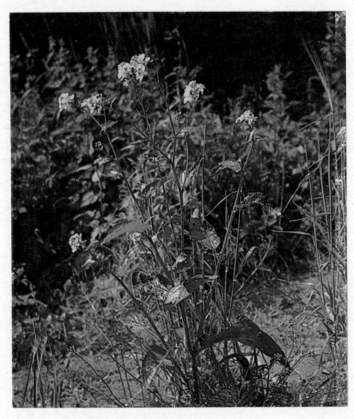

Mustard

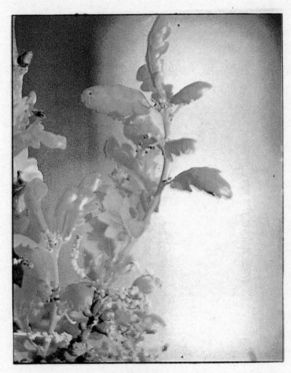

Oak

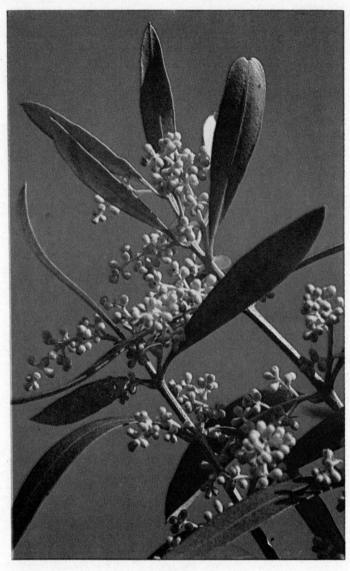

Olive

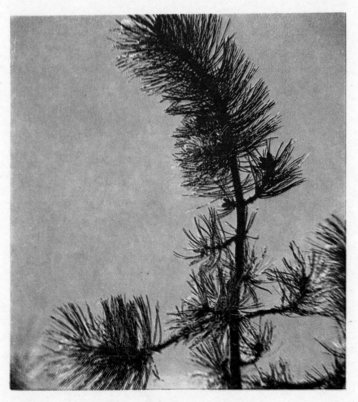

Pine

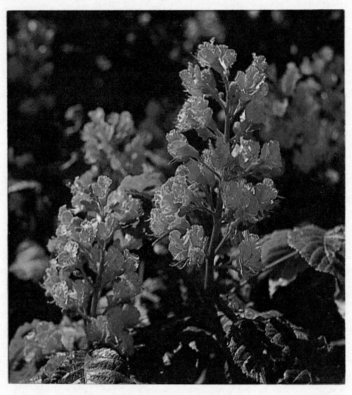

Red Chestnut

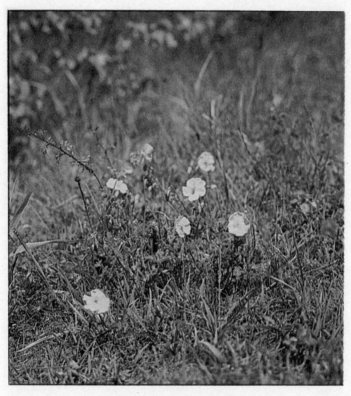

Rock Rose

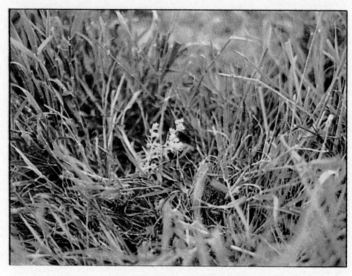

Scleranthus

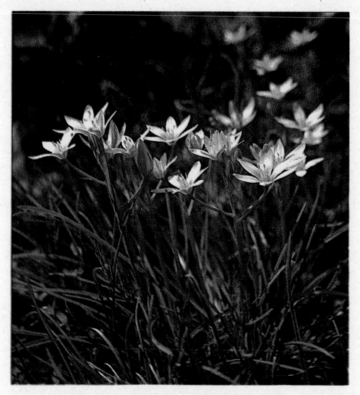

Star of Bethlehem

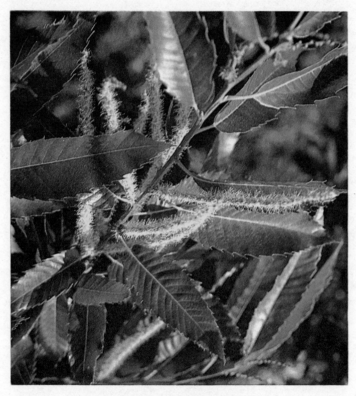

Sweet Chestnut

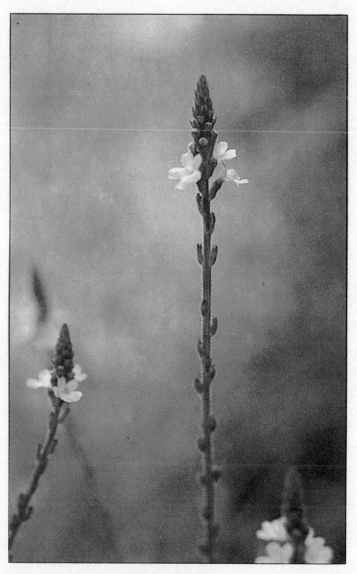

Vervain

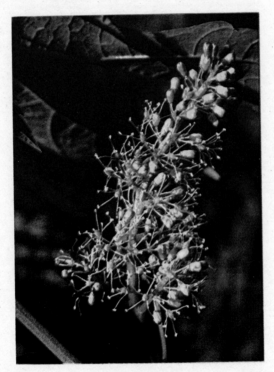

Vine

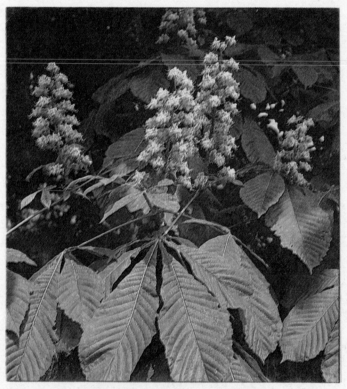

White Chestnut

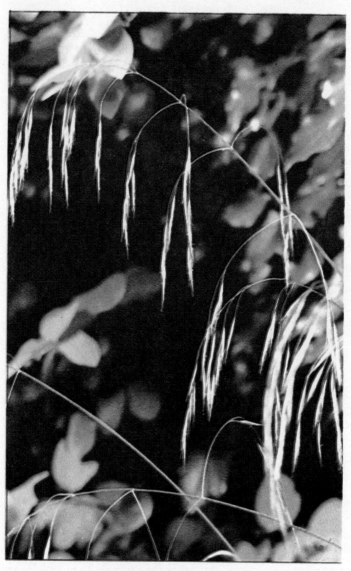

Wild Oat

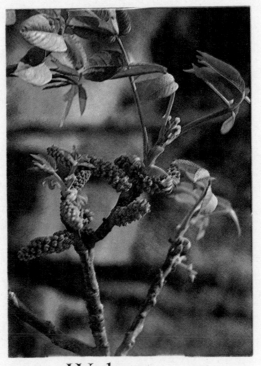

Walnut

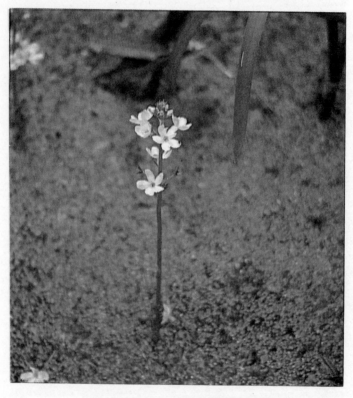

Water Violet

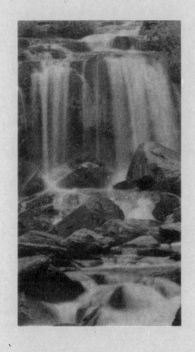

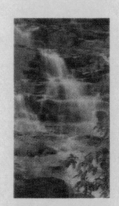

ROCK WATER (27)

(SELF REPRESSION AND DENIAL)

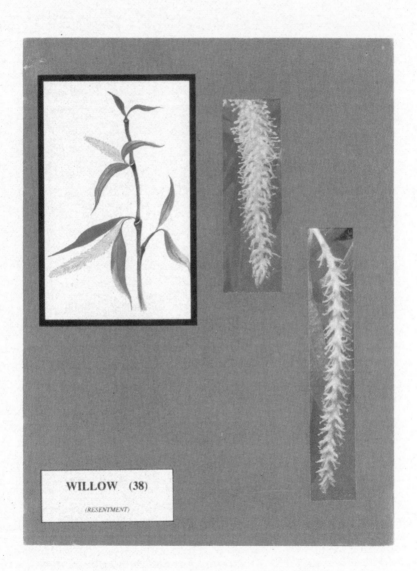

WILLOW (38)

(RESENTMENT)

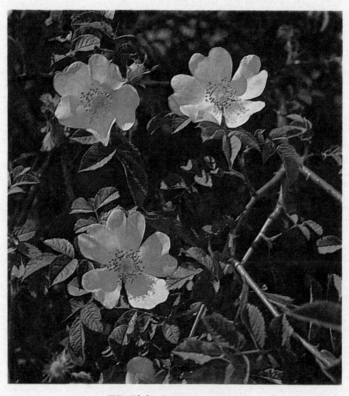

Wild Rose

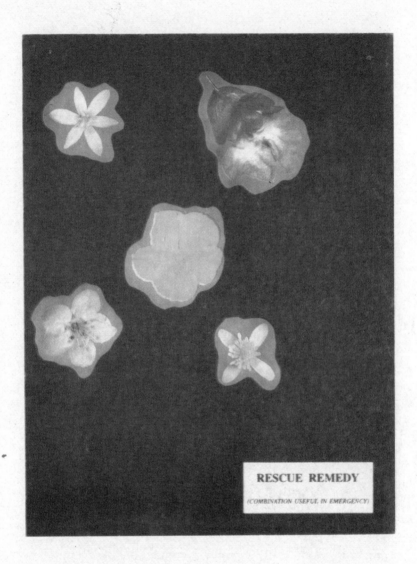

RESCUE REMEDY

(COMBINATION USEFUL IN EMERGENCY)

INTRODUCTION

*B*ook One explains two methods of alternative medi cine, namely homeopathy and Bach Flower Therapy, and shows how they work together to achieve cure.

Alternative medicine offers homeopathic medicine and Bach Flower Therapy as two holistic approaches to the healing of mind and body. Classical homeopathy, as founded by Dr. Samuel Hahnemann, uses remedies taken from nature and from some chemical compounds that stimulate the defense mechanism of the mind/emotions and body totality to achieve cure. One remedy at a time, individually selected according to the patient's need, is the treatment method of classical homeopathy, as compared to other approaches within the field which prescribe combinations of homeopathic remedies for recognized states of illness. This thesis deals with classical homeopathy, which is considered the mainstream in homeopathic care, and, therefore, the word "classical" will not be used in the subsequent text when homeopathy is referred to.

Whereas homeopathy is prescribed on the totality of

symptoms of mind/ emotions and body, the Bach Remedies are indicated according to specific mental/emotional symptoms and aim directly at healing those mental/ emotional imbalances that underly illness and hinder the progress of healing. As the mind/emotions balance under the impact of the Bach Remedies, the physical sites affected by emotions begin healing as well. Bach Remedies can be prescribed in single dose or in combination; often there are several imbalances which need to be addressed. This system of healing was founded by Dr. Bach, who was also a homeopath, and it is considered a branch of homeopathy, yet it has a unique approach to reaching and healing the deepest aspects of self and soul, even beyond the power of homeopathy. Thirty-eight remedies taken from flowers, bushes, trees, and a special source of water aim at restoring all mental/emotional imbalances possibly experienced by man.

The combination of these two holistic approaches in the healing of mind and body yields outstanding practical results. Close observation of the healing process, stimulated by both healing methods, led to new insights into the special workings of Bach Remedies within homeopathic treatment. Bach Remedies were found to heighten receptivity of the vital force to the healing effects of homeopathic medicines. An explanation of how this works will be given, plus a history of discovery of both methods of cure and an analysis of how cure happens in either system. Two true case presentations, done under medical supervision, will exemplify this new dynamic of cure. Twelve sample cases, presenting all thirty-eight Bach Remedies and homeopathic remedies specific to the case, will highlight the combined treatment method further.

WHY USE BACH REMEDIES CONCURRENTLY
WITH HOMEOPATHIC REMEDIES?

> ⚘ *The Significance of Homeopathy and How the Bach Remedies Fit in*
>
> ⚘ *The Helpful Effects of Bach Remedies During Homeopathic Treatment*

THE SIGNIFiCANCE OF HOMEOPATHY AND HOW THE BACH REMEDIES FIT IN

Homeopathy heals the totality of the human being, that is, mind, emotions, and body. The innate defense mechanism is strengthened by homeopathic medicines so that healing of symptoms is made possible from within. Homeopathy stimulates the mind/emotions and body totality to cure itself, whereas conventional medical treatment aims at doing it for the body by use of selected medicines that do not directly encourage the defense mechanism to help itself.

The homeopath takes the patient's case by closely investigating symptoms expressed by the vital force on all three levels of being, namely, mind, emotions and body. The mind is analyzed in its functional strength, clarity and purpose, and in its angles of perception and judgment. Emotions are strongly interwoven with the mental state, yet they more fully account for the force and dynamic of the person, expressing the longings and disappointments, the joys and needs. The body reflects the effects of mind/emotions; it is the physical representation of our inner selves. The vital force, being the innate higher principle or life spark that governs the defense mechanism, expresses imbalances through symptoms which are experienced by the patient, usually on all three levels, and then shared with the observing homeopath. The homeopath collects all symptoms, studies the overall picture and determines a homeopathic remedy that is known to be curative with the patient's combination of symptoms. If the remedy is chosen correctly, healing is speedy and effective in body, mind, and emotions also. Homeopathic cures can be miraculous; they can turn one's whole life around. Undoubtedly, homeopathy will be the medicine of the future, establishing itself worldwide.

Where then do the Bach Remedies come in? Whereas homeopathy aims at curing the overall symptomatology of the body, mind and emotions, the Bach Remedies more specifically aim at releasing mental and emotional imbalance. They work more deeply and lastingly than homeopathic medicines in the mental/emotional area which, through the Bach Remedies, is stimulated by innate healing impulses to rebalance itself. Bach Remedies also heal in the physical realm. There is an immediate lightening in the area of the body that is negatively influenced by specific blocked emotions. Organic damage can also be released over time, but not as speedily as with homeopathic remedies. If both methods are combined, they complement each other and yield outstanding results. One method is making the other more effective if both are used concurrently.

These combined effects, although beneficial for all types of diseases, are most easily recognizable in the treatment of chronic disease or milder chronic discomfort that originated in mental/emotional imbalance. Mental/ emotional and physical illness resulting from accidents, or degenerative defects, or old age symptoms, excepting those old age symptoms of psychosomatic origin, are more directly helped by homeopathic treatment, since these medicines more powerfully affect the physical body. In these cases of mostly physical causation, however, Bach Remedies also aid in the process of recovery and help clear the mental/emotional side effects of the trauma or degenerative defect. The attitude that one holds toward one's illness or impairment may impede healing and delay overall progress of recovery, especially should one feel powerlessness, hopelessness, anger, fear, denial, or shame about one's plight. The Bach Remedies can work successfully on this mental/emotional impediment so that the overall organism and one's consciousness is freed to attend to the curative process and allow the homeopathic remedies to do their optimal work.

THE HELPFUL EFFECTS OF BACH REMEDIES DURING HOMEOPATHIC TREATMENT

The foremost contribution of Bach Remedies during homeopathic treatment is the deepening of mental and emotional healing which is of vital importance during the process of cure.

It is generally acknowledged that disturbing mental/emotional factors trigger acute or chronic states of illness, whereas health in mind/emotions furthers health throughout the organism. Not only alternative medicine, such as homeopathy and Bach Flower Therapy, but also modern medical science, through the field of psychosomatic medicine, has explored the special connection between mind/emotions and body during illness and health.

Bach Remedies, when given during homeopathic treatment, help release the mental/emotional imbalance that triggered the illness in the beginning, persisted throughout the course of illness and propelled it further. Not only chronic disease states but also acute illnesses are greatly helped by the added use of Bach Remedies, especially if strong mental/emotional factors exist or were initially responsible for the breakdown in health. In general, healing is furthered and relapse into former mental/emotional patterns prevented as homeopathy and Bach Flower Therapy work together to achieve cure. Once healing is established, Bach Remedies, if taken for temporary imbalances, safeguard mental health and emotional happiness, and they render previous homeopathic cure more lasting and effective.

I have also observed a special catalytic effect of Bach Remedies that goes beyond emotional balancing itself, especially in long term homeopathic treatment of chronic discomfort or chronic disease. If only Bach Remedies are given at the beginning of the treatment, the vital force is energized and stimulated in a new way, since negative blockage of mind and emotions, which takes up valuable energy, diminishes. A strengthened vital force, more able to organize itself, will bring to the forefront the first aspect or layer of health disturbance that is most responsible for the present state of illness or discomfort. Homeopathic treatment usually involves clearing several layers of symptomatic expression before lasting cure is reached. This first important layer is not necessarily the one on "top" of all layers but may arise from deep within the economy, where it created the most influential disturbance in the overall health. Depending on the case, this process of emergence may take days or weeks until the layer is fully visible. This first main remedy picture, crucial in the overall cure, will be presented in a coherent, unified way, ready to be percieved by the homeopath, and ready to be released most effectively by the indicated homeopathic remedy. Real progress of cure is now possible, since the Bach Remedies heightened the receptivity of the vital force to the healing effects of homeopathic medicines.

A homeopathic remedy picture is usually discernible right at the beginning of treatment in varying degrees of clarity. A clear case calls for the immediate use of a homeopathic remedy that is given with or without the addition of Bach Remedies. Often, however, symptoms seem "disorganized," or there is a lack of clarity of physical symptoms and over emphasis of mental/emotional symptoms. The homeopath may then want to give the first discernible remedy right at the beginning of treatment along with the Bach Remedies. This would be beneficial, since the Bach Remedies would help the homeopathic remedy to work better and also further the emergence of new layers. Except in an urgent case or a clearly discernible case, it may be of benefit, however, to begin treatment with Bach Remedies only to allow the vital force to determine the first crucial layer to be released. Bach Remedies serve as catalysts; they open the case and set in motion the unraveling of innate health disturbances or layers.

As the layer emerges, the remedy picture becomes clearer by increased accuracy, not by severity of symptoms, especially on the physical plane. Under the influence of the Bach Remedies, symptoms mobilize into coherence, and, should new minor symptoms arise, they are usually on the periphery, pointing to a more complete recognition of the indicated remedy. On the physical plane, symptoms have been present before, but they are often not highlighted as clearly by the vital force in terms of coherence of the first important remedy picture to be released, especially if imbalances were expressed mostly on the mental/emotional plane which represents the first outlet or expression for the vital force. Without the catalytic effect of Bach Remedies, physical symptoms often point to several remedies or layers, making initial prescribing difficult. As Bach Remedies release mental/emotional disturbance during initial treatment of the case, a balancing or release effect from over-emphasis in the mental/emotional plane to the physical plane is observable, while the vital force is freed to express itself more accurately in terms of physical imbalance. This explains how the catalytic effect toward coherence of symptoms, especially physical ones, is achieved. Since homeopathy addresses the physical realm very effectively, the homeopathic medicines can now do their work best. Possible short-term initial aggravation of symptoms, which can occur, especially after a single high dose of a homeopathic remedy, is also greatly diminished when Bach Remedies are given simultaneously. Overall, prescribing becomes easier and more beneficent, since the homeopathic picture of the case has become more accurate and the vital force can respond more promptly to the indicated remedy.

Homeopaths may consider that, due to the healing of the mind and emotions in response to the Bach Remedy intake, the homeopathic remedy picture may be less complete, since mental/emotional imbalances are important factors of overall symptomatology. It is true that mental/emotional symptoms will be less acute, yet the tendency and disposition towards certain mental/emotional imbalances will remain in essence, being integrated into the overall coherence of symptoms. In some cases, a "flareup" or non-alarming highlighting of the mental/emotional imbalances as well can be observed, as the homeopathic picture presents itself fully, although the mind/emotions had been improving steadily. I assume that possible physiological imbalances that may have developed over time in response to some states of mental/emotional imbalance are being highlighted, along with other physical symptoms, during this crucial "flareup" period. As this concomitant physical disturbance comes to the fore, the mind/emotions may relive their related state of imbalance again in fuller impact. Should a homeopathic remedy not be given at this point, the Bach Remedies themselves would rebalance mental/emotional well-being and lead toward physical cure as well, but at a slower pace than homeopathic remedies. Bach Remedies are known to effectively release physical discomfort or even disease due to psychosomatic origin, if given time to do their optimal work.

The homeopathic remedy, when given during this crucial time of highlighting of symptoms, works most powerfully on the physical side effects wrought over time by the mental/emotional imbalance, while simultaneously stimulating mental/emotional healing and clarity further, and also, similar to the Bach Remedies, touching at higher levels of consciousness. The vital force is now freed of its main health disturbance and stimulated further to release remaining innate health imbalances or homeopathic layers, while the same Bach Remedies, for safeguarding progress, or newly indicated Bach Remedies are continued and the curative action of the first homeopathic remedy remains.

In order to understand this process, homeopathy and Bach Flower Therapy will be explained; how they were discovered, how they work, and how both methods combine in treatment. Furthermore, since recognition of the indicated Bach Remedies is crucial for cure, all thirty-eight Bach Remedies will be analyzed by use of creatively presented case material. Throughout this work, several homeopathic remedies will also be highlighted in their main keynotes and characteristics, also in regard to their complementary function for Bach Remedies.

2

HOMEOPATHY: DISCOVERY AND HOW IT WORKS

> 🐝 Hahnemann's Discovery of the Homeopathic Law of Similars by Use of Cinchona Bark
>
> 🐝 Provings and Preparations of Homeopathic Medicines
>
> 🐝 Possible Explanations, Scientific and Philosophical, of How the Remedies Act After Avogadro's Number
>
> 🐝 The Case of Beatrice: Case Taking Techniques and Determination of the Indicated Homeopathic Remedy

HAHNEMANN'S DISCOVERY OF THE HOMEOPATHIC LAW OF SIMILARS BY USE OF CINCHONA BARK

Homeopathic medicines, when given to a sick person, work by stimulating the defense mechanism to cure. The remedies initiate the healing process in body, mind and emotions. Cure is usually thorough, swift and lasting, and the patient often feels so uplifted and regenerated that even his former healthy self does not compare to the newly found wellness he experiences. How do the medicines work to achieve such an effect?

Samuel Hahnemann (1755-1843), physician, in his medical searches for effective medicines, read about a special healing substance prepared from Cinchona bark that was used by the natives of South America to treat malaria. Hahnemann was impressed by the astounding curative ability of Cinchona bark, and he decided to test this healing substance on himself, although he was in good health. His goal was to determine and observe the effects of this substance on the organism. To his surprise, after a few days of repeated intake, he developed symptoms of fever, such as those which occur in malaria. As soon as the drug was discontinued, those symptoms disappeared and he was well again. He concluded: "Peruvian bark, which is used as a remedy for intermittent fever, acts because it can produce symptoms similar to those of intermittent fever in healthy people."[1]

How can this phenomenon be explained? How can the healing agent itself produce in a healthy body those same symptoms of sickness that it cures in a sick body that was infected by a parasitic sporozoite which causes malaria? At the time, Hahnemann himself did not understand how this works, but based on his observations he further formulated a new law, namely the homeopathic law of similars: *Similia Similibus Curentur* (let like be cured by like). The very name "homeopathy" means "likeness of feeling" in Greek language. He further concluded that Cinchona bark is the one specific agent furnished by nature and best suitable to heal those matching symptoms that the vital force expresses during malaria or that type of intermittent fever. He later found out that *China (Cinchona officinalis),* as he named the remedy, has a wide range of action beyond malaria and was indicated to cure many more specific physical and mental/emotional symptoms in acute and chronic diseases, all of which fit the overall character and symptomatology of the remedy *China.*

Here is a question that comes to mind: Based on Hahnemann's experience of becoming ill from this medicine, one wonders why the sick person does not get sicker also upon receiving the powder gained from the healing bark. Firstly, one has to differentiate between the crude, fresh substance and the medicinally prepared substance. Cinchona is known as poisonous, and it would certainly lead to intestinal poisoning and further severe symptoms, should it be taken in crude, unrefined form straight from the bark, no matter if the person is initially healthy or sick. The powder he used, however, had already been prepared and refined medicinally by the knowledgeable South American Indians who had discovered the plant's healing power and experimented with it over the centuries. Hahnemann had tested this refined, dried substance, not the fresh, highly poisonous juicy extract from Cinchona bark; still, even the refined substance, if taken repeatedly over several days, had enough harmful content to create temporary symptoms in his initially healthy body. This minimally harmful content, however, does not harm the sick person but restores health instead.

This can be explained by the fact that the sick body, infected by the parasite, had already expressed those very symptoms that the drug creates in a healthy body. The vital force could not respond further. Instead, it responded to the innate healing power that must be contained in the plant and had been activated by medicinal refinement and preparation, such as by drying and grinding or trituration. This innate healing power achieves cure by resonating in a fortifying and healing way with the symptoms which are the defense mechanism's attempt to express and ward off the disease.

Hahnemann, inspired by his findings, was convinced that a new avenue to the treatment of disease had been found, and he set out to research and test more remedies which, if taken repeatedly by a healthy person, would mirror symptoms of known or hitherto unidentified disease states and cure them.

PROVINGS AND PREPARATIONS OF HOMEOPATHIC MEDICINES

Hahnemann selected more remedies from nature, mostly plants known to affect or disturb the organism, and he administered them to himself and other healthy people in small and refined doses. All participants took part of these *provings* of medicines on a voluntary basis, recording faithfully each new symptom caused by the medicines.[2] Hahnemann knew then to employ these medicines in the treatment of his patients whose disease states mirrored those artificially induced by provings but were contracted from natural causes such as from a virus, lack of nutrition, physical exhaustion, or mental/emotional chagrin. His healing record was excellent, and he further proved that a close link existed between the different expressions of the vital force during illness and those substances of nature that are matched in their medicinal effect to heal the diverse states of illness, each unique with a specific set of physical and mental/emotional symptoms. As if planned by higher intelligence, nature provided all substances necessary to cure all possible states of sickness, as they can be experienced by living organisms, that is, people, animals and vegetation as well.

Over the years, Hahnemann extracted healing power from many different sources of nature, not only from plants but also from animals, geographical matter and chemical compounds derived from nature. Many remedies were discovered accidentally, for example the remedy *Sepia (Sepia officinalis)* which is extracted from the ink of the cuttlefish. Hahnemann knew an artist who used this ink for his paintings and had the habit of licking the brush, subjecting himself to this special substance.[3] He complained to Hahnemann of several symptoms that Hahnemann in his ingenuity traced back to the brown ink. Upon Hahnemann's recommendation, the habit of licking the brush was discontinued and all symptoms disappeared. Should Hahnemann then find these same symptoms in other sick people, who had fallen ill from the usual natural causes, he knew to give the remedy Sepia. Many more remedies were discovered by way of *accidental provings* when people partook of substances and were unaware of their harmful content which would lead to acute or chronic states of illness.

Hahnemann further experimented with different ways of preparing medicines, and he soon discovered that the remedies had even more healing power the more they were progressively diluted and *succussed,* the latter denoting a vigorous pounding of the bottled diluted medicine onto a pliable surface. Conventionally, before being administered, all medicines undergo a process of trituration, extraction, distillation, dilution, mixing and shaking, which is the pharmacist's art of preparing his products. Hahnemann was aware that even this basic way of refining medicines released and activated their inner healing power, as in the case of Cinchona bark. Continued dilution and succussion, a process called *potentization,* progressively activated the curative power further, and new results in treatment were achieved.

Dilutions occur according to a ratio of 1:10, 1 part in 10 (for decimal potency or x potency), or 1:100 (for centesimal potency or c potency). At each step of the dilution, the remedies are succussed for at least ten times and higher vibrational healing power is released.

This is how it works: One drop healing substance in tincture is bottled with 9 drops of a solution of 20% alcohol/80% distilled water (x dilution) or with 99 drops of the alcohol/water solution (c dilution) and succussed. Out of this dilution, another single drop is taken and added to another set of 9 or 99 drops of the alcohol/water solution and succussed. As the number of dilutions and succussions increases, we move up on the scale from 1x or 1c to 2x or 2c, then on to 3x or 3c, and so on. The last drop or drops, as soon as the desired potency has been reached, are added to 99 parts of ethyl alcohol, then shaken one more time and stored. Lactose pills are then minimally impregnated with the alcoholic fluid, dried and sold as medicines. In regard to preparing insoluble medicinal substances, one part of the substance is triturated in 9 or 99 parts of pure lactose for one hour to yield the first decimal or centesimal triturated potency. This process is continued until the substance becomes soluble in alcohol/water, and regular dilutions and succussions carry on the potentization process.

The process of potentization can be done by hand, except for the high potencies which only have been done recently with the help of machines. The c potency especially is often raised to a level of one thousand dilutions and succussions and is then named 1M potency; fifty thousand times of dilutions and succussions are designated 50 M, and CM denotes one hundred thousand steps of dilutions and succussions on the c potency scale.

There also exists the millesimal series of potentization based on a dilution ratio of 1:1,000. This series, however, has never been employed widely within homeopathy. During his later years, Hahnemann developed a fourth method of potentization which is named the LM method and described in the sixth edition of his major work *Organon of Medicine* (paragraph 270). Nowadays, the LM method is not as commonly used as the two standard methods but it has its place in modern homeopathy. Remedies prepared by this method were to have even more vibrational healing power, while working more gently than the other two methods. Basically, the LM method works according to the centesimal potentization, except for a few important changes. At each step of potentization, the drop saved from the previous potentization is diluted in distilled water according to a ratio of 1:500. One drop of this dilution is then further diluted with 99 drops of 95% alcohol and succussed one hundred times. This whole process begins with a 3c potency, prepared according to the centesimal scale, which is then prepared as the LM1 potency and progressively potentized to LM30, the highest potency commonly used.

Hahnemann was aware that the material content of the healing substance was reduced gradually as dilutions and succussions increased, yet the healing effect remained or rather increased. Avogadro (1776-1856), an Italian chemist of Hahnemann's time, determined the exact place on the scale, namely 24x, corresponding to 12c on the c potency scale and to a LM4 potency, that marks the last dilution and succession containing any detectable molecules of the original healing substance. This place on the scale is referred to as *Avogadro's num-*

ber.[4] How, then, can remedies still be effective or even increase in healing power beyond Avogadro's number? What is the nature of the substances' inner healing power, and how is it rescued beyond Avogadro's number?

POSSIBLE EXPLANATIONS, SCIENTIFIC AND PHILOSOPHICAL, OF HOW THE REMEDIES ACT AFTER AVOGADRO'S NUMBER

One must assume the existence of inner carriers that are linked up with the atoms and contain the substances' inner healing power. These carriers are not detectable with current technological instruments, but they are assumed to be embedded in the crude shell or material cloak of the healing substance. As the material structure is refined and altered during medicinal preparation, these carriers are activated and can be of benefit to the diseased or unwell human organism. Progressive dilutions and succussions activate the inner healing power further, while breaking down and reducing material content.

One must assume further that the inner healing carriers, due to the dilutions and the repeated vigorous shaking, leave the molecular structure of the original substance altogether and are being released into the medium, namely distilled water and alcohol or distilled water only, where they adhere to its molecular structure. The healing carriers now travel with the water, imprint on it, raise its vibrational level, and in this way are rescued beyond Avogadro's number when material content of the substance is no longer detectable. This explains the scientifically proven effectiveness of homeopathic medicines beyond Avogadro's number and has been further verified by an important French scientific study.[5]

In what way do these medicines stimulate the body to cure itself? It is understood that the inner healing carriers inherent in the medicine release a vibrational healing message throughout the totality of the organism, permeating all bodily tissues and the psyche as well. These healing vibrations resonate with, support and strengthen the body's own vibrational rate which it employs to express and ward off disease. The defense mechanism is being strengthened and receives the message of how to cure the present state of illness; the healing vibrations elevate the body's vibrations to a new state of health.

As potency increases, the intensity of the vibrational rate increases also. A 200c potency is considered more effective in healing power than a 12c potency. However, each organism reacts differently to a strength of potency; some may respond with great benefit to lower potencies, whereas others show instant results from high potencies. As a rule, a single dose of a 200c or 1M potency is more likely to cure an entire acute or chronic state of illness than lower potencies which usually have to be given repeatedly in order to achieve good results. Being on a higher vibrational level, potencies of 200c and higher are also known to touch the higher realms of mind and emotions more effectively than lower potencies. In some cases, lower potencies seem to reach the physical structures and tissues in a very effective way, while touching the mind/emotions also.

James Tyler Kent (1849-1916), one of the most important founders and developers of homeopathy in this country, presented a philosophical explanation of the remedies' effectiveness.[6] As a proponent of higher potencies, he was confronted with the immaterial quality of homeopathic medicines and in turn with the immaterial parts of the human being, those being the inner dynamics and principles resonating with the healing vibrations of the medicines and from there reaching the physical structures as well. Leaning on Hahnemann's description of the "spiritual vital force" (*Organon*, paragraph 9), Kent explained these intrinsic truths to the scientific minds of his colleagues in the following way:

The immaterial vital principle or vital force animates the material body. This vital principle is endowed with formative intelligence which forms and operates the economy of the human, animal, vegetable, or mineral. Kent also referred to this intrinsic force as "simple substance" which is immaterial yet substantial in its presence and effects. In his own words:

This simple substance gives to everything its own type of life, gives it distinction, gives it identity whereby it differs from all other things. The crystal of the earth has its own association, its own identity; it is endowed with a simple substance that will establish its identity from everything in the animal kingdom, everything in the mineral kingdom.

This simple substance is alive; it adapts the organism to its environment, constructs it and conveys harmony. The essence or healing power of homeopathic remedies rests in this simple substance, in this unique identity of the natural substance used for medicinal purposes. The more the remedy is potentized, the more this simple substance's healing power is activated and released.

Each simple substance is again divided into subunits of hierarchical substances that form a whole. In the human economy, there is a continuous unraveling of degrees of life substance, from inner substances of will and understanding to the outermost degrees of the coarser tissues. Kent differentiated the soul as the highest substance which spreads throughout the being and becomes activated as the vital principle or vital force, caring for all parts of the body, while keeping operation of mind and will in order.

The different potencies of homeopathic medicines are designed to reach the various levels of the units of simple substance, from the highest potencies affecting character, soul and understanding to the lowest potencies addressing primarily the physical cells. These medicines then restore the lost balance within the expression of simple substance, and the diseased state is diverted. As immaterial realms are increasingly addressed within the human hierarchy of simple substance, the remedies themselves lose their physical properties after the 12c or 24x potency, or after Avogadro's number. In this way, the released and highly activated simple substance of the remedy is able to resonate with the highest realms of man's simple substance or inmost identity. Nonetheless, the higher potencies act powerfully on tissues as well, just as the human soul animates the totality of being.

Kent's insights, still of profound value today, plus the astounding results of homeopathic medicines, helped to convince the scientifically oriented minds of his colleagues in the founding years of homeopathy.

THE CASE OF BEATRICE: CASE TAKING TECHNIQUES AND DETERMINATION OF THE INDICATED HOMEOPATHIC REMEDY

There are several hundred known homeopathic medicines and more are continuously being discovered. Mastery of homeopathy is based on knowing these remedies, understanding how to recognize states of sickness and applying the matching healing remedy. Some remedies are more commonly asked for during prescribing, covering a large range of symptoms and applicable to many people; they are called the *polychrests*. Other remedies have a smaller range of action and specifically deal with rare or isolated symptoms; they are considered *small remedies*. More research is necessary to explore the action of some of the smaller remedies further.

Homeopathy is an individualized medicine, with each remedy fitted to the individual case. It is the skill and art of the homeopath to prescribe the correct remedy, to choose out of a group of possible or similar remedies the one best suited to the case at hand.

An example of a possible case follows:

Beatrice is in her early forties and complains of extreme irritability, nervousness and restlessness. Her teenage children have been unresponsive and uncooperative, while her husband has resorted to strong disciplinary measures that create more disturbance in the household. To protect herself from the turmoil, Beatrice has retreated into a self-protective state, where she shuns confrontation and tries to calm down her easily overwrought and irritable self. Furthermore, she lacks a satisfying, enriching occupation beyond house and children that would give new joy and creativity; instead, she finds herself absent-minded and removed from the tasks and people at hand, while she is imagining and wishing for some new adventure in her life, possibly in the area of a glamorous job, love, or fame, although she does not seriously consider such steps.

Her physical complaints are as follows:

She experiences a recurring headache in the vertex (top of head) and from temple to temple, with a feeling of pressure in the head. Her features are sunken and pale, somewhat yellowish. She appears rather thin. She has digestive troubles with complaints from fruit which makes her stomach ache and gives diarrhea. After eating, especially after meat intake, a weight seems to stay in her stomach, making her feel uncomfortable. Water and other fluids do not agree with her but make her feel slightly nauseous, though she feels quite thirsty and feels she should drink. She also complains of occasional abdominal distention Her skin is dry and she feels extremely irritable when touched lightly, although a firm hug relieves. She is nervous, exhausted, and restless. Her nights are difficult, with sweats and tossing about.

Because of the irritability, restlessness and sensitivity to disorder, the sunken, yellowish features and thin appearance, the aggravation from fruit and water, the dry skin, exhaustion, sweats and difficult nights, two outstanding remedies that cover those symptoms come to mind, namely *China (Cinchona officinalis)* and *Arsenicum album.* Both are polychrests. The homeopath will be aware of both remedy pictures and select the one most appropriate, while keeping in mind that other remedies beyond those two could be of interest also. For example, the remedy *Sepia (Sepia officinalis),* also a polychrest, is worth considering as an additional or third possibility. It covers the dissatisfaction and irritability in the face of family and chores, yet in the Sepia state one is usually more aggressive and critical rather than retreating into a dream world as Beatrice did. People in the Sepia state also may retreat to protect themselves, but they are usually not inclined to build dream castles, and their active engagement is more easily stimulated. On the physical plane, Sepia also shows nervousness, restlessness and yellowish features, yet it does not cover the marked aggravation from fruit. In the Sepia state, one enjoys all kinds of fruit and craves acidic fruit especially, whereas Beatrice was averse to it. In the Sepia picture, the extreme irritability to touch is also missing, although the symptom may be present to some degree as well. Furthermore, important keynotes that would support the choice for Sepia are missing, such as bearing-down sensations all over the body and the typical recurring aggravation of irritability and fatigue between 3 and 5 P.M. For all these reasons, Sepia is ruled out as a first or second choice, but it is kept in mind.

During these searches and processes of elimination of possible remedies, the homeopath may consult with a homeopathic repertory which lists symptoms and the indicated remedies that are known to cure such symptoms. Complete remedy pictures are presented in various textbooks that list important mental/emotional and physical characteristics, called the *materia medica* of remedies.[7] Originally, these symptoms have been gathered from provings or from accounts of symptoms being cured by the remedy. In each individual case, those symptoms listed in the materia medica are encountered in varying degrees of quantity and intensity. The major mental/emotional and physical symptoms of the remedies China and Arsenicum album follow.

CHINA (Cinchona officinalis)

The remedy China restores the fluid regulation of the body. It makes sure that fluid is properly absorbed by all tissues and circulated throughout the body. In an acute case, China should always be given after loss of vital fluids has occurred, such as in major blood loss, prolonged sweats, or if fluid intake had been curtailed due to emergency situations. It is indicated in intermittent fever or malaria when loss of vital fluids is also a factor.

Similarly, in a chronic case, the body slows down in its ability to absorb fluids, either because there was a major loss of vital fluids in the past that the body has not recuperated from or for reasons that lie mostly on the psychological plane. Often there may be some unhappiness in interpersonal relations, devotion and love may not be experienced or given in a fulfilling, enriching way. There may also be lack of devotion to a satisfying life task, or the demands of living are too high, the work or daily chores may be too strenuous, too irritating and exhausting. In general, life's "juices" are not flowing. Genetic factors also play a role; a China tendency may run in families. In addition, the body type may be a key factor; thin, nervy people are more likely to be in need of China than robust people.

The *generalities* or general symptoms of the remedy China are: Irritability of mind and body, great sensitivity to touch or noise, debility, periodicity of symptoms (especially in fevers), thirst, tendency to night sweats, anemia, liver disturbance. Many of these symptoms are due to the great sensitivity of all tissues; the nerves and other cells are not properly supplied with fluids and nutrients; fatty tissue may be reduced.

In regard to body parts, the specific symptoms are as follows:

MIND/EMOTIONS: Irritability; disinclined to take other people's orders; tendency to be averse to conversation and social interaction, yet there may exist romantic longing, or other kinds of aspirations, or planning for fulfilling times with increased imagination and tendency to build dream castles that are removed from reality. Depending on the person, the imaginations may center around mental constructs of a theoretical or intellectual kind.

HEAD: Sensation as if brain were loose in the head and painfully striking against the skull. Pain in vertex and temples, with sensation of pressure; scalp sensitive.

EYES: Sunken appearance; blue color around eyes, yellowish color of sclera (white part of eye), pressure in eyes.

NOSE: Coryza; easy bleeding from nose.

FACE: Yellowish complexion and drawn appearance (liver disturbances produce yellowish color of sclera and skin).

STOMACH: Hungry yet food does not appeal, since previous meal seems to lie undigested in stomach, especially meat. Fruit and all acidic foods disagree (stomach lining and other tissues are too sensitive). Water or fluids are not tolerated well or absorbed properly, and there may be nausea and bloating after drinking. Yet, there may be thirst. Pressure point felt above stomach, at lower end of sternum, worse while sitting and when bending over, with cardiac anxiety.

ABDOMEN: Flatulent colic, better bending double. Pain in liver region, with swelling, jaundice. Gastroduodenal catarrh.

STOOL: Undigested, yellowish. Diarrhea after fruit; weakness after stool.

RESPIRATORY: Influenza, with debility. Cough after meals. Breathing difficult, suffocative catarrh. Asthma.

HEART: Irregular heart beat.

BACK: Sharp pains across kidney region.

EXTREMITIES: Weariness of limbs and joints, averse to exercise, yet restless because of general irritability; sensitive to touch.

SKIN: Tendency to dry skin.

SLEEP: Not refreshing, with anxious dreams. Night sweats.

FEVER: Periodic rise and fall of temperature (intermittent fever), malaria.

The remedy picture of Arsenicum album is similar in action to China, yet it has its characteristic keynotes of mental/emotional and physical symptoms.

ARSENICUM ALBUM

The Arsenicum album patient has burning pains throughout his body and a sense of nervous, restless energy. There is great sensitivity to external impressions with heightened sense of beauty and appreciation, while there is irritability in face of disorder, noise, disharmony and commotion. In an acute case of food poisoning, as the body is trying to purge itself through vomiting and diarrhea, Arsenicum album is usually the indicated remedy.

Typical chronic Arsenicum album patients are also concerned with purifying themselves. There is anxiety about health, and there is the ceaseless endeavor to cleanse body, mind, and the immediate environment as well. They are often perfectionists, setting themselves and others high standards. If standards are not met, they can become disappointed or critical. They want to be able to control their lives and those of others also; there is worry and fear in face of those things out of their control, and this may cause a deep-seated sense of lack of security. Thin, wiry types that like to work hard are more likely to be in need of this remedy than robust, relaxed types.

The generalities of Arsenicum album plus specific symptoms pertaining to parts of the body are: Easy exhaustion, irritability, restlessness. Chilliness, except for head which can feel hot. Burning pains that are better from warm applications. Digestive disturbances; thirst for sips, prefers warm drinks. Aggravation of symptoms at midnight; periodicity of symptoms.

MIND/EMOTIONS: Sensitive to disorder and confusion, irritability and tension, many worries and fears (of death, of robbers, of being left alone, of not having enough money), can be possessive with people and things. High achiever mentality.

HEAD: Icy feeling of scalp, although head may feel hot from within; sensitive scalp. Throbbing pains, often on one side, chiefly above one eye, at root of nose, and in occiput. Inclination to vomit from headache.

EYES AND NOSE: Burning and acrid flow especially during colds.

FACE: Sunken features, can have yellowish color.

STOMACH: Anxiety felt in stomach. Sight and smell of food do not appeal; nausea. Bad effects from water and watery fruit. Stomach is very irritable, seems raw; yet, craving for sour, acidic things, also for creamy things.

ABDOMEN: Enlarged and painful liver and spleen. Bloating. Bad effects from food poisoning.

STOOL: Dark stool, excoriates skin around anus. Dysentery.

RESPIRATORY: Cough worse lying down, fears suffocation. Asthma.

HEART: Palpitation, with accelerated heart beat in morning.

BACK: Weakness in small of back.

EXTREMITIES: Pronounced restlessness, cramps, burning pains.

SKIN: Dry, rough, scaly.

SLEEP: Restless, with sweats, nightly aggravation at midnight.

FEVER: High temperature; intermittent, periodicity, worse at night, with sweats.

China is the indicated remedy; it covers the physical and mental/emotional symptoms more specifically, yet there are many overlapping symptoms that would be covered by both remedies, as already shown above. The main physical symptoms indicating China are: Great irritability when touched, but better from firm pressure; this in an important keynote of this remedy. Her head pains and stomach troubles resemble the China picture more closely than the Arsenicum album picture. Furthermore, Beatrice had trouble from all fruits, not just watery ones, as would be the case with an Arsenicum album patient. Her sensitivity and dislike were especially to acidic fruits, whereas the Arsenicum album patient would crave them. Her thirst and feeling that she should drink indicate the lack of proper fluid absorbency that is cured by China. In addition, her restlessness was not as extreme as in a typical Arsenicum album case, and there was no marked aggravation at midnight, this time of aggravation being an important keynote of Arsenicum album.

Beyond the physical symptoms, the main differentiation lies in the mental/emotional realm. Beatrice shows the typical China picture of lack of fulfilling relations and lack of devotion to tasks at hand, with the building of dream castles that are removed from reality. In comparison, the Arsenicum album patient is more fastidious and task-oriented, more interested in the present moment. There may also be fear and worry which spurs them to action, both of which Beatrice did not experience particularly. Usually, Arsenicum album patients do not retreat from their environment but rather endeavor to control all details, sometimes interfering with other people's lives as well. Beatrice accomplished her daily chores sufficiently, but not with the same incentive for order and the need to control. In regard to her children, she also relegated control and discipline to her husband, while she retreated.

The remedy China will cure all physical complaints, restore her mental and physical ease and well-being, while opening her mind again to the people and tasks of the present moment.

In this case, despite the important physical symptoms, it was the mental/emotional picture that clearly led to the correct prescription. The mental/emotional state constitutes the *essence* of the remedy around which the physical symptoms develop, unless causation of the illness had purely physical reasons.[8] Hahnemann himself discovered that, notwithstanding important physical symptoms, the individual mental/ emotional state is a crucial guiding light, if not the most important guide, to the selection of the correct remedy (*Organon,* paragraphs 210-213). Similar to Edward Bach, the founder of Bach Flower Therapy, Hahnemann recognized the individuality of each case and the importance of the mind/emotions in the origin, symptomatic expression and treatment of disease.

In Beatrice's case, healing would be deepened even further, if the mental/emotional causative components of her illness were identified and treated with additional Bach Remedies. Specifically, her mental/emotional picture consisted of irritability, helped by the remedy *Impatiens,* absent-mindedness and building of dream castles, helped by *Clematis,* mental/ emotional and physical weariness, treated by *Olive;* and for the lack of direction and joyless approach to her daily demands of living, *Wild Oat* would be indicated. These remedies would help restore healing not only in the mental/emotional realm but initiate physical recuperation as well, while deepening the effect of the remedy China. This combined approach to cure would also stimulate more actively the emergence of possible additional underlying layers of health disturbance so that these could be treated and a longer-lasting, deepened cure be achieved.

The description of the discovery, theory and practical application of the Bach Remedies follows.

⌘

BACH FLOWER THERAPY: DISCOVERY AND HOW IT WORKS

- Bach's Discovery of the Importance of the Mind/ Emotions During Disease and Cure, and the Development of the Seven Bach Nosodes

- Bach's Exposure to Homeopathy and the Replacing of the Bowel Nosodes with Plants

- Bach's Complete Identification of the Mental/Emotional Imbalances in Man and the Finding of the Matching Healing Remedies

- Discovery of the Sun Method and the Boiling Method of Preparation and the Presentation of the New System of Healing to the Public

- Medicinal Preparation and Curative Action: Bach Remedies in Comparison with Homeopathic Remedies

BACH'S DISCOVERY OF THE IMPORTANCE OF THE MIND/ EMOTIONS DURING DISEASE AND CURE, AND THE DEVELOPMENT OF THE SEVEN BACH NOSODES

Even in early life, Edward Bach (1886-1936) combined a deep compassion with all who suffered with a reverent love for nature. During his late teens, he became determined to help people overcome illness. He enrolled himself in Medical School and devoted himself to studying all known forms of diseases and their cure. He was not introduced to homeopathy during his studies.

During his medical studies, he observed the patients' individual personalities and their responses to treatment closely, and he noticed that the mental/emotional condition would influence the course of recovery and affect the efficiency of the administered medicines. He concluded that mind and emotions played an important role in the processes of disease and cure, and they should be taken into consideration during diagnosis and treatment. A further observation during his studies was that treatment was often prolonged, complicated and painful, and he felt that a gentle approach to cure should be found. This new approach to cure was to strengthen the whole personality, including the body.[9]

After completion of his medical training and branching into bacteriology, he began to study closely the mental and physical differences of the seven major types of personality that he had identified and observed during his medical training. His goal was to determine how the mind/emotions and body affected each other; specifically, he was interested in identifying those physical symptoms that were commonly experienced by people of the same type of personality. The most marked distinction between different types was found in the intestinal flora, or bacterial bowel lining, known to reflect the overall health of the organism. Each type of personality had its own specific intestinal flora, indicating that intestinal floras not only mirror physical health but also have an affinity with the type of personality and its major mental/emotional tendencies.

Bach developed seven vaccines from the bacteria of these intestinal floras and administered them successfully to the seven different types of patients, each patient according to his type, which was determined by a bacteriological examination, and a mental/emotional and physical assessment. By cleansing the system from within, Bach was able to raise his patients' overall health, including mental/emotional health which he had hoped to affect. These vaccines were named the *Seven Bach Nosodes,* a *nosode* meaning a medicine made from the products of the diseased state itself or from the inciting virus or bacteria. A list of the Seven Bach Nosodes with their major mental/emotional and physical indications can be given. Each nosode matches one type of personality with its specific tendencies toward mental/emotional and physical imbalance.

1. PROTEUS

Irritability, anger, internal grief. Edematous appearance, cramps, migraines, gastroduodenal ulcers, kidney problems.

2. DYSENTERY

Fear, apprehension, lack of confidence, heightened sensitivity. Delicate appearance, chilliness, insomnia, cyclical headaches, chronic indigestion, duodenal ulcers, loose bowels.

3. MORGAN

Depression, anxiety, introspection, grief. Red/blue congested appearance, rheumatism, asthma, eczema, hypertension, liver and gall bladder problems.

4. FAECALIS ALKALIGENES

Irritability, impatience. Yellowish appearance, nausea, liver troubles, constipation.

5. COLI MUTABILE

Changeability of mood. Increased warmth, increased mucosa, respiratory troubles.

6. GAERTNER

Hypersensitivity, nervousness, fears. Emaciated appearance, restlessness, deficient digestion and assimilation, food allergies, enuresis.

7. BACILLUS NO. 7

Mental prostration and mental weakness, non-alertness. Edematous condition, pale appearance, worse humidity, thyroid trouble, asthma, lack of muscle tone, constipation.[10]

This treatment was accepted enthusiastically among professionals and patients alike, mainly due to a new theory of the origin of chronic disease that had arisen in London during that time (early twenties). This new theory pointed to intestinal toxemia, caused by non-lactose fermenting organisms, as the leading cause of chronic disease. Accordingly, the Bach Bowel Nosodes were administered to cleanse the system from within and help the body ward off symptoms of chronic disease. Usually, traditional forms of treatment were employed as well to further healing. While studying patients and their healing response, Bach, however, became increasingly convinced that the true origin of chronic disease lay in the mental/emotional imbalance with the intestinal toxemia arising therefrom. He saw the Bach Nosodes as a first step towards consideration of the mind/emotions during treatment, since they were prescribed according to personality traits, and not only physical symptoms. He realized that the current use of the nosodes neglected this important aspect of his work; instead of concentrating on the mind as the causative factor, the nosodes were recognized and used towards the cure of physical disease only; the cart was put in front of the horse. He formulated the theory that all chronic diseases start in the mind and emotions, unless obvious external factors were responsible. He felt that much physical suffering could be prevented if remedies, akin to the nosodes, were found that were prescribed on mental/emotional characteristics, affected the mind directly and reestablished harmony in the person before chronic physical symptoms of disease could develop. At this time, the nosodes constituted a first incomplete step toward this goal, and he felt his search had just begun.

BACH'S EXPOSURE TO HOMEOPATHY AND THE REPLACING OF THE BOWEL NOSODES WITH PLANTS

During this time of research and successful treatment of patients, Bach became a great admirer of Hahnemann and his principles of homeopathy. He was impressed by Hahnemann's consideration of the patient's individuality during diagnosis and treatment and the special attention paid to the mental/ emotional state during prescribing. He was astounded to find homeopathic remedies affecting the mind directly, while curing the body. He believed that his Bach Nosodes, which were also indicated by physical as well as mental/ emotional characteristics, were curative in a similar way and could be of service within the homeopathic framework. Specifically, he assumed that the outward manifestations of the *miasm psora,* which had been identified by Hahnemann as a major layer of health disturbance commonly experienced by the general population over many centuries, were also expressions of intestinal toxemia and hence were curable by the administration of the Bach Nosodes, these being equal to or surpassing the healing power of the indicated homeopathic remedies.

Although Bach was impressed with the efficiency of homeopathy and its curative effect on mind/emotions and body alike, he did not abandon his search for more remedies that would benefit the mind/emotions directly. He felt that a new approach to healing, even more finely tuned to mental/ emotional states than homeopathy, was necessary and that homeopathic cure would actually be enriched further. The contact with homeopathy gave him inspiration and incentive to follow his own course further. He directly integrated many positive aspects of the homeopathic method in his own work. In his treatment of patients, for example, he decided to adopt the gentle homeopathic administration of medicines by pellets and forgo the syringes that he had used for his vaccines. From then on, all seven Bach Nosodes were prepared and administered as oral medicines. Furthermore, Hahnemann's foremost use of natural medicinal substances, with only occasional use of nosodes, inspired Bach to start a search towards replacing the Bach Nosodes, which were products of disease, with natural and pure healing plants from nature that would have a similar healing effect.

Specifically, he was interested in addressing and uplifting more directly the mental/emotional state that he felt was responsible for the intestinal imbalance and other symptoms of disease. It was his goal to search for a system of healing that would prescribe on mental/emotional states only and was directly derived from the beauty and purity of nature. This new system was to work gently without possible aggravations or contact with harmful substances, however minimal they might be.

He experimented with plants and soon found *Ornithogalum umbellatum* (Star of Bethlehem) to be almost identical in healing effect with the Morgan nosode which is indicated for individuals with depression, anxiety, introspection and grief. Three further plants, namely, *Mimulus guttatus, Impatiens glandulifera* and *Clematis vitalba,* were found similar to the other nosodes in healing effect. Specifically, Mimulus helped individuals belonging to the Dysentery and Gaertner groups which show fear, apprehension and nervousness as outstanding characteristics. Impatiens helped the Proteus and Faecalis alkaligenes types who suffer from irritability, anger, impatience and nervous strain, whereas Clematis helped those characterized by non-alertness and sleepiness as found in the Bacillus No. 7 group.[11] Compared to the nosodes, Bach found these plants to have a similar healing effect on the overall organism plus an actually heightened effect on the mental/emotional state. He began to consider the true possibility of healing potential stored in certain plants that could directly and specifically stimulate certain unbalanced mental/emotional states toward harmony and cure. These initial four plants proved to be important mental/emotional healers and were the forerunners of his new system of healing. Potentized and actualized further with a new method of medicinal preparation that he discovered later, Star of Bethlehem became the healing remedy for grief and states of shock, Mimulus was prescribed for fear and shyness, Impatiens for impatience and nervous strain, and Clematis for absent-mindedness and dreaminess.

BACH'S COMPLETE IDENTIFICATION OF THE MENTAL/ EMOTIONAL IMBALANCES IN MAN AND THE FINDING OF THE MATCHING HEALING REMEDIES

In view of the curative power of the first healing plants, Bach abandoned his work as a bacteriologist, including the use of the Bach Nosodes, and concentrated his efforts on identifying the foremost mental/emotional imbalances found in man, while collecting and researching possible corresponding healing plants. From his experience as a medical practitioner and from his continued close observation of his own and other people's psyche, he determined twelve outstanding states of mind, or twelve typical tendencies of personalities, that were basic to all humanity. He integrated the seven types of personality that he had identified initially into his new perspective and used these twelve basic states of mind, or types of personality, as building blocks for his new system of healing. These major mental/emotional states and their respective healing remedies, the latter which he had found and identified through his extensive searches in the outdoors and the laboratory, were:

1. Fear and shyness (Mimulus).

2. Terror (Rock Rose).

3. Mental torture or worry (Agrimony).

4. Indecision (Scleranthus).

5. Indifference or boredom (Clematis).

6. Doubt or discouragement (Gentian).

7. Overconcern for welfare of others (Chicory).

8. Weakness, too willing servitor (Centaury).

9. Self-distrust (Cerato).

10. Impatience (Impatiens).

11. Overenthusiasm (Vervain).

12. Pride or aloofness (Water Violet).[12]

Over the years, further study and personal experience of mental/emotional states served him to identify twenty-six additional states of mind which were gradually complemented with healing plants from nature. Initially, the twelve type remedies, or twelve *healers,* as Bach termed them, were complemented by seven adjunct remedies, or *helpers.* Whereas the healers address major parts or character traits of the personality, the helpers deal with long-standing states of mental/emotional suffering that have become entrenched in the character as a whole and have begun to overshadow the true personality. These healers and helpers, however, are not only prescribed for chronic states of mind but also for temporary upsets. They are given whenever indicated. These helper remedies were discovered in the following order:

13. Hopelessness (Gorse).

14. Despondency from overwork (Oak).

15. Self-centered talkativeness (Heather).

16. Hard master onto oneself, with an urge to inspire others (Rock Water).

17. Lack of motivation and incentive (Wild Oat).

18. Mental/emotional and physical weariness (Olive).

19. Domination of others (Vine).

The last nineteen remedies discovered were concerned mostly with temporary states of the mind/emotions that arise due to the circumstantial experiences of life. These mental/emotional states can be a part of the personality for prolonged periods of time but are not considered typical character traits. The remedies were mostly gained from bushes and trees.

20. Fear of losing mental balance (Cherry Plum).

21. Vague fears and foreboding (Aspen).

22. Fear for the other's welfare (Red Chestnut).

23. Mental fatigue (Hornbeam).

24. Longing for past happiness, nostalgia (Honeysuckle).

25. Feelings of powerlessness (Wild Rose).

26. Lack of mental tranquility (White Chestnut).

27. Depression and gloom (Mustard).

28. Immaturity of mind/emotions, failure to learn from mistakes (Chestnut Bud).

29. Vexations and jealousy (Holly) (later added to the helpers by Bach).

30. Easy impressionability (Walnut).

31. Shame or feelings of uncleanliness (Crab Apple).

32. Resentment and bitterness (Willow).

33. Sadness, grief, shock (Star of Bethlehem).

34. Despair and faithlessness (Sweet Chestnut).

35. Being overwhelmed (Elm).

36. Guilt and self-blame (Pine).

37. Low self-confidence (Larch).

38. Intolerance and criticism (Beech).

Bach felt that these thirty-eight remedies span the whole arena of mental/emotional suffering experienced by man. He divided these remedies into seven groups which represent seven major areas of consciousness where mental/emotional imbalances can occur. Each group, except for the group of *For Despondency or Despair,* contained one or two of the basic type remedies.

1. **FOR THOSE WHO HAVE FEAR:**

   Rock Rose, Mimulus, Cherry Plum, Aspen, Red Chestnut.

2. **FOR THOSE WHO SUFFER UNCERTAINTY:**

   Cerato, Scleranthus, Gentian, Gorse, Hornbeam, Wild Oat.

3. **NOT SUFFICIENT INTEREST IN PRESENT CIRCUMSTANCES:**

   Clematis, Honeysuckle, Wild Rose, Olive, White Chestnut, Mustard, Chestnut Bud.

4. **LONELINESS:**

   Water Violet, Impatiens, Heather.

5. **OVERSENSITIVE TO INFLUENCES AND IDEAS:**

   Agrimony, Centaury, Walnut, Holly.

6. **FOR DESPONDENCY OR DESPAIR:**

   Larch, Pine, Elm, Sweet Chestnut, Star of Bethlehem, Willow, Oak, Crab Apple.

7. **OVERCARE FOR WELFARE OF OTHERS:**

   Chicory, Vervain, Vine, Beech, Rock Water.

Over several years, Bach collected these thirty-eight remedies during extensive searches, mainly in the countryside of

England. Most plants and trees grow naturally on English soil, except for Vine, Olive and Cerato. Bach discovered the strikingly blue flowers of the bush Cerato in an English ornamental garden, although the bush is native to Tibet. On his travels through Europe, Bach detected the medicinal properties of the climbing bush Vine in Switzerland and those of the Olive tree in Italy. All Bach Remedies are gained from plants, except for Rock Water which Bach drew from a well in England that he knew to carry medicinal healing power.

When testing plants for healing properties, he used samples from wild flowers, vines, bushes and trees, prepared them in his laboratory and administered them to himself and others to determine their healing effect on the mind/emotions and the concurrent or subsequent effects on the body. Oftentimes, he would experience a negative mental/emotional state himself with concurrent physical symptoms, all of which were then relieved by a certain plant that he was testing. He was drawn to many plants by their outward appearances or characteristics which, he felt, mirrored certain mental/emotional states experienced by man. For example, the quivering of the Aspen tree reminded Bach of fear, trembling and foreboding; the white tufts growing on the Clematis plant seemed light and airy, and they would often float through the air like clouds, reminding of states of dreaminess or absent-mindedness, of being "in the clouds"; the Impatiens plant was marked by sudden explosions and scattering of seeds, pointing to states of impatience; the sharply pointed leaves from the Holly tree spoke of vexation and aggressiveness, while the red berries signaled warmth and love; traditionally, the branches with red berries serve as Christmas decorations. Holly is one example of a plant speaking of the negative state, while also indicating the positive state in its outward appearance.

Throughout the ages, many medicinal plants or medicinal properties of animals had been discovered by observation of the so-called *Doctrine of Signatures* which teaches that nature points out its curative effects by mirroring certain aspects of illness or of the affected organs in the structural appearance, in the color, or in the biological behavior of the plant or animal. The plant *Drosera rotundifolia,* for example, being an important homeopathic remedy for coughs, shows flimsy, tiny hairs on its leaves, pointing to the small hairs, or cilia, in the respiratory tract that it regenerates during coughs. In most of his searches, Bach was guided intuitively by the plant's signature to the inherent healing potential, while further testing verified the exact medicinal property.

DISCOVERY OF THE SUN METHOD AND THE BOILING METHOD OF PREPARATION AND THE PRESENTATION OF THE NEW SYSTEM OF HEALING TO THE PUBLIC

The flowers and their petals were of special interest to Bach who believed that the highest, purest healing energy was stored in the delicate petals and corresponded with the subtle, higher vibrations of man's consciousness. As the flowers direct, express and "head" the plant, so does man's head, cognitive perception and consciousness direct and express the overall organism and personality. Flowers also bring forth renewal, procreation and fruits, just as their healing essences bring new growth and fruits of consciousness. He experimented with several methods of preparation, always concentrating mostly on the flowering parts, until he had extracted the highest healing potential. Twenty of the remedies were gained by the sun method of potentization of petals; the remaining eighteen were prepared by boiling whole parts of the plant, bush or tree, including the flowers. Most remedies gained from trees were prepared by boiling whole twigs so that healing power stored in the wood could be extracted also, along with the healing power of the flowers. In both of these methods of preparation, water and heat were combined to extract the highest healing potential.

Bach had gained the idea of using the sun method of potentization by observing the sun's action of shining through and warming dew drops on flower petals, and he had wondered about the sun's power to activate and release healing energy from the petals into the water. Upon experimentation, he found this to be true, and he decided to prepare most of his tinctures right in the field by placing freshly plucked flowers into a bowl of sunlit water and leaving it for several hours to the sun's action. In this way, potential loss of healing power that could occur due to lengthy transportation was avoided. This water, imbued with healing power, was then brought to his laboratory, preserved with alcohol and poured into stock bottles.

The following twenty remedies, which included the twelve type remedies, were gained by the sun method of potentization: Agrimony, Centaury, Cerato, Chicory, Clematis, Gentian, Gorse, Heather, Impatiens, Mimulus, Oak, Olive, Rock Rose, Rock Water, Scleranthus, Wild Oat, Vervain, Vine, Water Violet, White Chestnut (blossoms). The water gained from boiling the plants and twigs was strained and likewise preserved and stored, resulting in the following eighteen remedies: Aspen, Beech, Cherry Plum, Chestnut Bud, Crab Apple, Elm, Holly, Honeysuckle, Hornbeam, Larch, Mustard, Pine, Red Chestnut, Star of Bethlehem, Sweet Chestnut, Walnut, Wild Rose, Willow. Only two drops from the stock bottles, along with fresh water and 1 teaspoon of brandy or vinegar, are necessary for each 1 ounce (30 ml) bottle of prepared medicine, from which four drops are taken four times a day. Depending on the state of illness, these drops are taken for short periods of time, as in acute illness, or for weeks or months, as in a chronic case.

As soon as the new system of healing was complete, Bach concentrated his efforts on teaching the use of the remedies to professionals and lay people alike. He recognized that the new healing method was profound, encompassing all possible mental/emotional states and going to the very root of 'isease, yet it was clear enough to be learned, understood and used by professionals and lay people alike. He wished for each household to have a set of the remedies, which were affordable over-the-counter medicines, so that emotional and concurrent minor physical imbalances could be treated even in the home, by simply observing the mood of the patient. He taught four basic ways of using the remedies:

1. PREVENTION
   Keeping strong in mind/emotions and body by treating mental/emotional states as they arise.

2. STOP ILLNESS AT ONSET
   Threatened acute or chronic illness can be diverted by treating those mental/emotional states accompanying the onset of illness, no matter if a contagion or an emotional imbalance or both started the illness.

3. HELP DURING ILLNESS, ONCE ILLNESS HAS BE-GUN
   Overall cure is furthered by lifting the emotions, by easing pain and discomfort during the illness, while actually leading to or even realizing cure of the physical complaint as well. In severe cases, a physician has to be consulted.

4. HELP WITH CHARACTER TRAITS THAT BRING
    UNHAPPINESS

Dispositions of character found undesirable can be trans-
formed into positive aspects that allow for increased personal growth and improved interpersonal relations.[13]

MEDICINAL PREPARATION AND CURATIVE ACTION: BACH REMEDIES IN COMPARISON WITH HOMEOPATHIC REMEDIES

The scientific medical community did not accept Bach's
teachings readily, since no active medicinal ingredient, except
simple herbal content, could be isolated. The astounding far-
reaching curative effects of the remedies were made known to
the medical community but ignored, as has happened in regard
to homeopathic remedies also. Both methods of healing have
an assumed healing carrier.

The healing essence of homeopathic remedies is released
through initial preparation of medicines and ensuing progressive dilutions and successions during which the healing essence
is carried over to the medium after Avogadro's number. Similarly, the Bach Flowers' healing essence is activated during sun
potentization or boiling of plants during which it is released
into the water by means of an assumed carrier. This process, as
tested by Bach, brings out the remedies' full healing potential,
making progressive dilutions and successions unnecessary.

Bach Flower Essences are stored in delicate and more accessible parts of the plant and are more easily released during
medicinal preparation than most homeopathic healing essences.
Many homeopathic remedies are gained from crude material
substances, including the heavier elements, and extensive tritu-

ration plus breaking down of molecules through dilutions and succussions is necessary to extract inner healing potential. The unique addition of the heating method during preparation of Bach Flowers, which is not used during preparation of homeopathic medicines, may further account for the more simplified and yet effective method of preparation of Bach Remedies. Furthermore, the very target area of the Bach Remedies' healing essence differs somewhat from the target area of the homeopathic medicine, although both are considered to be in the class of homeopathic healers, working on the mind/emotions/body totality. When compared with homeopathic remedies, the Bach Remedies aim more specifically at delicately distinguishable states of consciousness which they cure by more subtle and more finely tuned vibrations, these being released by a more subtle, delicate method of medicinal preparation.

These subtle healing vibrations released by the Bach Remedies, corresponding with the subtle vibrations of mind and emotions, consequently initiate or even complete healing of the body as well, in a gentle yet deep-reaching way. Homeopathic remedies, on the other hand, work more powerfully and directly on the material, physical body, while simultaneously furthering mental/emotional well-being.

In regard to the frequency and strength of administration of homeopathic medicines, some diseases, mainly those with mostly physical symptoms, may be cured with the repeated intake of low-potency homeopathic medicines. Other diseases or states of discomfort are more easily accessible with a few doses of high-potency homeopathic medicines which can act powerfully and efficiently on the totality of the organism. Without nearing the subtle, unique effect of Bach Remedies, homeopathic remedies become more refined with potentization and effectively touch the higher domains of consciousness, should this be the major seat of disturbance. The higher potencies act powerfully, however, not only on states of consciousness but on the physical plane as well, and, consequently, should not be repeated too often. The vital force may overreact to such profound boosts of health; this same effect may occur with low potency remedies.

Bach Remedies, in comparison, are always given repeatedly, four times a day over a period of days, weeks or months. Mental/emotional change may come gradually, and the personality has to grow towards new insights, resolutions and actions, all of which are furthered best by repeatedly sending selected healing impulses towards those areas of the personality where imbalances have occurred. Bach Remedies can target gently specific emotions, character traits, or areas of consciousness without possible disturbing side effects, whereas homeopathic medicines have to be considered in their powerful total effect on the organism and the possible side effects if repeated too often.

Homeopathic remedies, not only after having been given repeatedly but also when given for the first time, especially in high potency, may cause an initial, usually non-alarming aggravation of symptoms, as the vital force highlights the trouble spots and all healing power focuses on the problems at hand. Bach Remedies, on the other hand, send repeated gentle impulses that work without aggravations, although a highlighting of or a deepened awareness of the unbalanced mental/emotional state that is being treated may occur initially.

As far as overall cure is concerned, homeopathic remedies act by stimulating the defense mechanism to cure itself, by teaching the totality of the organism how to function normally again. Positive healing vibrations transform the negative vibrations of the diseased state. In a similar way, the Bach Remedies teach the conscious personality and the higher mind, which also regulates the operations of the vital force, how to reestablish harmony in the specific areas of the personality and the body that have become unbalanced and unwell. Specifically, the Bach Remedies vibrate with and stimulate the higher mind's positive potential which is then released to counterbalance and cure the specific unbalanced mental/emotional state.

This vibrational healing pattern originates from the inner spark within the higher mind, this spark being the inner fountain of inspiration and wholeness that can be experienced independently of the Bach Remedies, mainly through personal awareness, repeated reflection, faith and devotion. This inner core of wholeness, however, is greatly stimulated by the Bach Remedies, while the importance of personal awareness and devotion to higher values remains. Bach said of the healing plants used that they "have the power to elevate our vibrations and thus draw down spiritual power, which cleanses mind and body, and heals."[14] Likewise, homeopathic remedies work best when the inner self is open to higher values and healing works from the inner wellspring to the outward manifestations of disease, in a combined effort of the remedy's action and the personal desire for growth, wholeness, and for positive change of attitude towards the world, if indicated.

Bach himself was aware of the importance of the patients' active participation in the healing process. Specifically, he encouraged his patients, who often felt overwhelmed by the strength of their unbalanced emotions, to envision and strive for the desired mental/emotional attitude, such as love instead of hate, courage instead of fear, patience instead of impatience, rather than trying to battle against the wrong within. His goal was to help lessen preoccupation with the wrong or negative aspect and to guide the mind towards positive aspiration. This active devotion enhances the effect of the remedies, and, in a combined effort of the conscious personality and the remedies' repeated impulses, positive vibrations are able to flood the personality and wash away imbalance and negativity. Should active devotion to change not be engaged in, or in case the patient is too young to comprehend, the remedies still act by unconsciously furthering change; and, with time, the conscious mind according to its development will also be able to distinguish and experience the new attitude and well-being.

Since mind/emotions and body work as a unit, the Bach Remedies' curative action also reaches those sites of the body where imbalances of the mind/emotions had impinged upon. A knot in the stomach, for example, may be the direct result of apprehension and worry. Depression may lead to a general slowing down of bodily functions. Negative thought patterns, especially if persisted in over an extended period of time, are communicated through the nerves to the corresponding sites of the body, where they express the disturbance. As the mind/emotions lighten, as wholesome thought patterns begin to grow, the body lightens and rejuvenates also. Positive nerve impulses, stimulated by the healing impulses of the Bach Remedies, release healing within the affected tissues. Parallel homeopathic remedies, indicated to treat the specific symptoms at hand, will greatly aid in this process, especially if organic damage exists.

The two methods are indispensable to each other and greatly enhance overall cure. The Bach Remedies, if given initially, actually highlight the affected tissues and prepare them for release so that indicated homeopathic remedies are easily distinguishable and work most effectively. This same effect holds true when Bach Remedies and homeopathic remedies are given concurrently. Under the healing impact of the Bach Remedies, the now unhampered vital force continually initiates healing of the tissues, as the mind/emotions as cause of the illness release and the full curative effect of the homeopathic remedy becomes possible. Relapse into former thought patterns with concurrent physical symptoms is prevented, as Bach Remedies help safeguard mental/emotional health and work preventively, as imbalances begin to assert again.

These are new insights into the special workings of the vital force during treatment with both homeopathic methods. These insights are based on close observation of my personal case and some cases within the homeopathic study group. Specifically, one of the first cases, where both methods were used, alerted me personally to the catalytic effect of Bach Remedies during homeopathic treatment. Bach Remedies were not introduced until the middle of treatment when they initiated dramatic changes in the case with new results of cure being obtained. Following, find the case of *Francisca,* presented in present tense for immediacy and making vivid the many steps of prescribing; all data are correct, except for the change in name.

My personal case will follow, demonstrating the catalytic power of the single use of the Bach Remedies in releasing a crucial homeopathic layer.

⌘

4

THE CASE OF FRANCISCA: ILLUSTRATING THE COMBINED EFFECTS OF HOMEOPATHIC REMEDIES AND BACH REMEDIES

INITIAL COMMENTS

Although an array of Francisca's overall symptoms, idiosynchrasies and personality traits was taken, only those symptoms of the case are listed here that were most crucial and sufficient in determining the correct choice of remedy. Symptoms manifest themselves mostly around her headache which is her main complaint, with only minor concomitants in other parts of her body. These concomitant symptoms are important, however, along with the mental/emotional state, in determining the correct remedy. Variations of symptoms throughout the case give good examples of the materia medica or typical symptomatology of the indicated remedies. One can see how the case moves through different layers of health disturbance, each time asking for a new remedy, until the core of the main complaint is reached and real cure becomes possible.

VISIT 1, JUNE 8, 1988

Francisca, age forty-four, needs treatment for bad headaches that render her unable to pursue her tasks. Main symptoms of her headaches with concomitant symptoms are: Heavy, dull, throbbing pain in whole head with feeling of pressure; intensified pains around right eye. During the headache, there is no thirst but dryness of mouth. She feels chilled, wants to lie down and withdraw; yet, after doing so, becomes weepy and desires company. When she finds some strength, she goes for a slow walk in the fresh air, and her pains lessen. Except for getting a headache after eating too much butter, she knows no cause that may elicit her headache. No pattern of daily recurrence around certain hours or other signs of periodicity can be distinguished.

Important general mental/emotional symptoms are: Francisca feels some internal uncertainty which makes it difficult for her to commit wholeheartedly to people and a definite career path. She has a difficult time making decisions and occasionally feels depressed. Overall, she enjoys company, is friendly, outgoing and fun to be with.

All major symptoms point to the remedy *Pulsatilla nigricans* which is given twice in the 200c potency. Pulsatilla nigricans is considered a mostly female remedy, often indicated for women who tend to be changeable in mood and physical symptoms, with possible hormonal imbalances that could also be responsible for headaches and other typical Pulsatilla nigricans symptoms.

VISIT 2, JULY 1, 1988

After an initial aggravation, her condition is improved; her headaches are less painful, yet not alleviated completely. During this visit, she also reports a new sense of well-being in mind and body, which is not constant but surprises her from time to time. There is a new feeling of lightness about her and a growing certainty about her life's endeavors. Pulsatilla nigricans 200c is repeated to clear her headaches further and give her an additional stimulus to overall health.

VISIT 3, JULY 26, 1988

Twenty-six days later, she returns reporting headaches of a somewhat different nature. They are less severe than her previous headaches but still cause hardship and concern. Etiology and main symptoms of the headache are: After carrying her heavy backpack and straining back and neck, a headache comes on.

Not eating regularly also causes headaches to appear. There is a feeling of compression or squeezing of the head with throbbing pain. Furthermore, she experiences thirst for cold water and a short amelioration of the pain by applying a hot washcloth to the head. She feels cold and depressed, wants to withdraw and lie down. The headache is better after sleep when she wakes up with sweat on her face and on the back of her neck and head.

General mental/emotional symptoms are: Her mental/emotional outlook has improved further with uncertainty diminishing and a new resolution to take control of her life forming. She is upset when headaches delay her activities and make her slow down. *Calcarea carbonica*, known to be the chronic layer of Pulsatilla nigricans and matching the overall symptoms, is prescribed in the 200c potency and given in single dose. As compared to Pulsatilla nigricans, which is usually marked by uncertainty of attitude and occasional feelings of dependency, Calcarea carbonica is usually characterized by a more resolute, work-oriented attitude.

VISIT 4, AUGUST 11, 1988

During the fourth visit, she reports somewhat improved conditions but no overall cure of her main complaint, and there are no additional physical symptoms to report. The somewhat slow process of cure has disheartened her, and an array of emotions is now asserting itself. She feels resignation, depression and helplessness in view of her still recurring, though less intense headaches, and in view of her relationship, career and future ahead. There is lack of incentive and motivation to apply to a definite career path, with feelings of inadequacy and projection of failure.

At this point in the case, Bach Remedies are prescribed to help her cope with her emotions. *Gentian* is chosen for discouragement, *Wild Rose* for her feelings of helplessness and resignation, and *Wild Oat* for lack of motivation and incentive in view of her career. *Larch* is also indicated for anticipation of failure and *Mustard* for depression, yet the first three remedies are considered predominant and chosen over the other two, so as not to send too many impulses at once to the vital force. In addition, Calcarea carbonica 200c is given again to help clear remaining physical symptoms, although the mental/emotional picture seems to be steering away from the typical Calcarea carbonica mentality which is usually more resolute and work-oriented. However, periods of discouragement and lack of motivation can be part of the Calcarea carbonica state also.

VISIT 5, AUGUST 19, 1988

After only eight days of Bach Remedy intake, she returns prompted by the need to report an astounding new set of symptoms mainly on the physical plane. Her mental/emotional outlook had greatly improved, although a tendency to occasional feelings of discouragement and resignation has remained. Main physical symptoms are: Her headaches have further diminished in intensity but still show main characteristics. However, instead of the overall sense of compression and squeezing of the head, the pressure is now felt mostly on top of the head. There is also a new symptom of pain in the left temple. Further new symptoms are: Strong craving for fruit and fruit juice; there is inability to eat a heavy meal at night; need for frequent urination at night, although she feels that not an overly large amount of fluids had been consumed during previous hours. Her chest feels weak; there is a dry, tickling cough, although she does not have an acute cold. Her menses had been more profuse than usual. She also reports that after bathing a skin rash appears on her thighs and that athlete's foot has flared up between her toes. She feels chilly and somewhat weakened. *Phosphoricum acidum* 200c is prescribed. The initially prescribed Bach Remedies are continued to safeguard mental/emotional healing.

The remedy Phosphoricum acidum was clearly indicated for the physical symptoms and the tendency to resignation, and a single 200c dose effectively cleared all physical symptoms, while further improving her mental/emotional well-being. Her headache, however, was cleared for only three weeks when it returned with new and distinct symptoms that indicated the last remedy necessary to cure the case.

In regard to the overall progress of the case, it was apparent that the Bach Remedies had stimulated a more rapid emergence of an important layer of health disturbance that had been undermining her health and was largely responsible for her painful headaches. The first homeopathic remedies given had already worked through to this layer which initially appeared on the mental/emotional plane without the manifestation of distinct physical symptoms. Phosphoricum acidum is one important remedy for the specific mental/emotional state of resignation and lack of motivation. As the Bach Remedies were treating these mental/emotional components and as Calcarea carbonica stimulated the unraveling of the emerging layer further, the physical symptoms of the new layer became manifest and were ready to be released by the indicated remedy.

It was clear that such rapid progress of cure could hardly have been made without the additional prescription of Bach Remedies. An astounding fact was also that the mental/emotional picture of Phosphoricum acidum, which characteristically shows discouragement, feelings of powerlessness and lack of motivation, had improved under the impact of the selected Bach Remedies and was present only in tendency when Phosphoricum acidum was indicated so strongly on the physical plane. This observation gave the idea of the release effect that occurs when Bach Remedies help the vital force to express important health disturbances less in the mental/emotional realm but more clearly on the physical plane, where they can be released most effectively by homeopathic remedies.

VISIT 6, AUGUST 25, 1988

During her sixth visit, Francisca shares with me a meditative vision which symbolizes her new feeling of freedom, hope and well-being. In this vision, she was working in a steam ship when she peeked out of the window and saw land ahead of her. The land in sight gave hope, promised new horizons and adventure, while the water around her seemed to energize her whole being.

She has not had any headaches since Phosphoricum acidum had been given and was in good spirits about the progress made. The Bach Remedies, Gentian, Wild Rose and Wild Oat are continued to further safeguard her mental/ emotional well-being.

VISIT 7, SEPTEMBER 1, 1988

She has been free of symptoms until shortly before her seventh visit. She reports new feelings of depression and melancholia that were elicited by temporary circumstances in her life and further fed by reminiscences of unhappy times during her college years, now dating back twenty years. Since she has no new additional physical symptoms, the Bach Remedy *Mustard,* indicated in depression, is prescribed to help her cope with this setback, while Gentian, Wild Rose and Wild Oat are continued. It appears that Francisca's psyche, stimulated by present circumstances and the curative effect of the Bach Remedies and the homeopathic remedies, is releasing and bringing to consciousness those unhappy or traumatic times of the past that have not been "digested" properly and have accumulated in the unconscious mind. While being worked through within the unconscious mind, they may have accounted for mental/emotional and physical chronic discomfort and caused the possible emergence of a new layer of health disturbance. As she shares her memories, she finds new understanding and insights, and, with the addition of specifically selected Bach Remedies, healing of past experiences begins to happen.

VISIT 8, SEPTEMBER 9, 1988

She returns, reporting her first headache since Phosphoricum acidm had been given. Her depression, however, which has caused her much concern, has lifted. The headache reappeared on a day of feeling stressed and weary, out of sorts, with neglect of eating regularly. Symptoms of the headache were similar to her former symptoms, yet with new distinct keynotes: There was pain in the forehead and vertex, plus feelings of tightening and squeezing in the head with the urge to clamp her jaws together. Her neck and shoulders were stiff and tense. She felt chilled all over, especially her hands and feet, and she had cold sweat on her body, particularly on the forehead.

Apparently, a new remedy picture or layer, which was being highlighted during acute attacks, had crystallized. Likely, this additional chronic layer of health disturbance had been stimulated by the clearing of the Phosphoricum acidum layer, the added administration of Mustard and the concurrent revival and healing of traumatic past experiences through psychotherapy. Reportedly, the headache had returned with distinctive symptoms, as the depression had cleared under the healing impact of Mustard, showing the previous dynamic of emergence of physical symptoms, as the mind/emotions begin to balance. *Veratrum album* 200c is prescribed in single dose. It was hoped, this one-time high dose would eradicate the tendency to acute Veratrum album headaches. Veratrum album fits the physical symptoms of the acute attacks, has the etiology of exhaustion, and also shows the mental/emotional characteristics of melancholia and depression which already had been lightened by the Bach Remedies. The Bach Remedies Gentian, Wild Rose and Wild Oat are continued; Mustard is discontinued, since the depression has lifted.

VISIT 9, SEPTEMBER 17, 1988

During her next visit, she reports one more headache of the same nature, yet with new and intensified concomitant symptoms which came on after she had done her best in her job under pressure. Despite her efforts at work, she had felt unappreciated and exploited. She had not expressed her emotions but had continued to work hard; this may explain the severity of the ensuing attack. During the acute pain, she experienced the concomitant symptoms of diarrhea and vomiting with coldness, sweat and intense discomfort all over her body.

This recent headache with concurrent symptoms of diarrhea and vomiting had actually shown an even more pronounced picture of Veratrum album. The initial single dose of 200c had not been sufficient to clear this layer and prevent the acute attacks. The vital force signaled the need for additional attention. The potency strength may not have been appropriate in regard to the acute attacks and Francisca is given, in addition to the single 200c dose and the Bach Remedies, a vial of 12c Veratrum album to take repeatedly, if necessary, whenever a headache would come on.

On the mental/emotional plane, some typical Veratrum album symptoms were asserting more strongly as well. The single 200c dose had not been able to clear the layer but had brought it to the fore more distinctly so that homeopathy could cure more deeply, once repeated. This incident shows her willingness to work hard for others and give much at her own expense, with potential chronic effects of exhaustion and threatened breakdown. To help her not repeat this pattern, Francisca is also prescribed the Bach Remedy *Centaury*, for being a too willing servitor. In addition to states of melancholia and depression, this attitude can be part of the mental/emotional picture of Veratrum album, especially the wish to serve others, while simultaneously desiring to impress them with one's own efforts and point of view. As her own point of view had been thwarted during her efforts at work, her body then had expressed what could not be conveyed successfully through normal communication.

VISIT 10, SEPTEMBER 23, 1988

Francisca reports one more headache which was alleviated completely by the administration of Veratrum album 12c. Overall, her outlook on life is good. Centaury has helped her to feel strong and willing to grant herself rest instead of pushing herself to her limits in response to the demands of others, while neglecting her personal needs and path in life. Overall, the remedies Gentian, Wild Rose and Wild Oat also helped her to find more inner ease, freedom and purpose.

Since then, she has had no major headaches and no other major physical complaints. Only minor headaches caused by eyestrain during work on a computer came on from time to time and were alleviated by the homeopathic remedy *Ruta graveolens* in low potency. The low potencies proved very effective for Francisca; generally, they are prescribed with clear instructions for self-management when acute attacks threaten, while the high potency prescriptions, given under direct supervision, more deeply initiate cure by addressing the present layer of health disturbance in its mind/emotions and body totality. With this twofold approach of potency selection and administration, indicated primarily in chronic cases with acute complaints, plus the healing effect of the Bach Remedies, the vital force can be brought to health very effectively, as seen in this case. Overall, Francisca considered herself cured and even her mental/emotional outlook was thoroughly lifted. The Bach Remedies were discontinued gradually, while the effects of cure remained.

CONCLUDING REMARKS

As one looks over the case, one notices that the main complaint had been cured gradually, in a ladder effect, with each remedy lessening the intensity of pain, until the headache was healed with lasting results. Several layers underlying and causing the headache had to be cleared, until the layer mostly responsible for her headaches appeared, with the acute attacks showing forth as a pinnacle of the overall health disturbance. On close examination, one realizes that Veratrum album symptoms had been present in a nutshell throughout her slightly different attacks, especially the chilliness, prostration and sweat, yet they had been overshadowed by the other layers and their specific symptoms. Homeopathic remedies began the unraveling of the different layers. The added administration of Bach Remedies helped release layers even more effectively, especially the crucial underlying Phosphoricum acidum layer, by treating the layer's mental/emotional symptoms, which were present initially and accessible, while stimulating a coherent remedy picture to appear with distinct physical symptoms as well. These symptoms were rather minor, yet distinct enough to lead to a clear homeopathic picture. The homeopathic remedy was then more empowered to clear this newly emerged layer effectively so that the acute headache layer could be reached and cure be completed.

This case and my personal case, which follows, were crucial in demonstrating this dynamic interplay of homeopathic remedies and Bach Remedies.

⌘

5

MY PERSONAL CASE: HIGHLIGHTING THE CATALYTIC EFFECTS OF BACH REMEDIES TOWARDS THE EMERGENCE OF A CLEAR HOMEOPATHIC PICTURE

> 🐜 *Initial Treatment with Bach Remedies*
>
> 🐜 *Sudden Emergence of a Coherent Homeopathic Picture*
>
> 🐜 *Interpretation of Results*

INITIAL TREATMENT WITH BACH REMEDIES

I reached for the Bach Remedies during a demanding time in my life when I prepared for two important exams, while simultaneously taking care of small children and keeping up with home duties. The important exams loomed ahead and made me feel slightly unnerved, although I felt confident that all would go well. I decided to take *Mimulus* to stay calm and not give in to anticipatory fears. Mimulus typically treats uneasiness or fear of the mind in anticipation of events ahead that may be dreaded to some extent but need to be tackled.

To keep up my positive approach and enhance the feeling that all would go well and that the tremendous study load could be mastered, I added the remedy *Larch*. This remedy keeps up the feeling that one's capacities are at their best and that "one should go for it." It safeguards the trust that one has in one's own potential and one's successful active engagement. Larch also helps to stay focused on the duties of the present moment, and these relate to the people one is with as well as to the tasks that one is engaged in. Staying focused in the present was important in regard to upholding the happy engagement with my children, when I was with them during the day, and in regard to concentrating on the study load during the evening, both being crucial for positive outcome of events.

To stay strong, active and mentally concentrated, I chose the additional remedy *Hornbeam*. Hornbeam encourages maximum learning potential and keeps the mind and body energized during demanding times. It would help to keep my mind clear during those regular study hours in the evening when the children were sleeping.

These remedies were taken regularly for the three months preceding the first exam. They helped me to stay well and to concentrate on my various duties. I did not notice any outstanding physical symptoms or unusual activity of the vital force until after the first exam was over.

SUDDEN EMERGENCE OF A COHERENT REMEDY PICTURE

As the hurdle of the written exam was taken, I felt like relaxing for a while and catching my breath before the upcoming hurdle of the oral exams. I felt I had done well in the written portion and hoped for the best. The oral exam ahead, however, did not allow for much relaxation and I set to work again, although I felt drained and without much energy. I also noticed small symptoms that appeared without warning and they surprised me. The good effects wrought by the Bach Remedies seemed overruled, atleast momentarily, by something important that the vital force had to express. All emerging physical symptoms were familiar to me to some extent; I had experienced them off and on throughout my life. Now, they seemed to come up simultaneously, forming one coherent impression of overall symptomatology.

At this point, I was not yet aware of the catalytic effect of Bach Remedies in producing coherent remedy pictures; this awareness ripened fully after having observed several cases with this same dynamic of symptomatic expression. This case was crucial, however, in demonstrating the single power of the Bach Remedies in eliciting a clear picture of symptomatic expression.

As I looked at my symptoms, I decided to take my own case, feeling that this unusual occurrence of symptoms needed attention.

These were the main symptoms:

MIND/EMOTIONS: Increased weariness in mind and body, with a desire to rest and not have to struggle. Increased irritability.

HEAD: A slight feeling of tightness between eyebrows and higher up on the forehead with concurrent unpleasant feelings of being in a bad mood, or of being easily annoyed. These feelings seemed to originate in this tightness around the forehead. I was able to keep annoyance under control, but the tendency existed.

EYES: Slightly irritated lids, with a sensation of heat around the eyes.

NOSE: Discharge of mucus from the left nostril with some blood mixed in. Throughout my life, I had had the tendency to produce mucus, sometimes purulent, from nasal sinus cavities. This time, the mucus was only slightly yellowish.

STOMACH: A gnawing, almost painful feeling, especially when the stomach was empty. Great craving for ham. Increased thirst and increased hunger.

ABDOMEN: Slight feeling of extension, although no extension was noticeable from the outside.

KIDNEY REGION: A dull ache across the back in kidney region.

BLADDER: Increased urination.

Initially, none of the well known remedies came to mind. This seemed to be a new or unusual remedy in my case history as well, arising from deep within. The tendency to increased urination made me think of such remedies as *Phosphoricum acidum, Argentum nitricum, China (Cinchona officinalis),* or *Arsenicum album.* I searched the literature and the repertory for confirming symptoms, but none of these remedies seemed to fit quite right. The marked craving for ham finally led me to an unusual remedy, namely *Uranium nitricum,* which is listed in Kent's repertory under "desires raw ham" in the section on the stomach. I had eaten cooked ham but probably would have found raw ham equally appealing. One might want to add "cooked ham" to this rubric. Upon further examination, this remedy seemed to have potential. It did cover the main symptoms. The literature on Uranium nitricum is not extensive, but I gathered enough information to confirm the remedy.

A single dose of 200c had astounding results. For the first few days after taking the remedy, however, I felt no reaction. Then, all symptoms were highlighted, and I felt that my vital force was truly responding. Subsequently, all symptoms left and never returned, and this dates back five years. Here are the curative results:

My usual cheerfulness returned, and the tendency to irritability with concomitant pressure in the forehead gave way to a friendly, open feeling and a clarified sensation around the forehead. The irritation around the eyelids disappeared. The sinus cavities, which had shown a tendency to long-lasting infections throughout my life, cleared up and since then have been free of disturbance, this administration of Uranium nitricum dating back five years. Furthermore, the tendency to coughs and bronchial infections, which had been occasionally active throughout my life, vanished. The temporarily strong craving for ham was normalized, the hunger pains healed, and the slight abdominal feelings of extension had left. The dull aching across the kidney region and the tendency to increased urination were healed. I also noticed a vitalizing effect throughout my whole being. Tasks seemed enjoyable again, there was new incentive to go on with my various duties. Furthermore, there was new strength of body posture, as if liberated or freed of pressures.[15]

The Bach Remedies were slowly discontinued, since I felt well in mind and body. Soon the last exam was passed successfully and life went back to normal.

INTERPRETATION OF RESULTS

I knew that a crucial layer had been released, one that was largely responsible for my individual tendencies to health disturbance. Each person has certain "weak spots" or recurrent troubles that can be eradicated as soon as the main layer underneath is elicited and cured. I bel..eved that the Bach Remedies had in some way furthered this process of manifesting the crucial layer. Three months of continued Bach Remedy intake had mobilized the vital force in such a way that a layer from deep within came to the fore, ready to be acknowledged and released. The remedy picture was clearly presented, and one single dose of the indicated homeopathic remedy took hold of the economy with an optimal, most efficient curative effect.

As uranium rests deep within the earth, this layer arose from deep within the economy. It is generally understood by students and practitioners of homeopathy that those layers cured by the potentized heavier elements or minerals used within homeopathy tend to lie at the bottom of a case, whereas the more accessible top layers use remedies mostly from the plant kingdom, although this succession may not be existent or apparent in each case. As plants form the outer accessible layer of the earth, the top layers within a case are often treated with remedies gained from plants. In my case as well, the plant remedy *Hydrastis canadensis* was indicated months after Uranium nitricum had been given. This remedy took hold with lasting results, since the underlying disturbance had been removed first and since the unraveling effect of the previously administered Bach Remedies had continued.

The usual way to do homeopathy is to treat those symptoms that are visible on top, with the hope and intent of peeling off each layer, until the bottom layer is reached. The case of Francisca was initially treated in this same manner. It was noticeable, however, that accelerated and deepened progress of cure was achieved by the added use of the Bach Remedies which furthered the emergence of the crucial underlying layer, Phosphoricum acidum, and led to the correct prescription of Veratrum album, a plant remedy healing the remaining and clearly expressed manifestations of Francisca's headache. The Bach Remedies appear to stimulate the vital force to bring to the fore the remedy most responsible for the overall manifestations of ill-health. The process of cure is reversed; the bottom layers tend to be released first, with the top layers following.

Cure begins by analyzing the mind/emotions and determining the present needs. As the mental/emotional disturbances are being addressed by the Bach Remedies, the vital force is freed of major negative energy expense in the mental/emotional realm and can set to work in the overall economy. As mind/emotions and body work as a unit toward release, the physical symptoms accompanying the mental/emotional complaint emerge for coherent treatment as well. A unification of all curative forces occurs, with coherence of overall symptomatology appearing. The Uranium nitricum picture, in my case, was stimulated by the remedies Mimulus, Larch, Hornbeam, all of which deal with strengthening the mind so that extra mental demands could be coped with. Hornbeam may have been most responsible for the release of the Uranium nitricum picture which typically shows the mental/emotional symptoms of weariness and irritability due to fatigue and overexertion of the mind. Along with the continued effect of the Bach Remedies, this homeopathic remedy helped to strengthen mental powers of concentration and vitality.

Concomitant physical symptoms were released as well, together with deep-seated tendencies to health disturbances. The overall economy found new strength and vitality, and the vital force was enabled to reach with healing impulse into areas of the economy other than the original Bach Flower prescription had targeted for. Bach Remedies stimulated a snowball effect of curative release which was carried to new heights by the added use of homeopathic medicines.

It is apparent that consideration of the psychological state with correct recognition of mental/emotional states is crucial for overall cure. The thirty-eight mental/emotional states as described by Bach and their respective healing remedies are worthy of in-depth study so that diagnosis and prescription become as simple and clear as possible and maximum curative release can be triggered and achieved.

6

BACH'S SEVEN GROUPS OF REMEDIES AND THE
SPECIFIC INDICATIONS FOR EACH REMEDY

INITIAL COMMENTS

Bach divided the thirty-eight mental/emotional states of mankind into seven groups that represent seven areas of consciousness where imbalances can occur. Each group lists several remedies that heal those specific imbalances within one group. How these remedies differ within the group and how their main indications and therapeutic goals are to be viewed will be explained in this chapter, which gives a good introduction and quick overview in regard to the thirty-eight remedies.

Emphasis is on seeing how the mind/emotions behave in each one of these states of imbalance.

GROUP 1: FOR THOSE WHO HAVE FEAR

Rock Rose:

Rock Rose heals acute states of extreme fear and terror and their after-effects. During an acute state, there may be feelings of great danger, sometimes with the urge to run, and the mind is racing also. There may be fear of death.

In chronic cases, Rock Rose treats sensitive nervous systems and states of chronic anxiety.

Goal: Courage, self-transcendence, true heroism.

Mimulus:

The mind goes forward anticipating fearful events and shrinking away from them with a sense of dread. Mimulus treats concrete fears of known objects, situations, or people.

Goal: Facing feared events with courage and trust.

Cherry Plum:

In the negative Cherry Plum state, the mind is struggling to hold down threatening impulses from the unconscious, as it knows them to be wrong and does not want to engage in them. There is anticipatory fear that the impulses will win, and reason and control will give way.

Goal: Learning to understand the true meaning of the impulses arising from the unconscious, and learning to integrate them into the conscious mind in a healthy, non-threatening way.

Aspen:

The mind is in a fearful state with a sense of foreboding without knowing what exactly threatens. There is free-floating anxiety and a feeling of being vulnerable to outside forces that are sinister and out of one's control. Vague eerie feelings and superstitions are easily stimulated.

Goal: Faith that one is safe and guarded.

Red Chestnut:

The mind goes out to a loved one with fear that something bad or dangerous might befall this loved one. Typically, the loved one is removed and out of the immediate watch care of the one in fear, and there is the feeling that the situation is out of control and one cannot guard the threatened one. With this state, there may be great nervousness and agitation.

Goal: Releasing the other to his destiny with faith.

GROUP 2: FOR THOSE WHO SUFFER UNCERTAINTY

Cerato:

Within oneself, there is uncertainty and lack of decisiveness. One's own ability to make decisions is not trusted and others are often asked for advice. Often there is lack of inner assuredness or lack of self-confidence.

Goal: Inner assuredness and wisdom; increasing intuitive powers.

Scleranthus:

Uncertainty results from having to choose between two options, usually of some magnitude, and not being able to make up one's mind. There is dread of making the wrong decision, of having to let go of one option which might have been the better one in hindsight. Typically, there is flooding of the mind with details and arguments, and one loses perspective.

Goal: Lifting the mind to a higher vantage point so that a new perspective and overview can be gained. Reliance on inner wisdom.

Gentian:

Uncertainty extends into the area of action and doing. In the negative Gentian state, one is easily discouraged and often gives up an activity when obstacles arise.

Goal: Faith in one's ability and perseverance. Faith in general.

Gorse:

In the negative Gorse state, there is loss of certainty and hope that anything can be done to be saved or to save oneself from the undesired condition one is in.

Goal: New hope.

Hornbeam:

Uncertainty lies in the inability to focus the mind with clarity and power of concentration to the tasks at hand. The mind, and to some extent also the body, seems tired, prone to procrastination and bent on avoiding prolonged effort.

Goal: Mental clarity and joy of attending to one's tasks.

Wild Oat:

In the negative Wild Oat state, there is uncertainty in the area of motivation and incentive in regard to choosing a current activity or a whole life path. There may be a passing interest in various activities which are abandoned, since certainty of endeavor and true satisfaction are missing. Daily chores may be accomplished with a sense of boredom or with aversion.

Goal: Rekindling of joy and incentive while engaging in current activities deemed necessary or worthwhile. Inner certainty in one's quest for actualization of one's potentials.

GROUP 3: NOT SUFFICIENT INTEREST IN PRESENT CIRCUMSTANCES

Clematis:

One does not believe that happiness can be found in the present, and the mind wanders with longing to a time in the future when fulfillment is hoped for. There is daydreaming and absent-mindedness.

Goal: Trust that happiness is to be found here and now and that one can reach for it.

Honeysuckle:

In the negative Honeysuckle state, one dwells with nostalgic feelings in the memories of happiness once experienced in the past, believing that the present or future will never duplicate that happiness.

Goal: Trust that the present and future promise and hold new happiness. Gratitude for previous happiness.

Wild Rose:

The present denotes hardship and unhappiness that one feels powerless to rise above. As a consequence, one loses interest in the present and experiences apathy and lack of involvement.

Goal: To feel empowered again in regard to changing one's lot.

Olive:

Mind and body are too exhausted to attend with full capacity the tasks at hand. There is great fatigue with an urge to avoid oneself from involving in the present circumstances and give in to the need to rest.

Goal: To strengthen and revitalize the mind/emotions and body.

White Chestnut:

The mind is preoccupied with worrying thoughts of a serious nature that have more impact than the circumstances of the present moment and remove the person therefrom.

Goal: To increase serenity of mind so that worrisome thoughts can be kept at bay and free the mind for devotion to the present.

Mustard:

The mind is overshadowed by depression and gloom, making it almost impossible for the person to find joy in the present circumstances.

Goal: To bring light and incentive to the mind so that life appeals again.

Chestnut Bud:

The mind is unsettled and impulsive, too restless to attend to the circumstances of the present. As a consequence, there is lack of depth-involvement with issues at hand, and life's lessons and experiences may not be grasped in their deeper meaning.

Goal: To become calm and to deepen the understanding and learning of life's lessons.

GROUP 4: LONELINESS

Water Violet:

Loneliness of mind and heart arises by removing oneself from people and putting oneself above them, instead of tuning in to their inner natures and bonding with them.

Goal: Spontaneous affection, easy opening up towards others, "we are all created equal."

Impatiens:

Inner loneliness exists because one is quick in thought and action and urges others on to follow, without taking their inner needs, their personal pace and individual natures into account.

Goal: To allow others to unfold according to their individual pace; patience based on inner kindness.

Heather:

Inner loneliness comes from not connecting fully with others and their personal needs. Instead, one is overly concerned with one's own affairs and needs, and one gives in to the strong urge to talk about them.

Goal: To become a good listener and tune in to others' problems, which leads to de-emphasis of one's own concerns.

GROUP 5: OVERSENSITIVE TO INFLUENCES AND IDEAS

Agrimony:

The mind is overly sensitive to discord and disharmony in the environment, especially since there is already internal restlessness and worry, plus the effort to find peace within one's own mind.

Goal: To strengthen inner peace so that outside discord is not too disturbing.

Centaury:

Oversensitivity comes from being too open and receptive to the expectations and demands of others, enhanced by one's desire to love and serve.

Goal: To keep one's own needs in mind, while upholding one's good intentions and joy of service.

Walnut:

The mind is overly sensitive to all impressions and influences from the outside, especially during transitional stages of life when the person leaves behind a definite structure of living and is open to new impressions.

Goal: To give inner stability, reduce vulnerability to impressions that may disturb inner balance and deter from the state of being true to oneself.

Holly:

The mind/emotions and body are overly sensitive to upsetting circumstances within the environment, or to personally perceived circumstances of threat, that create vexations, irritation, and the need to "fight back." Emotions of a strong and vehement nature are easily stirred up and may turn the person away from kindheartedness, if only temporarily.

Goal: To stay focused on love and kindness; forbearance.

GROUP 6: FOR DESPONDENCY OR DESPAIR

Larch:

Shaken self-confidence, possibly leading to despondency and despair, arising from lack of those joyful and devoted experiences with people and tasks that would improve self-esteem and knowledge of one's capacities. Preoccupation and worry about self may further prevent healthful engagement and stabilized self-esteem.

Goal: Creating a balanced and sturdy self-confidence by reducing focus on oneself and devoting oneself to other people and tasks.

Pine:

Despondency and despair center around guilt feelings that one feels unable to rise above. Self-blame and regret may be high.

Goal: Resolve to not repeat the same fault and forgive oneself. Self-forgiveness comes easier when one learns to forgive others with similar faults.

Elm:

The mind feels overwhelmed by tasks or happenings, and a state of despondency or despair may come on, since one does not feel empowered or in charge enough to get a handle on things.

Goal: To give inner calm and a new overview so that tasks can be mastered one at a time.

Sweet Chestnut:

Despondency and despair arise from not seeing meaning in life and giving one's thoughts to faithlessness and nihilism.

Goal: To have faith and trust in a meaningful universe and be open to guidance by one's inner truth and love.

Star of Bethlehem:

Sadness, grief, or the bad effects from trauma cause despondency or despair.

Goal: To soothe and comfort the heart and release trauma.

Willow:

Despondency and despair arise from the perception of not being dealt with fairly and feeling resentment towards those at fault or towards fate in general.

Goal: Forgiveness and gratitude for the good aspects of one's life.

Oak:

Despondency and despair come from working very hard and not making satisfying progress or gaining rewards. There is a tendency to stoicism and feats of willpower.

Goal: To balance work and recreation in a healthful way. To work "playfully."

Crab Apple:

The mind concentrates on one's internal or external aspect of the personality considered unclean or shameful, with feelings of helplessness and possibly guilt, and, as a consequence, one feels despondency and despair.

Goal: To create healthy self-acceptance.

GROUP 7: OVERCARE FOR WELFARE OF OTHERS

Chicory:

One overly attends to others in a rather self-centered way without fully taking the others' inner needs into account, especially their need for independence. One seeks closeness with those one cares for. There is easily aroused self-pity, if one's efforts are not recognized or wished for.

Goal: True tuning in to the others' inner world and respect for their wishes. Ability to turn self-pity into continued true devotion.

Vervain:

One is convinced that certain ideas or views are right, and one ardently tries to convert others to one's own viewpoint, which leads to overcare for others' welfare.

Goal: To be open-minded to different views and allow others to determine their own views and opinions.

Vine:

Overcare for others' welfare exists in one's tendency to influence and control others, even if they do not wish for it.

Goal: To let others determine their own course of action. To allow oneself to be led, instead of being the leader, should the situation call for it.

Beech:

One sets up ideals of people's behavior, their demeanor and position in life and criticizes those that do not measure up. Overcare for others' welfare exists, if this attitude is openly expressed and attempts are made to fit the other into this ideal image.

Goal: To develop tolerance and learn to appreciate others for what they are, seeing their strengths, rather than evaluating them by their shortcomings.

Rock Water:

In the negative Rock Water state, one is a hard master onto oneself and believes oneself to be a good example to others. This brings the urge to inspire and convert them, leading to overcare for others' welfare.

Goal: To be more reasonably lenient and gentle with oneself. To cultivate the attitude of "live and let live."

GROUP 8: RESCUE REMEDY

Bach also discovered a unique combination of five remedies which aim at restoring balance and calm to a person in acute emergency situations. Rescue Remedy is of great value immediately after accidents or similar moments of shock and panic when there is faintness, trembling, or other failing of normal physical functioning.

Here are the contributions of the five remedies that together give a unique synergistic effect:

Rock Rose to counteract terror and panic; *Cherry Plum* to balance intense tension and the fear that events and one's own life, including one's mental power, are out of control; *Clematis* to reduce faintness or coma; *Impatiens* to counteract inner turmoil, tension and impatience; and *Star of Bethlehem* to reduce shock, trauma, sadness and to prevent the trauma's possible long-lasting effects on mind/emotions and body from imprinting.

Rescue Remedy can also be used as a daily remedy in chronic situations of intense nervousness and tension when the vital force needs to recharge and recuperate.

⌘

7

PRESENTATION OF THE THIRTY-EIGHT BACH REMEDIES BY USE OF CASES, WITH ANALYSIS OF COMPARATIVE HOMEOPATHIC REMEDIES

INITIAL COMMENTS

While homeopathic remedies treat whole aspects of the personality that may contain several mental/emotional tendencies, the Bach Remedies "dissect" the overall mental/emotional picture and aim at specifically treating each recognizable mental/emotional imbalance. This explains why cases usually need several Bach Remedies, given at once or gradually, to encompass the totality of the mental/emotional picture. By aiming at specific areas of the personality, the Bach Remedies also have a more intensified curative effect in that particular area than a homeopathic remedy that could not reach the target area as specifically. Homeopathic remedies, however, effectively address the totality of symptoms on the physical and mental/emotional planes and gives a powerful boost to the overall progress of cure.

Twelve cases, creatively presented, will describe the thirty-eight mental/emotional states and their respective healing remedies. Case material is derived largely from actual case observation, from real life observations of people's mental/emotional imbalances and from insights into the dynamics of the psyche. Each case is treated with three or four remedies that address the overall picture of the mind/emotions. The cases are presented from the prescriber's viewpoint. Focus is on prescribing accurately, with insight and care, so that cure can be predicted with assurance. For this reason, the cases are not followed up or investigated further in this presentation; cure is entailed in the accuracy of analysis, prescription and prediction.

Homeopathic remedies complementing the case are analyzed for the purpose of comparative study. These homeopathic remedies mirror in their own symptomatology the tendencies towards those mental/emotional imbalances treated by the Bach Remedies. Usually, several homeopathic remedies are potentially applicable in the treatment of certain psychological states, and exact prescribing hinges on recognizing the minute details in the physical area and in the mind/emotions as well. Each case is unique and should be assessed with a fresh point of view. In this sense, the homeopathic remedies chosen for the twelve sample cases should not be regarded as general complementary remedies for those specific mental/emotional states described in the case.

The cases presented do not overly deal with physical symptoms but concentrate on portraying, recognizing and treating the mental/emotional states of imbalance. The cases mostly represent people with only minor or hardly noticeable physical complaints, except for case Two. One homeopathic remedy that contains the same psychological dynamics plus matches the physical symptoms will be presented for comparative study purposes as well and in some cases similar homeopathic remedies are referred to in addition.

In regard to prescribing, to warrant additional homeopathic treatment in cases of mental/emotional emphasis, some major physical keynotes should be apparent, however subtle. In case one starts treatment with Bach Remedies only, one has to be aware of the highlighting effect of physical symptoms, however subtle, which could arise, as the vital force tries to make known the homeopathic remedy it needs by releasing emphasis of symptomatic expression from the mind/emotions to the physical plane. In cases of chronic disease with mental/emotional imbalance and concomitant physical symptoms, this release effect will be more pronounced in symptomatic expression on the physical plane, and homeopathic treatment is definitely indicated; in severe states, homeopathic remedies should be given along with the Bach Remedies at the beginning of the treatment, to give faster relief. In lighter cases of chronic physical disease or discomfort, the Bach Remedies alone are able to cure symptoms, since healing of the tissues can begin as the mind/emotions clear and the concomitant physical symptoms are being highlighted and focused on by the vital force. Bach himself was able to cure even pronounced or long-standing states of chronic illness with the Bach Remedies only.[16] If homeopathic remedies are added to the treatment, they greatly enhance, accelerate, or even complete cure of both, physical complaints and the mental/emotional imbalances as well.

Each case will represent one of the twelve types or twelve outstanding mental/emotional states which Bach found basic to mankind. The twelve respective Bach Remedies, or *healers,* in addition to two or three supporting remedies, are analyzed in their healing potential, as they lighten in combined action the person's mental/emotional difficulties that arose in response to a concrete acute or longer-lasting chronic circumstance of life. At the beginning of each remedy presentation, Bach's own description of the indications for each remedy, marked by empathic understanding and clarity, is given.[17] The plants will be explored in their expressive potential, as they indicate the negative or positive or both of the mental/emotional state in view of the Doctrine of Signatures.[18] The flowering periods given may vary in length according to regional climate.

CASE 1. MIMULUS, CRAB APPLE, LARCH, WILD ROSE (SILICEA)

Doris, eighteen years old, is concerned about her skin, especially her facial skin. She has a mild case of acne that she feels is beyond help, since she has tried, rather inconsistently, a few ways of improving it without apparent success. She has resigned herself to this unwanted condition which greatly affects her overall life experience.

The feeling that her skin is unattractive and unclean hinders her enjoyment of life and her social contact with others. She fears that others, especially the other sex, find her undesirable or would appraise her negatively, preferring women with a healthy complexion. She feels like retreating and turning her face away when others look at her closely, and she fearfully anticipates social events. Often her fear of mixing with the world takes hold of her, and she wants to stay home, behind closed doors.

She does not share her feelings openly with others but rather hides them, being afraid others will put her down because of her insecurities. She feels vulnerable inside and is afraid of intimacy with a partner and of people in general invading her space too closely. During the interview, she appears somewhat nervous yet willing to share her emotional state openly. She also shows intent to get a handle on her emotional hindrances; she especially does not want to be afraid of being observed or appraised by others. She is hoping to gain inner strength, confidence, and improved feelings of inner and outer beauty.

The Bach Remedies *Mimulus* for fear, *Crab Apple* for shame, *Larch* for low self-worth and *Wild Rose* for resignation are indicated to lighten Doris' emotional burden, improve her skin and help her reach her overall goals.

On the physical plane she shows a tendency to suppuration, sore throats, sweat on head and feet, sluggish posture, and chilliness.

MIMULUS (Mimulus guttatus)

Group: For Those Who Have Fear.

Preparation: Sun method, use of flowers.

Flowering Period: June through August.

Indications by Bach: Fear of worldly things, illness, pain, accidents, poverty, of dark, of being alone, of misfortune. The fears of everyday life. These people quietly and secretly bear their dread, they do not speak freely of it to others. *(Twelve Healers)*

Mimulus was chosen as the main remedy or type remedy because of her tendency to shyness and because fear had become too prevalent in her life. Specifically, Mimulus was to counteract her nervousness in social situations, her fears of appraisal and rejection by others, her dread that others will find out about her internal insecurities, and her fear that her skin condition is beyond help. Mimulus would enable Doris to enjoy life more and give herself more freely to others without feeling stifled by needless fears. It would help her foster devotion, courage and incentive to mix with the world without anticipatory fears and worry about unpopularity or rejection.

A general keynote of Mimulus is the looking ahead of the mind with anticipatory fears to a dreaded concrete situation. This can be fear of appraisal as in Doris' case, or it can be fear of concrete events such as exams, surgical operations, or impending poverty. In the negative Mimulus state, one cannot easily face these situations but rather feels like retreating from them. Under the action of the remedy, the fearful event ahead will appear less threatening and overwhelming, but more like a normal occurrence in the continuum of life that can be dealt with.

The "Common Monkey Flower" is the popular name of the Mimulus plant, which is native to North America. Interestingly, in literature and legends, the monkey is seen as a symbol of fear. When one looks at the Mimulus plant closely, one could imagine the flowers that hang sidewise on the stem as tugged-in heads, indicating a shy, fearful, somewhat dejected look. Yet, the happy yellow color and friendly openness of the petals, plus the plant's tendency to grow in groups near soothing streams, speak of the healing quality brought to those troubled by fears and stifled by the tendency to retreat from people and the world. Mimulus creates an easily flowing consciousness without unnecessary fears and shyness, furthering enjoyment of people and life in general. The mind stays focused on the present, and the people and tasks at hand rather than envisioning or dreading fearful events or circumstances.

CRAB APPLE (Malus sylvestris/pumila)

Group: For Despondency or Despair.

Preparation: Boiling of clusters of flowers and leaves.

Flowering Period: May.

Indications by Bach: This is the remedy of cleansing.

For those who feel as if they had something not quite clean about themselves.

Often it is something of apparently little importance: in others there maybe a more serious disease which is almost disregarded compared to the one thing on which they concentrate.

In both types they are anxious to be free from the one particular thing which is greatest in their minds and which seems so essential to them that it should be cured.

They become despondent, if treatment fails.

Being a cleanser, this remedy purifies wounds if the patient has reason to believe that some poison has entered which must be drawn out. *(Twelve Healers)*

Crab Apple was chosen for Doris because her skin problem had become her foremost preoccupation or fixed idea, and because she felt her problem had to be cured before she could be acceptable to herself and others, and find happiness. She felt unattractive and stifled by the need to hide her flaws from others, indicating the Crab Apple sensitivity to appraisal. Social enjoyment, devotion to others and healthy self-forgetfulness were hampered by her preoccupation with her outer appearance and her feelings of imperfection. Doris also felt some despondency, especially since several treatments to improve her skin condition had failed.

The remedy Crab Apple would lessen preoccupation with her flaw and help her understand that her skin problem was not overly important and that attention should rather be focused on her goodness and love that benefit others and help her to accept herself. Crab Apple would act as a cleansing remedy in the mind and in the body as well, affecting her skin also. As one feels purity and self-acceptance, the body responds with efforts to purify and bring about beauty and health.

Generally, Crab Apple is not only indicated in preoccupation with physical flaws but also helps in healing concern and shame in regard to certain traits of character, habits, or thought patterns that are considered wrong, unclean, or imperfect. Often there are feelings of helplessness, as in addictions, and the need to hide the wrong or unclean aspect. By reducing preoccupation with defects, Crab Apple opens the mind and helps to initiate change towards more wholesome patterns, or, should imperfect aspects persist, it helps to restore feelings of self-acceptance and purity. In case wrong habits affect the welfare of others, everything must be done to turn defects into positive action, while the remedy works to release shame or guilt. Oftentimes, Crab Apple is also indicated for the receiver of the faulty action, who may feel soiled or have loathing towards the wrong suffered, as in extreme cases of abuse or sex offense.

Crab Apple, as the name indicates, takes care of those thoughts and faulty patterns that are needless, impure and stifle recognition of one's true values. It reestablishes feelings of inner and outer beauty and innocence. The tree itself expresses the idea of purity through its radiant white-pink blossoms which effectively stand out from the dark green foliage. The blossoms are delicately shaped, clean looking and beautifully scented.

LARCH (Larix decidua)

Group: For Despondency or Despair.

Preparation: Boiling of twigs with both male and female flowers.

Flowering Period: March and April.

Indications by Bach: For those who do not consider themselves as good or capable as those around them, who expect failure, who feel they will never be a success, and so do not venture or make a strong enough attempt to succeed. *(Twelve Healers)*

Larch was chosen to counteract Doris' feeling of inferiority due to her skin condition. She expected failure in interpersonal relations and lack of popularity and considered herself less desirable or successful than girls with beautiful complexion. Because she did not openly and easily give herself to others, she received little feedback as to her worth as a person, and this made her feel less desirable or capable of achieving recognition.

Larch would give her new self-confidence, including the confidence that she can improve her skin condition. Larch would also lessen the worries about herself and enable her to concentrate on "where the others are at." Self-esteem would grow as the others, feeling enriched and grateful for her attention, returned her focus and caring.

In the negative Larch state, as in Doris' case, one compares oneself with others and comes out the short end. The remedy increases awareness of one's positive potential and instills the feeling that "one can do it," may it be the accomplishment of a certain endeavor or project within one's job, school, or home life, or, as in this case, the achievement of recognition among peers and acceptance by others and by one's own self. The remedy Larch helps to shift the focus from personal concerns to concentration on tasks or people. As one devotes oneself to others and meaningful tasks, internal stumbling blocks are overcome, while the joy of service is activated. This joy is the experience of the positive Larch state; creative potential is released and success and self-confidence are achieved, as one is aware of people and the world benefiting from one's desire and deed to serve and accomplish.

The Larch tree speaks of a state of low self-confidence by its apparent inability to hold itself erect and by its drooping branches. During frosty winters, it survives without being able to draw water from the frozen ground, which is unusual for trees, and it needs to shed its leaves to survive. The tree revives as frost declines; water is again raised through the trunk, and slowly leaves and delicate red flowers begin to form. The tree may experience this refreshing rebirth in a similar way as the "larched-up" person enjoys a new sense of self-confidence and revival of personal effectiveness, plus renewed devotion to people and tasks. As the water creates new sap and renews leaves and blossoms, so does newly inspired confidence end the state of being "sapped" and yield the fruits and joys of service and accomplishment.

WILD ROSE (Rosa canina)

Group: Not Sufficient Interest in Present Circumstances.

Preparation: Boiling of flowers with leaves and stalks.

Flowering Period: June and July.

Indications by Bach: Those who without apparently sufficient reason become resigned to all that happens, and just glide through life, take it as it is, without any effort to improve things and find some joy. They have surrendered to the struggle of life without complaint. *(Twelve Healers)*

Wild Rose was indicated for Doris because she did not feel empowered enough to rise above her limiting conditions. Specifically, she was not able to gain self-acceptance and popularity, which was due, as she felt, to her skin that she conceived as unattractive. Since various efforts at improving her skin condition had failed, she felt powerless and uncertain in regard to solving this problem. Yet, she had the wish to handle her emotions more effectively, while still hoping to gain more beauty. Wild Rose was chosen to give her the necessary inner strength and dynamic to rise above her feeling of powerlessness and begin the process of actualizing her wishes and hopes. As the mind begins to activate new wholesome patterns of thought and action, the body also responds with renewed attempts to establish health in those areas that have been disturbed or unbalanced.

As the stifling attitude of "this is beyond help" no longer attaches to her skin condition, new attempts at healing ensue.

Wild Rose is also indicated in severe cases when limiting factors remain, as in permanent disabilities, terminal illness, or loss of a loved one. Despite restricting conditions, Wild Rose will give a new sense of freedom that arises from deep within the self. Wild Rose will also help the compassionate onlooker who wishes to help the sufferer, yet lacks the power or ability to do so.

The Wild Rose bush conveys the impression of liberated abundance, freedom of growth and beauty. These same qualities grow in a heart once resigned to limiting conditions; there is new incentive to change and increased zest for living.

Comparative Study of Applicable Homeopathic Remedy:

The remedy *Silicea,* made from flint, would match Doris' mental/ emotional symptom picture. Silicea is a substance that gives structure and support to plants and humans as well. If a person develops insufficient assimilation of this vital substance, problems related to stamina and vitality ensue. On the mental/ emotional plane, a person in need of Silicea is generally shy, nervous and suffers easily from anticipatory fears (Mimulus). There is also a tendency to anticipate failure and feel less capable than others or inferior to others (Larch). Fixed ideas, as Doris' assumption of being unlovable due to her skin, are also common in the Silicea state (Crab Apple). There can be preoccupation with internal problems and retreat from social situations. Often, there is a tendency to feel weakened within oneself or not fully empowered in one's potential (Wild Rose).

This dynamic is not fully expressed in each Silicea case but should be visible in tendency; depending on the person's strength of character, it is managed in varying degrees. People in need of Silicea are usually very sensitive to impressions, as well as being sensitive to the needs of others. They are often helpful people, appear generally refined and may be delicate in appearance. Although they appear flexible, they can also show obstinacy, mainly due to their tendency to have fixed ideas and preoccupation that are not easily shaken off. Some physical confirming symptoms would be: A tendency to suppuration; recurrent sore throats; increased sweat of scalp and feet; lack of physical stamina, sluggish posture, chilliness; in some cases, thinning of hair and white spots on nails; Doris had most of these symptoms.

Several other homeopathic remedies could apply in similar cases of acne and social shyness, such as *Calcarea sulphurica, Thuja occidentalis, Pulsatilla nigricans, Calcarea carbonica* and so on. The exact mental/emotional and physical analysis of symptoms decides the choice of remedy.

CASE 2. ROCK ROSE, GORSE, SWEET CHESTNUT, OLIVE (ARSENICUM ALBUM)

Jane, a lady in her late fifties, is admitted to the hospital to be under constant supervision during the terminal stages of her inoperable stomach cancer. She is of the nervy type and awaits death with recurring feelings of fright and a general state of tension. She is shaky, weak and almost unable to consume any food. She is unable to sit up in bed and is compelled to lie down. Every little effort exhausts her.

While she lies passively without any distracting occupation, her thoughts become overwhelming and she greatly suffers from death anxieties, hopelessness and deepest despair which is kept inside and hardly expressed. Her hopelessness centers around the terminal state of her illness and is aggravated by the absence of her son whom she would like to see before she dies, yet she knows he is deterred by an overseas war and unable to come home. She sees no meaning in her own suffering and also despairs over the unnecessary annihilation of life in the war, imagining with fright that her son may die also. She had viewed scenes of the war on television prior to being admitted to the hospital, and she had despaired over them and lost all faith.

The following Bach Remedies are chosen to uplift her emotions and ease her through the last struggles of life: *Rock Rose* for fear and terror, including fear for her son's life, *Gorse* for hopelessness, *Sweet Chestnut* for feelings of meaninglessness and faithlessness and *Olive* for exhaustion.

Additional physical symptoms are: Frequent vomiting and diarrhea, thirst for sips, restlessness despite great weakness, and aggravation at midnight.

ROCK ROSE (Helianthemum nummularium)

Group: For Those Who Have Fear.

Preparation: Sun method, use of flowers.

Flowering Period: May through August.

Indications by Bach: The rescue remedy. The emergency remedy for cases where there appears no hope. In accidents or sudden illnesses, or when the patient is very frightened or terrified, or if the condition is serious enough to cause great fear to those around. If the patient is not conscious the lips may be moistened with the remedy. Other remedies in addition may also be required, as, for example, if there is unconsciousness, which is a deep, sleepy state, Clematis; if there is torture, Agrimony, and so on. *(Twelve Healers)*

These above words give the indications for Rock Rose during emergencies, but Rock Rose is also prescribed in chronic cases of tension and nervousness which show recurring feelings of fright and terror. Especially if death is to be faced, there can be occasional attacks of panic and general fragility of nerves. Being of the nervy type and because of intense circumstances, Jane was in need of this remedy. It would help her calm down, gain strength and face the last stages of her cancer, the accompanying pain, and death calmly. It would also help her to feel less fright in view of her own son's possible death. She imagined her son to be under dangerous circumstances, and, fed by her own closeness to death, held great terror in her heart. As Bach said, this remedy also helps the onlooker as death threatens a loved one.

Red Chestnut is another remedy that treats fears for another person's welfare, and it would have helped her also. Rock Rose, however, because of her own closeness to death, covered her fears for her son's life as well. Oftentimes, five or more remedies seem indicated on taking the case. It is best to limit prescriptions to two, three or four remedies, so as not to send too many healing impulses at once.

In general, Rock Rose gives self-transcendence and courage during dangerous times, or when death is imminent. It is also of use during milder circumstance when there is debility or fragility of nerves, an easily frightened or startled state, a tendency to nightmares, or a past trauma of fright that continues to have an impact.

The area around the stomach becomes especially weak and tense in the negative Rock Rose state. This is also where Jane's stomach cancer had developed. She has had the tendency to fearful worry and easy agitation of nerves throughout the major part of her life.

The beautiful, delicate Rock Rose flower grows on rocky terrain, difficult for plants to take hold in, as if to speak of the courage and power for survival that it transmits to the psyche. The bright yellow color of the flowers conveys comfort, cheer, and the healing warmth of the sun.

GORSE (Ulex europaeus)

Group: For Those Who Suffer Uncertainty.

Preparation: Sun method, use of flowers with stalks.

Flowering Period: March through June, mostly.

Indications by Bach: Very great hopelessness, they have given up belief that more can be done for them.

Under persuasion or to please others they may try different treatments, at the same time reassuring those around that there is so little hope of relief. *(Twelve Healers)*

Jane had given up hope that her illness could be cured and that she would ever see her son again. Her state was of true hopelessness, where facts were against her and could not be changed. She was under conventional medical treatment, and homeopathic remedies that might have induced active tissue changes to some degree were unacceptable and not known to Jane, although she was open to treatment with Bach Remedies to aid her mental/emotional state. The remedy Gorse would help her overcome the intensity and severity of her state and direct her view to faith and hope for her soul's journey and a possible reunion with her son in the beyond, while hope for his survival in the war would be raised also. Although the body may be failing rapidly, Gorse opens the mind to new horizons and feelings of joyful anticipation.

Oftentimes, as Gorse gives new hope of recovery, even long-lasting chronic illnesses can be turned around. As faith and hope of recovery grow, our inner intelligence that regulates healing, or our vital force, is encouraged or freed to initiate cure. In situations of life perceived as hopeless, other than physical illness, Gorse will bring new faith and incentive to not give up and give one's best to the people and tasks at hand.

The Gorse bush begins to bloom during the last days of winter, unhampered by cold and snow, as if to point to the new life and hope it brings amidst hardship and cold severity. The spikes growing along the stem also remind of pain and adversity, while the golden-yellow, abundant blossoms speak of the sun's warmth and its life-giving sparks.

SWEET CHESTNUT (Castanea sativa)

Group: For Despondency or Despair.

Preparation: Boiling of male and female flowers and leaves.

Flowering Period: July.

Indications by Bach: For those moments which happen to some people when the anguish is so great as to seem to be unbearable.

When the mind or body feels as if it had borne to the uttermost limit of its endurance, and that now it must give way.

When it seems that there is nothing but destruction and annihilation left to face. *(Twelve Healers)*

Sweet Chestnut was indicated for Jane because of her deep despair, faithlessness, and sense of meaninglessness in view of her own upcoming premature death, the war victims' and possibly her son's annihilation. At times, her mind felt as if it could not withstand the great unhappiness and desperation, and she hardly knew how to express herself in words. Sweet Chestnut would enable her to have faith and look beyond material existence to eternal survival in the love of God. It would also ease her dread about the upcoming death struggle and the last stages of cancer.

Generally, people in need of Sweet Chestnut tend to keep emotions of despair within and suffer in silence. After the death of a loved one, a negative Sweet Chestnut state can come on in view of the nothingness that prevails where once was a living and loving person. It is the remedy for extreme circumstances of agony when life itself seems to fall apart.

The Sweet Chestnut tree speaks of a tortured mind by means of its furrowed dark trunk that grows in twisted curves. It reminds the onlooker of convulsions, agony and a state furrowed with darkness and despair. On the other hand, the sweet nuts inside their prickly shell speak of nourishment for the soul and survival that can be experienced even under harsh or prickly circumstances. The feathery, showy plumes of catkins that branch out in all directions denote new life and softness where once was harshness. The branching out may symbolize the mind as it devotes itself to new ideas and turns to the outside world, away from internal preoccupation and the "dark night of the soul."

OLIVE (Olea europaea)

Group: Not Sufficient Interest in Present Circumstances.

Preparation: Sun method, use of flowering clusters.

Flowering Period: May or June, mostly.

Indications by Bach: Those who have suffered much mentally or physically and are so exhausted and weary that they feel they have no more strength to make any effort. Daily life is hard work for them, without pleasure. *(Twelve Healers)*

Jane was completely exhausted in body, mind and spirit. Physical illness and mental anguish had weakened her considerably. She was almost unable to sit up in bed and feed herself; she could hardly talk, and she had lost her mental/emotional strength and her spiritual faith. Olive would revive her in all parts of her being. Simple activities would be possible again without weakening her. This would lead to new occupations, including reading and conversations with others, which would help dispel her gloomy thoughts and give new incentive and joy.

Generally, the negative Olive state can be recognized by a person's inability to persevere with simple tasks. Normal chores of living are begun and then discontinued because exhaustion takes over. Even in less extreme states of exhaustion, Olive is of great service to all in need of recharging and revitalizing the body, mind/emotions and inner spiritual core. It is an important remedy for burn-out syndrome, weariness with prolonged tasks and exhaustion during chronic or acute illness.

The Olive tree, native to the Mediterranean, is known for its ability to bloom in abundance, generation after generation, even when it is bent and hollow with age. This suggests the energy and vitality it brings even to those bent by hardship, age or sickness. The tree, when cut back, renews itself with three or four young stems, symbolizing the renewed life it brings to those "cut back" by exhaustion and fatigue. The liveliness of Mediterranean people may be fueled by the regular intake of Olive oil which may contain traces of the plant's revitalizing power.

Comparative Study of Applicable Homeopathic Remedy:

In case Jane had accepted homeopathic remedies, *Arsenicum album* would have been a good choice, since physical symptoms agreed in addition to her mental/emotional symptoms. The remedy, even if death was imminent, would have eased her psychological state and lightened her physical discomfort and pain. In the mental/emotional realm, Arsenicum album is indicated in states of fear of death (Rock Rose), hopelessness and despair (Gorse and Sweet Chestnut), and general weakness and exhaustion (Olive).

Some confirming physical symptoms are: Restlessness and disquiet felt within and all over the body, also when lying; burning pains; difficult nights with aggravation at midnight; thirst for sips, frequent vomiting and dysentery; Jane had most of these symptoms.

Arsenicum album, indicated for nervy, easily worried people with stomach problems, may have been a predominant remedy for Jane throughout her life.

CASE 3. AGRIMONY, CHESTNUT BUD, PINE (SULPHURICUM ACIDUM)

James, a man in his forties, loses his job due to a minor mistake that had extensive consequences and caused his company to lose a major business deal. He is of the cheerful, jovial kind with a tendency to hide inner cares and worries so that others would not be troubled by them. Staying cheerful also helps to avoid disputes with his wife who is well-meaning but easily upset. He is considered the peacemaker within the family and by his former group of colleagues. Even now after his mishap, he seems quite happy and outgoing, although he feels increasingly troubled inside and worried about finding a new job, keeping himself busy, and continuing to support his family.

While looking for a new job, he feels restless and unoccupied. The lack of structure in his life bothers him, and everyday he sets himself goals of accomplishing certain tasks around the house, in the community, and on the job market so he would have a sense of accomplishment, purpose and progress. When things seem to stagnate and completion is delayed, he feels uneasy, blames himself and worries that things would not be done on time. This causes him to speed up the next day so that he rushes into his activities, trying to do too much at once.

In his thoughts, he rushes too, being way ahead of the tasks of the moment, imagining the many things he had to do and wishing them completed. This causes him to lose concentration on the task at hand and the restful devotion to the present moment he had once enjoyed. He speeds up inside, rushes his activities, pressures himself and blames himself when things are left undone. He is aware that rushing is unhealthy and that mistakes are made more easily, yet he is caught unaware repeatedly by the impulse to jump into his tasks without calm planning or reasonable foresight. He recognizes this unhealthy pattern and blames himself for not being able to rise above it. Guilt feelings also center around the loss of his former job, the hitherto fruitless job search, and the fact that he presently is not a professionally occupied and money-earning member of society.

To cope with internal pressure, keep up his cheerful attitude and not burden his family with his worries, he drinks increased amounts of alcohol, although he knows that he is possibly harming himself again after he had tried so hard the year before to reduce the amount of drinking; yet, he had never indulged heavily in this habit. As of late, he has become increasingly unhappy, feels his tasks are joyless, and finds his restlessness and inner need to rush increasingly unbearable.

Agrimony is indicated for worry, *Chestnut Bud* for rushing ahead, and *Pine* for feelings of guilt.

Additional physical symptoms are: He bruises easily, suffers from occasional heartburn and experiences stiffness and cramping in the neck and arms. He also reports a state of internal restlessness that resembles trembling or fluttering.

AGRIMONY (Agrimonia eupatoria)

Group: Oversensitive to Influences and Ideas.

Preparation: Sun method, use of flowering stalks.

Flowering Period: June through August.

Indications by Bach: The jovial, cheerful, humorous people who love peace and are distressed by argument or quarrel, to avoid which they will agree to give up much.

Though generally they have troubles and are tormented, restless and worried in mind or in body, they hide their cares behind their humour and jesting and are considered very good friends to know. They often take alcohol or drugs in excess, to stimulate themselves and help themselves bear their trials with cheerfulness. *(Twelve Healers)*

Being the peacemaker, James portrays the Agrimony type. Agrimony was also indicated because of his inner restlessness, the tendency to be cheerful on the surface, and the attempt to spare his family unnecessary upset and preoccupation with his cares. The typical Agrimony tendency to worry centered around finding a job and a new focus of task acomplishment, keeping himself busy in the meantime, getting current things done and keeping his family from worrying. The alcohol helped him to deaden internal pressure and keep up his cheerfulness. By not expressing his inner worries and pressures and by gliding over them cheerfully, he stifled his inner need for communication, which then resulted in increased nervous energy and restlessness. This is the etiology of Agrimony. The remedy would help James to share his inner cares; it would lessen his restlessness and the intensity of his worries, reduce the need for alcohol, and give him peace of mind/emotions and body.

Generally, in the negative Agrimony state, the unconscious mind is stifled and often the person is not in touch with his true feelings. Agrimony will heal the split and bring wholeness of experience and inner harmony. Worries and concerns become less intense under the influence of Agrimony, which opens up communication of inner needs and allows people to share their burdens with one another. Agrimony also soothes people in restless need for devoting themselves to a significant other or a meaningful task. In the negative Agrimony state, they do not quite know where to "put themselves."

In regard to the body, Agrimony brings peace and relaxation. It is especially indicated during times of physical pain when there is great torture and restlessness. Often pains are not expressed or shared with others, which increases the intensity of pain.

The yellow flowers that grow along the stem of the Agrimony plant speak of calmness, joy and unity, whereas the burs that remain after the petals fall off portray a less desirable or uncomfortable state. As one passes by the plant, these burs get caught in one's clothes and are carried along, similar to the cares

that one carries along wherever one goes, as happens in the negative Agrimony state.

Agrimony people are often brave people; it takes a great
effort to be cheerful on the outside, while inner cares worry and
burden. The remedy, by dispelling the often needless worries
and helping to regain the enjoyment of the present moment
and its people, will instill true inner peace and a genuine, deeply
felt cheerfulness that radiates with ease to the outside world.

CHESTNUT BUD (Aesculus hippocastanum)

Group: Not Sufficient Interest in Present Circumstances.

Preparation: Boiling of twigs with buds.

Growth Period: April, mostly.

Indications by Bach: For those who do not take full advantage of observation and experience, and who take a longer time
than others to learn the lessons of daily life. Whereas one experience would be enough for some, such people find it necessary
to have more, sometimes several, before the lesson is learned.
Therefore, to their regret, they find themselves having to make
the same error on different occasions when once would have
been enough, or observation of others would have spared them
even that one fault. *(Twelve Healers)*

Chestnut Bud was indicated for James because of his inability to learn from his perceived mistake in regard to drinking
and in regard to his urge to rush ahead in thought and action,
both of which he knew to be detrimental to his health. He was
giving in to impulsive urges from within which directed his actions and were not held in check by reason. These impulses
originated in his need for a satisfying task, which is in itself a
reasonable urge but may become unreasonable if pressure mounts

and dictates one's actions. Moreover, he was driven by the need to reduce self-blame and reestablish self-worth and integrity, which led him to engage in self-appointed tasks, often with unnecessary rushing and feelings of being not well centered, although the work helped to dispel his worries temporarily. Self-reproach and restlessness would resurface when definite progress, especially in regard to his job search, was not made, or when other tasks did not yield satisfaction and completion. The resulting uneasiness would urge him further to find meaningful occupation, while the tendency to rush ahead increased.

This pattern might not be broken until a new and fulfilling professional position could be found. In the meantime, James was trapped in this cycle, while knowing fully that he was undermining his mental/emotional and physical peace. This is where the healing power of Chestnut Bud comes in. Chestnut Bud would help him bridge this transitional time by furthering his reasonable insight over his unreasonable impulsiveness, helping him this way to understand how to break this cycle and how to regain inner peace and restful devotion to the present moment, while trying to reorganize his life.

The remedy Impatiens would have also helped James with his urgency and hurried state during task completion. However, it was not considered one of the predominant remedies, since he did not show the typical Impatiens tendency to urge other people on and become impatient with them. James was driven by the urge to speed within his own personality only, and he did not involve others impatiently. The result was rather an Agrimony state of trying to be cheerful and kind while being with others, although internal pressure existed. This pressure could have been treated by Impatiens also, even though the pressure was not put on others; each Bach Remedy has a wide range of action. Chestnut Bud also addresses the tendency to speed ahead in thought and action with the ensuing loss of calm receptivity to the present moment, although James managed to stay tuned into other people. Bach grouped Chestnut Bud under the heading of *Not Sufficient Interest in Present Circumstances.*

Chestnut Bud is an important remedy for all processes of learning, in school age children and grown-ups alike. For the growing child, learning capacity and power of concentration are greatly enhanced, especially if the indications were lack of seriousness about school matters, easy distraction during learning, and slow retention of the material learned. Generally speaking, Chestnut Bud balances inner impulses and easy distraction of the mind, fed by unconscious urges or unsettled matter, with reason, clarity, and good sense. This remedy also helps a person to grow in moral insights and strength of character; it overcomes the tendency to not learn from one's mistakes and repeat faulty behavioral patterns.

The remedy is gained from the Horse Chestnut tree which is known for its fast-growing buds that shoot up with great strength and vitality. This symbolizes the dynamic mind trying to express itself into full growth of consciousness and find balance between reason and unchecked spontaneous self-expression or impulsiveness. The fast-growing bud also reminds of the impulsiveness and fast pace of a mind unsettled and urged on by inner restlessness. This restlessness may be due to a developmental phase of life, as in childhood or adolescence; in some cases, it may be chronically entrenched in the character, or it expresses a passing imbalance during one's life due to unfavorable circumstances.

Interestingly, the remedy White Chestnut is gained from the whitish-red blossoms of the same tree after the buds have opened. To a preoccupied mind, White Chestnut brings peace and serenity, and Chestnut Bud furthers growth towards this stage also.

PINE (Pinus sylvestris)

Group: For Despondency or Despair.

Preparation: Boiling of twigs with both male and female flowers.

Flowering Period: May.

Indications by Bach: For those who blame themselves. Even when successful they think they could have done better, and are never content with their efforts or the results. They are hard-working and suffer much from the faults they attach to themselves.

Sometimes if there is any mistake it is due to another, but they will claim responsibility even for that. *(Twelve Healers)*

Pine was indicated for James because of his self-accusing attitude in regard to his job loss and the hitherto fruitless job search. He also blamed himself when tasks were left undone and progress was not made. Because a structured work environment was missing, he had become his own master in regard to appointment of small jobs and granting of approval upon task completion. Consequently, self-worth was low when things did not progress satisfactorily.

Larch would also have been a good remedy for James who also felt guilt and reduced self-worth when comparing himself with fully employed members of society. He was also somewhat disappointed by the slow progress made in his job search, yet his confidence did not seem severely shaken. Mainly, Larch was not chosen as a predominant remedy because his ability to tune into other people's feelings was high. In the negative Larch state, one often does not feel fully in tune with others, since self-worry is high. Larch, as well as Impatiens, could be added to a subsequent prescription, should the first three not be effective in balancing the case.

James' guilt feelings were also enhanced by his inability to get a handle on the drinking problem and his failure to control the inner urge to rush through his day, although he knew that both were detrimental to his health. The remedy Pine would address these issues and further relieve him of the nagging guilt feelings that surfaced when his wife had become upset for whatever reasons and when his role as the peacemaker of the family had failed. Pine would also hold in check exaggerated guilt feelings that often arose when he felt the need to share his burdens with his family, and he would feel free to share himself more openly, which would then relieve internal pressure and loneliness, and make him a happier person. The pressure around the drinking problem would lessen as well, which would make it easier for him to attend to the problem. Overall, Pine would help James to be more gentle with himself and forgive himself the temporary imbalances in his life.

In general, Pine is indicated for all people who unjustly blame themselves when things go wrong, such as in relationship issues and during joint work projects. It also soothes memories of one's childhood experience when punishment and guilt feelings served to perpetuate education. Should a true crime have been committed, Pine would lessen the severity of guilt without curtailing the moral lesson learned.

The pine tree speaks of comfort and warmth; especially at Christmas time, it cheers our homes and hearts by its refreshing

scent and evergreen appearance. The longevity of pines may symbolize the longevity of some of our guilt feelings which we often
carry through life. The pine tree has the power to release even
those feelings of self-reproach and guilt that reside deep in our
unconscious mind and have been collected over many years of
life experience.

Comparative Study of Applicable Homeopathic Remedies:

Sulphuricum acidum and *Tarentula hispanica* are two possible homeopathic remedies among others that treat great hur-
riedness, and the urge to stay busy and get things done (Agrimony, Chestnut Bud and also Impatiens). In comparison to
Tarentula hispanica, Sulphuricum acidum shows more guilt, occasional low self-confidence, lack of feeling appreciated and depressive feelings (Pine and also Larch), all of which are compensated for by hurried activity and satisfaction obtained from task
completion. Tarentula hispanica is marked by wound-up nervous tension and the sheer physical need to move. This remedy
also shows great sensitivity to seeing others in distress. On the
other hand, these patients can be very irate and resort to outbursts of vehemence. Both remedies treat conditions of inner
restlessness and lack of fulfillment of inner needs that assert a
driving impulse throughout one's being (Agrimony and Chestnut Bud).

Exact physical analysis decides the choice of remedy.
Sulphuricum acidum was the more clearly indicated remedy. It
typically may show some of the following physical symptoms:
Compressive pain in occiput and upper neck, especially right
side, and feeling of painful plug in right temple. Rapid breathing, heartburn, internal trembling and craving for alcohol;
cramping pains in arms and easy bruising with blue discolora-

tion. Most of these symptoms were experienced by James, except for the headache, although he did feel some tension in his upper neck in addition to cramping of the arms.

Tarentula hispanica shows nervous tension with intense headaches that resemble the effect of needles pricking the brain. Further symptoms may be vertigo; heart palpitations; restless, twitching legs; great sensitivity to music and bright colors.

CASE 4. SCLERANTHUS, WHITE CHESTNUT, MUSTARD (LYCOPODIUM CLAVATUM)

Monika, twenty-eight years of age, is a single woman from Austria who has studied for several years in the United States, with interruptions. She has enjoyed switching her place of study regularly and has gone back and forth between American universities and her own in Vienna. Now, towards the end of her studies, she knows she could make a living in either country, and the decision to choose one or the other presents itself. There is urgency in her planning, since studies are drawing to a close, parental funding is ending, and a job has to be found.

She has a strong inclination and longing to settle and work in one country from the start and build a permanent home, since the many years of travel have somewhat tired her and made her feel unfocused. The decision-making process weighs heavily on her, and, against her will, she finds her mind preoccupied to the point where concentration on her studies and enjoyment of life are curtailed. She also is assailed by occasional bouts of depression.

Since she knows of all the advantages and disadvantages for living in either country, she repeatedly weighs both options in her mind, trying to determine which one appeals to her most.

She reiterates the bonus points of one country and feels excited about the prospects when the other option reasserts itself again with its advantages, although she had tried to let go of it. As she then looks at this option, thinking it to be the right choice, the other option appeals again and so on. It seems difficult, almost impossible, to let go of one opportunity and scenery of life that she had once enjoyed.

This vacillating process is repeated continually and puts her mind into a tormented state, where recurring thoughts and internal arguments interfere with her interaction with people, her studies and duties of the moment. She also finds herself avoiding this topic with her friends and feels increasingly gloomy and depressed under the heavy burden of decision-making, which she has decided to carry alone. She thinks that her friends, although well-meaning, would advise her wrongly, curtail her freedom of choice and possibly complicate matters. Her friends do retreat from her, while letting her know that they care about her.

Her joy of living is stifled, all cheer and lightness gone, as she wrestles with this problem. Occasionally, she has been subjected to bouts of depression in her life, but never to such intensity.

Monika is prescribed the remedies *Scleranthus* for vacillating between two options, *White Chestnut* for mental preoccupation, and *Mustard* for depression.

She has only minor physical symptoms, except for her headache that bothers her from time to time. Her headache is characterized by compressive pain in both temples. She also shows increased physical and mental weariness in the late afternoon but picks up again after dinner. In regard to food, she has digestive troubles and gas pains from beans and cabbage, dislikes carrots, enjoys warm food over cold food, and is usually hungry during the late evening. She has dark circles around the eyes.

SCLERANTHUS (Scleranthus annuus)

Group: For Those Who Suffer Uncertainty.

Preparation: Sun method, use of flowering parts.

Flowering Period: May to September.

Indications by Bach: Those who suffer much from being unable to decide between two things, first one seeming right then the other.

They are usually quiet people, bear their difficulty alone, as they are not inclined to discuss it with others. *(Twelve Healers).*

Monika had suffered from occasional indecision all her life, but she had never felt so burdened by a particular decision-making process. Scleranthus was the main remedy indicated, since she shared the characteristic vacillation between two options and the tendency to bear the problem alone, although Scleranthus can also be prescribed when the problem is shared with friends. Typically though, the person in need of Scleranthus knows that only within oneself can the last decision be made, even if the problem is shared with others.

Scleranthus would help Monika to reduce the pressure and intensity of the vacillating process, while uplifting her mind to a higher vantage point, where she could make a clear decision without being caught up in all the details and multiple impressions that would impinge upon her and trap her. Scleranthus gives peace and fortitude of mind; it strengthens the inner core of certainty and gives the ability to move decisively through life;

it harmonizes and clarifies options and impressions, instead of being entangled by them. It is a good remedy for all who feel easily overwhelmed by details and multiple impressions and have a hard time finding their way out in decisive thought and action.

The Scleranthus plant grows in tangled formation, without the appearance of especially beautiful, colorful blossoms, as if the plant could not decide how to express itself, and reminding us of the tangled, indecisive mind.

WHITE CHESTNUT (Aesculus hippocastanum)

Group: Not Sufficient Interest in Present Circumstances.

Preparation: Sun method, use of flowers.

Flowering Period: May and June.

Indications by Bach: For those who cannot prevent thoughts, ideas, arguments which they do not desire from entering their minds. Usually at such times when the interest of the moment is not strong enough to keep the mind full.

Thoughts which worry and will remain, or if for a time thrown out, will return. They seem to circle round and round and cause mental torture.

The presence of such unpleasant thoughts drives out peace and interferes with being able to think only of the work or pleasure of the day. *(Twelve Healers)*

Monika needed White Chestnut to calm her indecisive, burdensome, recurring thoughts that eluded conclusion and would keep her from concentrating on her tasks at hand and from enjoyment of the present moment. White Chestnut would give her serenity, peace of mind and anchoring in the present by conquering the decision-making process and its dominating impact on her overall mental state. In the negative White Chestnut state, one typically feels that worrisome thoughts predominate and cannot be ruled out. White Chestnut will also bring clarity and relaxation to eyes and the forehead, where muscles tend to contract during worrisome mental preoccupation.

The mental worries in the White Chestnut state differ from the Agrimony type of worries, in that they are burdening the overall personality, also visibly on the surface, whereas the Agrimony type of worries are hidden behind a facade of cheerfulness. In the negative White Chestnut state, the mind is interfered with to a high degree and closed off to the entire world, whereas the Agrimony person manages to keep worries down and the mind bent on cheer and openness to the outside world. Cherry Plum is another Bach Remedy dealing with the intrusion of unwanted thoughts. However, the thought content in the negative Cherry Plum state is of a definite wrong or even dangerous nature and cannot be accepted by the consciousness. The more one pushes down the dreaded impulse, the more it may reassert itself, to the point where one fears all reason of mind to be threatened. Cherry Plum treats the fear of the mind losing control over dreaded thoughts or actions that threaten to take place. The negative White Chestnut state is a much lighter state of not being able to rule out worrisome, unresolved thoughts that are not shocking in nature but interfere with the full devotion to the present.

The White Chestnut tree speaks of majestic grandeur and beauty; the white blossoms portray calmness and clarity, those being the gifts it brings to the preoccupied mind.

MUSTARD (Sinapis arvensis)

Group: Not Sufficient Interest in Present Circumstances.

Preparation: Boiling of flowers.

Flowering Period: May to July.

Indications by Bach: Those who are liable to times of gloom, or even despair, as though a cold dark cloud overshadowed them and hid the light and the joy of life. It may not be possible to give any reason or explanation for such attacks.

Under these conditions it is almost impossible to appear happy or cheerful. *(Twelve Healers)*

Monika needed Mustard because the temporary process of vacillating between two options had taken her joy of life and put her in a gloomy frame of mind. The idea of having to let go of either country depressed her, while the inability to overcome the indecisiveness further deepened her gloom. She had suffered occasional bouts of depression throughout her life.

Generally, a negative Mustard state easily arises when the need for love and understanding has not been met. Often the person is not aware of this connection, feels overpowered by gloomy, depressive feelings, without understanding how to rise above them. It is possible that Monika's depression was enhanced by her turning away from friends during this crucial time and may also root in her state of being single. Mustard would help her find inner cheer and light and feel more inclined to interact with her friends, with whom she might share burdens and find support.

As one looks at a green field, interspersed with waves of golden Mustard flowers, one is reminded of the rays of the sun, and the light and warmth it brings to a mind darkened with gloom. Mustard will actually brighten the world to the perceiver, as if the consciousness had been empowered to give and receive more light.

Water Violet may also have been a good remedy for Monika, since she turned away form her friends, preferring loneliness and believing her own judgment to be best, all of which portray a potentially proud or aloof state which is treated by Water Violet. However, in face of this intense decision-making process and the internal pressures, pride was not quite apparent; yet, the remedy can be kept in mind for a possible later prescription. Wild Rose is another remedy that is lightly indicated in her case. She showed some inability to disentangle powerfully the web she was in; she was torn between two options that seemed equally appealing or important.

Comparative Study of Applicable Homeopathic Remedy:

The remedy *Lycopodium clavatum* was indicated. In the mental/ emotional realm, Lycopodium clavatum treats the tendency to vacillate (Scleranthus) and the tendency to have internal arguments and conversations (White Chestnut), including a possible bent to depression and disheartenment (Mustard, Wild Rose, the latter being only mildly indicated) plus the inclination to retreat from people in aloofness or defiance (Water Violet, also only mildly indicated). Aloofness or defiance may root in feelings of inferiority, though not visible in Monika's case.

Her physical symptoms matched the Lycopodium clavatum picture also: Lycopodium clavatum shows characteristic aggravation of symptoms between 4 and 8 P.M., which she had. The remedy also covered her compressive headache in both temples, her gastric sensitivity to beans and cabbage, her gas pains, plus dislike of carrots and preference for warm food over cold food, and the typical hunger feelings late at night. Her dark circles around the eyes would also improve under the healing impact of Lycopodium clavatum.

Typically, Lycopodium clavatum treats affections of the liver, however apparent, and general weakness of digestion, usually characterized by bloating. Symptoms and pains often move from the right to the left side, especially during acute states of sickness, but also in chronic complaints.

CASE 5. CLEMATIS, WILD OAT, STAR OF BETHLEHEM (BARYTA CARBONICA)

Nancy, six years of age, received a hamster for her birthday, whom she loved dearly. The mother is delighted to see her girl so actively engaged in play, since she knows of the child's tendency to daydream or not be actively engaged with her toys. When the hamster dies in an unfortunate accident, Nancy's world crumbles, and she experiences the first real grief of her young life.

The mother is beside herself, too; she is trying to explain to the weeping child that the hamster went to heaven, where she will meet up with him some day. This stifles Nancy's tears temporarily and she begins to look forward to a reunion in the future, while she feels that all joy of the present has gone. Mother decides not to buy a new hamster, since she wants to avoid tragedies of that sort, while Nancy confirms this decision by insisting that no hamster could ever replace her special friend.

Nancy's performance in school, her social interactions and her motivation to play suffer due to her disappointment that is not coped with. She sits unoccupied, often wishing she could meet her hamster in heaven. The tasks and toys at hand, and even peers, seem to give no joy or incentive. She starts a task or playful interaction and then discontinues, since her interest is low. She complains of boredom to her mother who begins to worry about her daughter.

The remedies *Clematis* for daydreaming, *Wild Oat* for lack of interest in play and school, and *Star of Bethlehem* for grief are prescribed.

Additional physical symptoms are: Tendency to colds and tonsillitis; during colds, there is usually swelling of upper lip, according to mother's observation. Often, the glands of her neck are enlarged. She has frequent hiccups and strong dislike for acidic fruits. Sometimes, she complains of pain or pressure in the larynx. Nancy is a somewhat small child for her age and appears shy.

CLEMATIS (Clematis vitalba)

Group: Not Sufficient Interest in Present Circumstances.

Preparation: Sun method, use of flowers.

Flowering Period: July to September.

Indications by Bach: Those who are dreamy, drowsy, not fully awake, no great interest in life. Quiet people, not really happy in their present circumstances, living more in the future than in the present; living in hopes of happier times, when their ideals may come true. In illness some make little or no effort to get well, and in certain cases may even look forward to death, in the hope of better times; or maybe, meeting again some beloved one whom they have lost. *(Twelve Healers)*

Nancy was of the Clematis type; she was often daydreaming and not actively engaged in play. Temporarily, the hamster had helped her to find interest and stay focused. Yet, upon the hamster's sudden death, she again relived her former absent-mindedness and disinterest in play, even in a more intensified way. Since the accident, more than before, she looked to the future as holding the key to her happiness, when reunion with her hamster would happen, and she was convinced that the toys, peers and joys of the present were worthless. The present held no incentive or fascination, and her mind wandered off into a place within herself where she gave herself to hopes for future enjoyments.

Clematis would focus her mind on the present, so she could absorb again the full effect of the beauty and enjoyment of life. Daydreaming and absent-mindedness disappear under the healing impact of Clematis; there is new vigor in mind/emotions and body, as if each facet of the personality and each cell of the body is revived.

People in need of Clematis often complain of feeling "spaced out" or not well centered, as if mind or body are not fully focused. There is usually a feeling of being unfulfilled in the present, or a sense that present circumstances are not pleasing or beautiful, or are too boring or too exhausting. The mind removes itself and is pulled by a longing for, or an interest in, more fascinating or complete experiences of love, life and occupation that are each person's heritage.

The Clematis plant shows white flowers with fuzzy parts that, in autumn, float through the air like small clouds, reminding one of a dreamy state or of a state of being in the clouds.

WILD OAT (Bromus ramosus)

Group: For Those Who Suffer Uncertainty.

Preparation: Sun method, use of flowering ends of spikelets.

Flowering Period: July and August.

Indications by Bach: Those who have ambitions to do something of prominence in life, who wish to have much experience, and to enjoy all that which is possible for them, to take life to the full.

Their difficulty is to determine what occupation to follow; as although their ambitions are strong, they have no calling which appeals to them above all others.

This may cause delay and dissatisfaction. *(Twelve Healers)*

Here, Bach pointed out the importance of Wild Oat in determining one's career or special calling in life. Yet, it is indicated during all phases of life when motivation and incentive to play or work are missing. Wild Oat brings new joy of experience, especially during those activities that are beneficial to us, and it helps to express inner potential so that one knows with clarity that certain activities or fields of interest harmonize more with oneself than others. Wild Oat also raises the overall readiness to feel motivation and incentive for tasks at hand, even for necessary tasks of duty such as school, work or chores, especially if boredom and dislike in face of these duties exist.

In the case of Nancy, the etiology for the intensified Wild Oat state resided in the grief; previously, she had shown occasional disinterest also, but not as pronounced. Now, Wild Oat was specifically indicated for her inability to find joy in almost any of her activities, after her favorite play experience was taken from her. The grief stifled her enjoyment of the present moment and made her see life as colorless and dull in comparison to the lively animal she had once enjoyed. Wild Oat would help her to feel motivated to play again, even if her hamster was not there, and school tasks would also appear interesting and fascinating.

The name "Wild Oat" reminds of liberation and new adventure within the context of leading to definite interests or goals that are beneficial to mankind and oneself, or it simply brings new motivation and enjoyment to daily activities. The remedy Wild Oat may also bring new direction and purpose to someone "sowing his oats" in unsettled activity.

The Wild Oat grass can be seen swaying gently in the breeze, as if to speak of dancing playfulness and lightness of step.

STAR OF BETHLEHEM (Ornithogalum umbellatum)

Group: For Despondency or Despair.

Preparation: Boiling of complete flowering parts.

Flowering Period: April to June.

Indications by Bach: For those in great distress under conditions which for a time produce great unhappiness.

The shock of serious news, the loss of someone dear, the fright following an accident, and such like.

For those who for a time refuse to be consoled, this remedy brings comfort. *(Twelve Healers)*

Star of Bethlehem would soothe and help heal Nancy's saddened heart, and it would also remove the trauma and the effects of the shock so that her memory would not lastingly be burdened with the shocking event and the ensuing sad feelings. Her occasional periods of weeping would end, and she would be consolable again after she had refused any help, since nothing could make her hamster come to life again. Star of Bethlehem would allow happiness to enter Nancy's heart again and help her to find joy and comfort in the people and play at hand.

Sometimes, Star of Bethlehem is indicated even when the grief dates back many years; it helps to reopen the heart that often closes down in shock at the reception of sad news. Hearts open over time but may stay burdened and heavy for a long time. Star of Bethlehem will help lighten the heart and bring release of old trauma and deep-seated wounds.

"Star of Bethlehem" is a fitting name, heralding comfort and peace in the same way as the real star of Bethlehem in Judea once announced the coming of Christ, the savior and comforter of all. The beautiful, six-petalled white flower radiates clarity, healing and light.

Comparative Study of Applicable Homeopathic Remedy:

Baryta carbonica was the indicated homeopathic remedy for Nancy. In the mind/emotions, it treats the tendency to be disinterested in play and school, with lack of motivation and incentive (Wild Oat), plus the tendency to daydreaming and absent-mindedness (Clematis), and it treats states of grief (Star of Bethlehem). Children in need of this remedy may also show stubbornness and a tendency to tantrums. Often, these children are shy and appear small for their age. The remedy is known to give developmental growth spurts in body and mind/emotions when indicated.

On the physical plane, Baryta carbonica typically shows, among other symptoms, a tendency to colds, usually accompanied by a swollen upper lip and tonsillitis with swollen glands. There is also a strong dislike for acidic fruit, a tendency to hiccups, and a pain or feeling of pressure in the larynx. All of these symptoms were experienced by Nancy.

CASE 6. GENTIAN, ELM, HORNBEAM (PICRICUM ACIDUM)

George is a twenty-two year old science student who usually enjoys his studies and manages well, yet is of late discouraged, overburdened and mentally fatigued. One of his papers that he had put a lot of effort into was rejected due to a minor oversight on his part and had to be redone. George feels disheartened in view of the minor mistake he had made and the consequence it had wrought, while the idea of having to redo the paper further discourages him. It is his last semester in school, and he is resolved to finish his last classes so that he can graduate on time.

As he looks at the numerous tests and papers ahead of him, he feels overwhelmed and unsure about his progress, mainly due to the present delay in fulfilling his assignment. Occasional feelings of being overwhelmed and discouragement had assailed him earlier as well, but he had felt he could manage and stay on top of things.

Trying to manage as much as possible his feelings of disheartenment and of being overwhelmed, George tries to fulfill his assignments, yet he feels his mental strength and power of concentration waning, and there is the urge to procrastinate or take a rest. Physically, he also feels lack of stamina and fatigue; he feels like giving up. The tasks ahead seem to grow above a manageable level and overpower him.

The following remedies are indicated: *Gentian* for discouragement, *Elm* for feeling overwhelmed, and *Hornbeam* for mental/emotional and physical fatigue and lack of power of concentration.

Additional physical symptoms are minor: A light headache in the back of the head that comes on during his studies; at times, there is temporary dizziness with noises in his ears. Generally, the brain feels tired. His eyes appear red, smarting and get tired during studying, and George has the urge to close them. Occasionally, the eyes secrete a yellow discharge. Further, there is a bitter taste in his mouth and not much interest in eating. His urine is scanty, with increased urging at night. There is also a burning sensation along the spinal cord, though he is generally chilly.

GENTIAN (Gentiana amarella)

Group: For Those Who Suffer Uncertainty.

Preparation: Sun method, use of flowers.

Flowering Period: From August to early October.

Indications by Bach: Those who are easily discouraged. They may be progressing well in illness or in the affairs of their daily life, but any small delay or hindrance to progress causes doubt and soon disheartens them. *(Twelve Healers)*

Gentian was indicated for George to counteract his discouragement and doubts in regard to managing his tasks, since the additional assignment had caused delay, stifled his sense of progress and caused a sinking heart. In general, George had a slight tendency to feel discouraged, indicating the Gentian type, but usually he has managed to see his tasks through.

Gentian would help George to muster his inner strength, courage and certainty, and he would have faith again in his abilities and the benevolence of circumstances.

The remedy Oak also deals with similar feelings of disheartenment when progress is not achieved despite efforts made; yet, in the negative Oak state, the despondency is of a more severe and stoic nature. The inclination to give up does not occur; on the contrary, one is determined to persevere, even to one's physical detriment. George wanted to persevere, too; but the willpower invested was less and he showed the recurring Gentian type inclination to slow down, take rest and give up, if only temporarily.

In general, Gentian helps all those who doubt their abilities and often do not even want to begin or learn a new task, anticipating lack of mastery, delayed progress, or failure; or, once started, they discontinue due to a minor hindrance or setback. Gentian renews faith in oneself and life in general and also invigorates faith in the care of a loving God.

The sturdy pink-purple plant, rich in blossoms, prefers to grow on hilltop grasslands, close to the sky, as if to point to a stout heart and the importance of faith in loving care from above. The many blossoms may speak of the fruits of service that come forward once disheartenment is eased away and creative potential is expressed more powerfully.

ELM (Ulmus procera)

Group: For Despondency or Despair.

Preparation: Boiling of twigs with flowers.

Flowering Period: February to March.

Indications by Bach: Those who are doing good work, are following the calling of their life and who hope to do something of importance, and this is often for the benefit of humanity.

At times there may be periods of depression when they feel that the task they have undertaken is too difficult, and not within the power of a human being. *(Twelve Healers)*

Elm treats feelings of being overwhelmed that assail during one's life task and in view of far-reaching tasks of significance that still lie ahead. One easily feels overpowered by the vastness and detailed nature of human, global problems or human suffering. Elm is equally indicated in treating feelings of being overwhelmed in view of daily tasks of life maintenance; small, seemingly unimportant details can burden as much as responsibilities on a larger scale.

In George's case, the feelings of being overwhelmed centered around the multiple papers and exams, the grinding out of school requirements. Due to a setback in progress, these tasks had become piled up in front of him, threatening to literally grow above and overpower him. This is the feeling typically experienced in the negative Elm state.

The remedy Elm helps to raise the doer again above the tasks to be done and gives a new perspective and feeling of staying on top of things. One also does not look at the totality or huge amount of tasks but concentrates on one task at a time, giving one's full devotion to the present task at hand.

The Elm tree characteristically shows a large, billowing crown that dominates the lower branches of the tree, reminding of the state of being below or overwhelmed by tremendous or multiple tasks. The healing essence gained from this tree cures by turning feelings of being overwhelmed into feelings of being in charge of one's tasks and enjoying them.

HORNBEAM (Carpinus betulus)

Group: For Those Who Suffer Uncertainty.

Preparation: Boiling of twigs with male and female flowers.

Flowering Period: April to May.

Indications by Bach: For those who feel that they have not sufficient strength, mentally or physically, to carry the burden of life placed upon them; the affairs of every day seem too much for them to accomplish, though they generally succeed in fulfilling their task.

For those who believe that some part, of mind or body, needs to be strengthened before they can easily fulfil their work. *(Twelve Healers)*

Hornbeam was indicated for George because of his mental and physical fatigue. Especially his mind had been strained and overtaxed to the point where his mental strength, clarity and power of concentration were curtailed. He felt he had not much stamina left and experienced a tendency to procrastination and an inclination to give up and rest. Hornbeam would help George to be revived in mind and body, while setting new incentive to complete his study load and enhancing his learning potential.

Hornbeam helps the mind to wake up to clarity and renews the power of focus; it gives a new light and strength in mind/emotions and body. It is a good remedy for school-age children, students and all those fatigued by prolonged mental study.

The name "Hornbeam" reminds of strength, vigor and a beam of light. The tree is known for its dynamic vitality.

Comparative Study of Applicable Homeopathic Remedy:

Picricum acidum was the homeopathic remedy indicated to help heal further the mental/emotional symptoms and speed up healing on the physical level. This remedy is generally known as the "student's helper," addressing mental overstrain and general exhaustion (Hornbeam), feelings of being overwhelmed and of dread (Elm), plus disheartenment with lack of willpower and disinclination to work (Gentian). The Picricum acidum state often is accompanied by anxiety in regard to exams, which would be helped further by Mimulus, but is also covered by Elm to some degree, as in George's case. George also felt some fear, but it was not one of the predominant mental/emotional states.

On the physical plane, Picricum acidum covered George's symptoms as well. Picricum acidum treats headache in the back of the head that comes on during studying, the occasional dizziness, roaring in ears, and general mental/emotional and physical fatigue. It would help freshen George's eyes, increase his appetite, heal the burning sensation along the spine and the light urinary troubles. The Bach Remedies can be considered as additional healers on the physical plane.

CASE 7. CHICORY, HONEYSUCKLE, RED CHESTNUT (CAUSTICUM)

Susan, fifty-one years of age, is experiencing the "empty nest syndrome." Her three children have moved out recently, and Susan feels with sadness that the happy family unit she once enjoyed will never be whole again and that her mothering role is now different and not as complete as before.

She had enjoyed taking care of her children and being closely related to the details of their lives, while she is aware that she might have been too concerned or overly wrapped up in details at times. Now, with the children gone, she feels empty-handed, left out and not fully appreciated for her many years of service and caring.

She also finds herself worrying about her children's welfare, feeling unable to assist or protect them, and dreading that something bad or harmful might befall them.

Susan develops increasing self-pity and feels stifled and un-fulfilled, since her main focus of active care and devotion is taken from her. Her former active engagement now is turned into men-tal preoccupation and worry. She tries to bridge this gap through frequent phone calls, trying to reassure herself that all is well with her children and that she is still important to them as a mother. Often, her children reassure her that too much worry and the frequent phone calls are not necessary. She also enjoys joint dinners and festivities that help her relive former happi-ness, while she knows with sadness that the past cannot return in its fullness.

Susan is prescribed *Chicory* for her tendency to overcare that is now stifled and accompanied by self-pity, *Honeysuckle* for longing for an irretrievable past state, and *Red Chestnut* for her fears that something dreadful might befall her children.

Her physical symptoms are minor: She has a tendency to eruptions around her nose and warts near her fingertips. There are frequent coughs and hoarseness. She has a strong dislike of sweets but craving for smoked foods. She suffers from constipa-tion and occasional left-sided sciatica.

CHICORY (Cichorium intybus)

Group: Overcare for Welfare of Others.

Preparation: Sun method, use of flowers.

Flowering Period: July to September.

Indications by Bach: Those who are very mindful of the needs of others; they tend to be over-full of care for children, relatives, friends, always finding something that should be put right. They are continually correcting what they consider wrong, and enjoy doing so. They desire that those for whom they care should be near them. *(Twelve Healers)*

Susan was a caring mother who had devoted herself to the lives of her children. She had been interested in each detail of their lives and had invested much effort in meeting their needs. This is not a negative Chicory state in itself, especially if the inner welfare of the children is of concern as well, which was the case with Susan. However, overcare for each detail can lead to the typical Chicory overcare, with possible neglect of the others' true emotional needs. In addition, a tendency to feel self-pity may develop, should the others not appreciate one's efforts, which is a typical Chicory state also. This is the twofold character of the negative Chicory state, and both sides were experienced by Susan.

At the end of many years of active devotion to her children, Susan mostly experienced the self-pity state; she felt unappreciated, left out and without the rewards that come from giving, receiving and mutual togetherness. Frequent phone calls and dinner invitations expressed her continued care and need for togetherness, while the children found her focus somewhat unnecessary and overbearing at times, which then increased her self-pity.

The remedy Chicory would help Susan to feel less need and demand for closeness to her children, while her genuine feelings of love and devotion would be deepened further. She would realize that her children's happiness can unfold without her overcare and that they are independent and taken care of by their own efforts. She would understand that her desire to care for someone can be focused to those people living in her vicinity, while she can hold her children with love in her heart and look forward to those special family reunions.

Generally, a negative Chicory state is also common during courtship or within an established man-woman relationship when one partner is rebuffed and retreats into a hurt state of self-pity, unable to continue the usual devotion. Chicory helps then to either forgive and make up or find joy in other people or tasks and not be rooted in one's hurt feelings. Furthermore, for all active caretakers with a bent to be overly involved, Chicory helps to let go of the need for control, and one learns to live and let live, while genuine caring remains. It is a good remedy for children and also for adults who tend to seek attention and then retreat and pout when not responded to properly.

The blue Chicory plant grows in abundance, with multiple flowers, by the wayside, reminding of the many opportunities for true devotion that come our way.

HONEYSUCKLE (Lonicera caprifolium)

Group: Not Sufficient Interest in Present Circumstances.

Preparation: Boiling of flowers with some leaves.

Flowering Period: June to August.

Indications by Bach: Those who live much in the past, perhaps a time of great happiness, or memories of a lost friend, or ambitions which have not come true. They do not expect further happiness such as they have had. *(Twelve Healers)*

Susan needed Honeysuckle to help her overcome her sadness in face of the disintegrated family unit and the realization that the happiness from the past will never return fully. A new life cycle had begun for all members of her family, while Susan still was unable to let go of the old and embrace the new. She kept her reminiscences mostly to herself and often found herself lost in thought, roaming through past memories, while the present held no perceived potential for happiness.

Honeysuckle would help Susan understand that her happiness was not only bound up with her children and her mothering role but could be fulfilled through other people, especially her husband, and other occupations also. Her hopes for new possibilities of further happiness in her life would be raised. Her happy memories and her enjoyment of family reunions would be treasured further without pain, and she would know deep inside that those fulfilled days of the past and the love for her children were hers to cherish forever.

Generally, Honeysuckle is often indicated, in addition to Star of Bethlehem, in states of grief when the death of a loved one is mourned and one knows full well that the happiness once had will never return during this life. Honeysuckle will shift the viewpoint from the past to the present and the future and the happiness still possible therein, while treasured memories remain without being overly engaged in or interfering in the here and now. Should the loss be tragic and the longing for the past be unbearable, Honeysuckle will still help to lighten the feelings of inevitability.

The Honeysuckle hedge is thick and abundant, with a very delicate, beautiful scent that stimulates longing and imagination; or one may notice a sweet, laden undertone reminding of nostalgia and melancholy, those being the mental/emotional states it cures.

RED CHESTNUT (Aesculus carnea)

Group: For Those Who Have Fear.

Preparation: Boiling of flowering clusters in full bloom.

Flowering Period: Late May and June.

Indications by Bach: For those who find it difficult not to be anxious for other people.

Often they have ceased to worry about themselves, but for those of whom they are fond they may suffer much, frequently anticipating that some unfortunate thing may happen to them. *(Twelve Healers)*

Susan needed Red Chestnut for her fears that something unfortunate or dreadful might befall her children while they were independently engaged in the world and away from her loving care. When the children were close to her, she had felt they were safe, and she had derived comfort and ease from the union, as she still did during family gatherings. Since her children were gone, she engaged in anxious imaginings and nervously anticipated the worst for them. In her thoughts, she reached out to her children, trying to be with them or protect them, while in actuality she was separated from them and felt powerless and out of reach.

This is the etiology of the Red Chestnut bond, arising from an intense love bond threatened by dangers and interrupted by distance. The remedy Red Chestnut would help Susan to release her children to their own destiny, while her genuine love bond would remain. She would have faith in her children's capabilities and safety, have more faith in God's or fate's care, and turn her nervousness and fear into trust and hope.

In other areas of life, Red Chestnut, if indicated, is a good remedy for young parents who hover over each step of the unsteady youngster engaged in exploring the dangers of the world. Here the Red Chestnut fears are present even though togetherness exists, since possible dangers threaten continually, as the toddler moves away even steps from one's immediate vicinity or is threatened in other ways such as by sickness. Generally, should a loved one fall ill or have an accident, a negative Red Chestnut state can develop in the onlooker and also in the understanding patient who is aware of the caretaker's concern.

The Red Chestnut tree shows beautiful raised clusters of red blossoms that stand out dramatically from the dark-green foliage, as if to radiate alarm and danger. The dark-green leaves, on the other hand, soothe and calm, as if to give shelter to the state of fear and alarm. The clusters point to the sky, reminding of the healing power of faith.

Comparative Study of Applicable Homeopathic Remedy:

Causticum was the remedy indicated; it covers the genuine concern with a bent to overcare, plus the feelings of self-pity or sorrow for one's unjustified lot, should others not appreciate the output of care (Chicory). Causticum further treats states of grief or coping with a loss (Honeysuckle), plus the exaggerated fears and concerns for others' welfare (Red Chestnut). People in need of Causticum are usually very sympathetic people; they often involve themselves in social or political service and have high ideals in regard to alleviating injustice on earth. This urge can also be expressed in one's endeavor to raise healthy, well-attended to, and emotionally happy children, as in the case of Susan.

On the physical plane, Causticum is marked, among other symptoms, by eruptions on the nose and warts near the finger-tips, contraction of tendons, a tendency to chest colds, consti-pation, incontinence of bladder, left-sided sciatica, dislike of sweets with craving for smoked foods, preference of wet weather over dry weather. Susan had most of these symptoms.

CASE 8. CENTAURY, WILLOW, HEATHER (PHOSPHORUS)

Kimberly is a young mother of twenty-eight years, engaged in the full-time duty of raising her children, a one-year-old and a three-year-old. She is a cheerful person and enjoys her mothering role very much, trying her best to give her children a beautiful, healthful life, while she tries to pamper her husband also. Furthermore, being outgoing and social, she is actively engaged in the community with fund raising efforts and planning and preparations of social events.

Although she finds it her joyful duty to love and serve others, her various tasks so demand her attention that, to her regret, she has little time to devote herself to favorite past time activities she once enjoyed, such as dancing, hiking, or reading books of interest. She also regrets her husband's frequent absence from the home, since he travels on his job regularly and is then not available for her own and the children's support and company. She finds herself working very hard and overtaxing her strength considerably, yet she is always urged on by her heartfelt impulse to enrich life for others.

Frequently, she urges her husband to find a different, more home-bound position within the company so that travels would end and he could assist her more in the home. Although this is possible for him, he does not seem particularly interested in the idea. This attitude hurts Kimberly's feelings and creates resentment. Since Kimberly is interested in making life pleasant for her husband and sparing him trouble, she is not inclined to stir up fights or heated disputes. While being interested in his welfare, she does not represent her own position forcefully enough, which results in increasingly unhappy feelings that are mostly held within. She feels misunderstood and does not understand her husband's lack of initiative in regard to improving their life style.

She experiences the strong urge to share her plight with others, to find understanding and sympathy. Her internal pressures find release when she talks to her girlfriends who give her a willing ear. Together they analyze the problem, trying to understand the husband's viewpoint and finding ways to improve the situation. No real progress is made with the problem at home, however, since her husband is not open to suggestion. This in turn increases her internal unhappiness, growing resentments and her urge to discuss the problem and find sympathy. Her girlfriends begin to tire somewhat under the impact of her incessant need to share this recurrent topic that evades solution. They are surprised to see Kimberly this concerned, since formerly she was more relaxed and more interested in listening to their problems than discussing her own affairs.

In regard to her marriage, Kimberly is aware that her output of love and service is not equaled, and she feels increasingly disillusioned with her life and somewhat weakened in her resolve and strength to give to her husband and others unceasingly. However, she does not want resentment to get hold of her and stifle her love of service which she enjoys.

The Bach Remedies indicated are *Centaury* for her willingness to serve others beyond her personal strength, *Willow* for her growing resentment that she tries to hold in check, and *Heather* for her urge to discuss the problem and find understanding.

Some physical symptoms of interest are: Kimberly suffers from occasional nosebleeds and also complains of heavy menstrual periods; she feels burning inside her stomach that instills a craving for ice-cold drinks and ice cream. She also has a craving for chocolate, salt and fish. There are further symptoms of tingling in her fingertips; weakness, and of late increased nervousness and fear of thunderstorms.

CENTAURY (Centaurium umbellatum)

Group: Oversensitive to Influences and Ideas.

Preparation: Sun method, use of flowers.

Flowering Period: From June to September.

Indications by Bach: Kind, quiet, gentle people who are over-anxious to serve others. They overtax their strength in their endeavors.

Their wish so grows upon them that they become more servants than willing helpers. Their good nature leads them to do more than their own share of work, and in doing so they may neglect their own particular mission in life. *(Twelve Healers)*

Kimberly was of the Centaury type, since her desire to enrich the others' lives went so far as to undermine her personal strength in mind/emotions and body. Household and children, plus added tasks in the community, took their toll. The desire to please her husband and not fight more vigorously for improvement of her home life, while trying to keep resentment in check, further weakened her inner stability and sense of authenticity. The inability to pursue favorite pastime activities also reduced her joy of living and prevented recharging of her stifled inner energies.

In the negative Centaury state, physical weakness often accompanies the emotional drain, as if the body signals the need to slow down and rest, reminding the person of his limitations.

Centaury would strengthen Kimberly on all levels and help her realize how to take care of her personal needs, while her worthy desire to love and serve would continue to guide her actions.

In some cases, the etiology of the negative Centaury state is not only rooted in the desire for service but also fueled by feelings of guilt or self-blame which are then corrected by the urge to go beyond one's share of work. Should the extra effort not be appreciated, feelings of resentment can develop which will lead the usually conscientious Centaury person to further guilt feelings. To reduce self-blame for thinking or enacting resentment, the Centaury person is then again spurred on to renewed service and attempts at making up with the other person, should there have been open disputes. This Centaury-Willow-Pine cycle is then repeated, should the other person be unkind or not truly understand or appreciate one's efforts. Pine was not indicated for Kimberly, however, since she did not blame herself for her recurrent feelings of resentment, and since she managed to keep strong feelings of resentment at bay, although this was not easy.

In regard to Bach's comments on the Centaury tendency to fail one's mission in life, it can be said that Kimberly was fulfilling her mission on a large scale; she had given herself wholeheartedly to her family life and was happy with her choice. She also knew that her talents would find further expression during her future work experience which she planned to resume part-time, once the children were in school. The negative Centaury state, however, can arise even while engaged within one's mission and its meaningful activities, since the demands may go beyond one's strength and one's call of duty. In regard to Kimberly, she simply needed to pay more attention to her personal

needs in order to overcome her negative Centaury state. Bach
meant that some people go so far as to unwittingly relinquish
their yet unrealized missions and personal ways of fulfillment
throughout their lives in service for others who are often not
aware or appreciative of the sacrifice. Although this is worthwhile and beneficial service, it may not be the best utilization of
their personal talents and could result in a lifelong tragic state of
lost potential and unfulfilled dreams. The remedy Centaury helps
one to be aware of one's error and gives direction and creative
strength toward one's personal fulfillment. One can now respond
to the so-called "call of destiny." True destiny ideally combines
the desire to love and serve with the expression and utilization
of one's creative potential, so as to give the world one's full benefit.

The beautiful pink Centaury flower looks delicate and ten-
der, as if to remind of the preciousness and sensitivity of the
service-loving person. The multiple flowers within one cluster
speak of generosity of attitude.

WILLOW (Salix vitellina)

Group: For Despondency or Despair.

Preparation: Boiling of male and female catkins with twigs.

Flowering Period: April and May.

Indications by Bach: For those who have suffered adversity
or misfortune and find these difficult to accept, without complaint or resentment, as they judge life much by the success
which it brings.

They feel that they have not deserved so great a trial, that it
was unjust, and they often become embittered.

They often take less interest and are less active in those things of life which they had previously enjoyed. *(Twelve Healers).*

Willow would help Kimberly to overcome her growing resentment against her husband's stubbornness and keep a forgiving, understanding heart, as was her wish. In her case, the potential for resentment was high, since she was giving towards her husband but did not receive the expected equal consideration in return. Willow would also help her express her concerns and disappointments more frankly. Furthermore, the remedy would reduce the preoccupation with the problem and lessen the intensity of her attitude towards the unresolved question, and she would learn to relax more about it and feel fortunate again.

Typically, a Willow state can come on when feelings of unhappiness that arise due to another person's neglect are not openly expressed, or, should those feelings be expressed, are not responded to or taken seriously, as happened in Kimberly's case. The person in the negative Willow state then tends to blame the other and holds him/her responsible for the unhappiness and lack of success. Often, the person's lot has truly been influenced detrimentally by another person's fault; whereas, at other times, the blame is placed unjustly and self-assessment should come first. In some cases, blaming gets out of hand and one imagines one's whole life going wrong due to the fault of another, which would be an extreme negative Willow state. Kimberly was aware of this dynamic also and decided to work on her growing resentment so that blame and unhappiness would not rule her. Willow was the remedy needed to give her the extra inner strength and power to forgive, as well as enable her to speak up at the right time when with her husband and not resort to pushing down hurt feelings that would have to be shared later with a third party.

Since Kimberly preferred to speak her mind in a mild rather than forceful way in order to keep her husband at peace, the remedy Agrimony could also be of interest in her case. However, Agrimony was not considered a predominant remedy because concerns were truly voiced and discussed with the husband and not pushed underground, and because these concerns were openly shared, acknowledged and dealt with during sharing time with her friends. Typically, Agrimony attempts to not deal in depth with problems but tries to glide over them cheerfully, while inner worries nonetheless remain.

In general, Willow is for all those who carry grudges, sometimes for a long time after the disputes or provoking situations have been settled. If individuals are not to blame for one's plight, Willow also helps with resentment and bitterness in face of missed opportunities and an unfavorable course of life. In the negative Willow state, self-blame is low; one seeks the cause of dissatisfaction outside of oneself, even if there is only fate itself to blame.

The Willow tree has flexible branches that bend like no other wood, symbolizing bending with forgiveness and bowing towards the offender. The fuzzy catkins speak of friendly feelings and warmth.

HEATHER (Calluna vulgaris)

Group: Loneliness.

Preparation: Sun method, use of whole sprigs.

Flowering Period: August and September.

Indications by Bach: Those who are always seeking the companionship of anyone who may be available, as they find it necessary to discuss their own affairs with others, no matter whom it may be. They are unhappy if they have to be alone for any length of time. *(Twelve Healers)*

Heather was indicated for Kimberly because of her strong need to share her hurt feelings which she felt she could not express adequately to her husband and which were not responded to properly by him. She craved sympathy and understanding and a willing ear that would truly listen to her, take her viewpoint into consideration and give her support.

In the negative Heather state, one feels lonely inside, often misunderstood or disregarded, and one wants to be heard. In extreme cases, should one not have close friends or family, any acquaintance may be talked to until internal pressure is relieved. The urge to talk usually is so great that one neglects to tune into the listener who may become overwhelmed by the flow of words or lose interest. Next to the need to express hurt feelings, the person in need of Heather is usually driven by self-preoccupation and craving for attention. One tends to see one's own problems as overly important and lose perspective for the listener's position.

Heather would also help Kimberly to express herself at the right time, while being with her husband, instead of carrying her burdens elsewhere. She would also be more available again to lend a willing ear to her girlfriends' problems, since internal pressure and the need to express her own plight would lessen.

Heather grows in abundance, spreading across the countryside much like a profuse flow of words. Its beautiful pink-purple color soothes and calms the onlooker, and it speaks of the inner peace and harmony it transmits.

Comparative Study of Applicable Homeopathic Remedy:

The remedy *Phosphorus* was indicated for Kimberly, as the Phosphorus state may be characterized by a cheerful, outgoing attitude and the desire for loving service that can be engaged in to the point of weakness and nervousness (Centaury). Phosphorus patients can easily feel resentment after such an output of affection, should others not respond equally or be mindful of a giver's needs (Willow), and these patients are prone to have a strong need to talk and share with others (Heather). To add to the picture of Phosphorus, there is also sensitivity to all impressions (helped by the remedy Walnut), mental weariness (Hornbeam), and, in some cases, a tendency to fearful nervousness (Mimulus and Rock Rose); these states were not strongly experienced by Kimberly.

On the physical plane, Phosphorus is marked by profusion also: There is easy and profuse bleeding of bright red blood, such as during nosebleeds and menses. It is considered a good remedy to stop hemorrhages in an emergency. Phosphorus can cure or improve many eye troubles such as cataract or glaucoma. Furthermore, it treats the burning in the stomach with craving for ice-cold drinks and ice cream. Typically, there is craving for chocolate, fish and spicy food. Tingling in the fingertips and heavy legs are further symptoms, along with fear and nervous agitation during thunderstorms. The Phosphorus patient is very sensitive to atmospheric troubles. Kimberly had most of these symptoms.

CASE 9. CERATO, WALNUT, ASPEN
(THUJA OCCIDENTALIS)

Tim is a seventeen year old high-school student who is regularly involved with his peer group, which asserts great influence on him. It is of great concern to him to be accepted as one of them and be considered "cool." He participates in all the trends and the popular activities, although he vaguely knows that some are detrimental to his physical and emotional health, such as taking drugs, which he does not do to excess, and seeing horror or violent movies.

The horror movies impress him too deeply and put him in an eerie state of mind with a sense of foreboding which he does not share or openly discuss with others, while the drugs enhance his discomfort and further lead to internal instability and susceptibility. All this is compounded by his inner insecurity and his lack of self-identity and purpose.

In general, he has a difficult time making up his mind and deciding for himself, in this way making himself dependent on the advice of others and an easy target for peer pressure and the influence of trends and fads. In his social interactions, he is also unsure of his appearance, mannerisms, and his position within the group, always wondering whether he is acceptable, attractive and lovable. Yet, there are undercurrents or plans within the group that he does not feel attracted to, that are hidden from him and somehow scare him, especially since he often cannot pinpoint where the group dynamics carry him. Not sure what to make of it all, Tim yields to peer pressure, although feelings of foreboding and uncertainty are high; yet, he enjoys being a part of the group's social interaction.

He is not sure how to manage staying in the group and yet be free from the influences that make him feel ill at ease. He is beginning to feel increasingly unhappy, insecure and not true to himself. Under the admonition of his parents, who are mostly concerned with his drug habit, he decides to atleast reduce the amount of drugs taken.

For his mental/emotional states, *Cerato* is indicated for inner insecurity and instability in making decisions, *Walnut* for being influenced too easily, and *Aspen* for vague fears and feelings of foreboding.

Predominant physical symptoms are: Shiny skin, slightly yellowish; chronic nasal catarrh and persistent mucus in his throat that has to be swallowed; stomach sensitivity, especially to raw onions and sour apples; feeling of increased mucus in stomach with sensation of pressure that extends upwards into the esophagus; a tendency to warts and history of gonorrhea.

CERATO (Ceratostigma willmottiana)

Group: For Those Who Suffer Uncertainty.

Preparation: Sun method, use of flowers.

Flowering Period: August to early October.

Indications by Bach: Those who don't have sufficient confidence in themselves to make their own decisions.

They constantly seek advice from others, and are often misguided. *(Twelve Healers)*

During this phase of his life, Tim was showing characteristics of the Cerato type, namely, lack of inner stability, easy susceptibility and indecisiveness. The negative Cerato state does not only arise during decision-making processes, as one might think on reading Bach's description, but can apply to any uncertainty of attitude or insecurity experienced within various life situations and one's own personality realm. In this sense, Tim showed insecurity about his social standing in the group, about his acceptability and popularity, and about his personal mannerisms and his appearance. His inner center of self-identity and his personal decisiveness and effectiveness had not yet fully manifested, as is often the case during teenage years. Tim had not yet found his personal sense of purpose and unique expression of potential.

He also showed the negative Cerato state in view of the direction of group dynamics that he often could not pinpoint, and he showed uncertainty about his personal way of reacting to the situation that often made him feel ill at ease, although the overall social interaction was enjoyable to him in many ways.

Cerato would help Tim to find his inner core of stability and direction, also for his adult years ahead; he would be able to make up his mind, trust his inner judgment and intuition and be less open to suggestion. His need to be a part of the popular group's various activities would reduce also, since self-reliance and independence would increase. He also would no longer be misguided into adventures that did not appeal to him, and he would learn to be his own master.

In general, a Cerato state can develop when loving approval from others is not present or not expressed adequately and the receiving person left uncertain, or when the others are uncertain themselves in their attitude towards the receiver. Children who are not supported lovingly or reassured in their being may develop a negative Cerato state. In complete acceptance and unconditional positive regard lies the best cure for the uncertain child. This would also foster the child's ability to love, which would reduce uncertainty further. This holds true for all in need of Cerato; the wholehearted concentration and devotion towards others reduces personal uncertainty and preoccupation with self and furthers cure. This activated focus would also lessen Tim's internal insecurities.

A further point is that persons in need of Cerato tend to hide their inner feelings of insecurity because they consider them troublesome and somewhat embarrassing.

The beautiful blue Cerato flower comes from Tibet, the land of wisdom and meditation. Just by looking at the strikingly blue flowers, one experiences certainty and clarity.

WALNUT (Juglans regia)

Group: Oversensitive to Influences and Ideas.

Preparation: Boiling of flowering stems with young leaves, use of female flowers.

Flowering Period: April and May.

Indications by Bach: For those who have definite ideals and ambitions in life and are fulfilling them, but on rare occasions are tempted to be led away from their own ideas, aims and work by the enthusiasm, convictions or strong opinions of others.

The remedy gives constancy and protection from outside influences. *(Twelve Healers)*

Bach's last paragraph on Walnut more specifically applies to Tim's case. The previous words also warrant to some extent the choice for Walnut, since Tim knew that certain group activities and group dynamics were detrimental to him and that his expectations for having a good time often were not met; yet, he was consistently drawn to the group. He was too easily influenced, not only by trends and group dynamics, but also by the horror films or films of violence that shook him up and imprinted fear-evoking content onto his consciousness. During drug experiences, he also felt open to impressions and shaken in his inner stability.

Walnut would help him find his inner balance and firmness, and he would not be so easily influenced and swayed by outside impressions. Relying on inner wisdom and finding strength therein, Tim's consciousness would learn to sort through rather involuntarily the impressions of life and give attention and devotion to those worthwhile and good. Walnut works like a protective shield filtering out those unnecessary impressions of detriment and meaninglessness that could deeply damage the soul.

Another aspect of Walnut is its function as a link-breaker; it enables people to let go of the past and start afresh, if so desired. This could apply to Tim also, should he wish to break with the group completely. It is a good remedy to help with the instability that occurs as a person goes through a change or transition of life. Changes such as moving away from home and having to find new friends may create temporary instability during a state of flux and reorganization, and Walnut gives protection from being unduly influenced by outside impressions and helps to rely on one's inner guiding light.

The Walnut tree is known for not mixing with the world around it; the fragrance acts as a repellent to insects and other plants.

In animal and pet care, crushed Walnut shells can be used as litter, this being a recent innovation. Animal refuse is merely sieved out and crushed shells can be reused for a long time, since they do not mix with or absorb particles or odors of the refuse.

These characteristics speak of the tree's power to shield from undue outside influence and of its power to retain one's identity.

ASPEN (Populus tremula)

Group: For Those Who Have Fear.

Preparation: Boiling of twigs with leaf buds, and male and female flowers.

Flowering Period: February to April.

Indications by Bach: Vague, unknown fears, for which there can be given no explanation, no reason.

Yet the patient may be terrified of something terrible going to happen, he knows not what.

These vague unexplainable fears may haunt by night or day.

Sufferers are often afraid to tell their trouble to others. *(Twelve Healers)*

Aspen was indicated for Tim because of his vague fears, his sense of foreboding and uncertainty that circled around the group's plans and secret endeavors. The horror movies and states of fear induced by drugs further made him ill at ease and unnerved him. He kept his fears to himself, which is typical for the negative Aspen state, since the reasons for fears cannot be pinpointed or explained. Furthermore, his inner uncertainty and indecisiveness (Cerato), plus his easy susceptibility to impressions (Walnut), made him more prone to develop the negative Aspen state, since fear-evoking impressions impacted fully, without being balanced or dealt with.

Aspen would help Tim to feel in charge of his fearful feelings, on top of them rather than being carried by them. Gradually, a sense of ease and safety would replace uncertainty and fearful foreboding, while reason would be stimulated to counteract eerie, threatening impressions.

The remedy Aspen fosters faith in a friendly universe that protects rather than threatens with the "big unknown." The branches and leaves of the Aspen tree tremble in a light breeze, reminding of a shaken, scared state which it has the power to cure.

Comparative Study of Applicable Homeopathic Remedy:

The remedy *Thuja occidentalis* applied to Tim's case. Thuja occidentalis is a cedar tree; its Latin name "arbor vitae" or "tree of life," hints at the life giving and healing quality that it brings. In the mental/emotional realm, Thuja occidentalis cures uncertainty and insecurity which may be felt in regard to one's appearance and behavior. It treats undue self-consciousness which may curtail the ability to be decisive and frank in one's dealings with others (Cerato); it also helps with easy susceptibility to influences and trends (Walnut), and vague fears and foreboding (Aspen).

On the physical plane, Thuja occidentalis heals the over-production of mucus; mucus is felt especially in the throat and seems to be produced in the stomach and along the esophagus, where also a disturbing pressure is felt that reaches all the way to the stomach. In this area of pressure, persons in need of Thuja occidentalis seem to hold the feelings of uncertainty and insecurity about themselves. The inner stomach lining is very sensitive and cannot tolerate sharp foods such as onions. Typically, there is also shiny facial skin and fleshy growth of warts. In the

negative Thuja occidentalis state, cells tend to overgrow and overproduce, not only on skin and mucus membranes but also in internal organs, where tumorous growth can develop. Thuja occidentalis is often indicated after a bout of gonorrhea, as hap-
·pened in Tim's case.

CASE 10. IMPATIENS, CHERRY PLUM, ROCK WATER (NUX VOMICA)

Robert, age thirty-two, has become impatient and tense since he has quit taking drugs one week ago. He finds himself being ill-tempered, short with people and less considerate of their needs. A slight tendency to impatience and nervousness had existed before but now is greatly enhanced by the unsatisfied craving for the drug and the physical and mental/emotional side effects of the withdrawal.

Since the craving for the drug is intense, Robert is almost constantly engaged in mental battles, trying to overrule the urge to reach for the drug with strong resolve and with the vehement pushing down of the inclination to engage in the habit that he had once enjoyed. When the craving comes upon him, he feels great fear and tension mounting in face of the possibility that he would give in to the urge for the drug, lose his resolve and give up the struggle of quitting his habit.

Despite these difficulties, he is resolved to see this process through and hopefully inspire some of his friends to follow his example, and he is proud of having come so far.

The following remedies are indicated: *Impatiens* for mental/emotional and physical tension that would impinge on others, *Cherry Plum* for fear of the mind losing control, and *Rock Water* for easing the struggle of being a hard master onto himself.

Physical complaints next to tension and irritability are: Severe frontal headache; tightness in nape of neck; ineffectual urging to vomiting and bowel elimination, with ravenous appetite and craving for meat.

IMPATIENS (Impatiens glandulifera)

Group: Loneliness.

Preparation: Sun method, use of pale mauve flowers.

Flowering Period: July to September.

Indications by Bach: Those who are quick in thought and action and who wish all things to be done without hesitation and delay. When ill they are anxious for a hasty recovery.

They find it very difficult to be patient with people who are slow, as they consider it wrong and a waste of time, and they will endeavor to make such people quicker in all ways.

They often prefer to work and think alone so that they can do everything at their own speed. (*Twelve Healers*)

Robert's usual slight bent to impatience was greatly enhanced during the first week of the withdrawal, and he showed the characteristics of the impatient type who is tense, driven, and wants other people to follow his pace. The remedy Impatiens would calm him in mind/emotions and body, diminish his nervy state, and reduce the impatient craving for the drug. It would give him patience with people and with the slow process of drug rehabilitation, while his body and mind would learn to live without the usual stimulation by the drug.

In general, the remedy Impatiens helps one to consider the pace of others and their needs; one becomes more aware and stops urging people to work and think faster. It is an excellent remedy for young mothers who have a tendency to impatience while dealing with their small children and the children's unique pace of growing and learning. It is a good remedy for all those tired of being driven and caught up in the fast pace of modern times and who wish to slow down and find restful peace. Furthermore, people who tend to have angry outbursts that come on suddenly would benefit from Impatiens.

The beautiful mauve flower is known for its sudden "outbursts" and thrusting of seeds that are scattered "impatiently" abroad. The leaves have toothed edges and are arranged in a sort of rigid way, reminding of a nervy, wound-up, or painful state. Yet, the delicate mauve petals and the soothing color speak of gentleness and quiet repose.

CHERRY PLUM (Prunus cerasifera)

Group: For Those Who Have Fear.

Preparation: Boiling of twigs with flowers.

Flowering Period: February to April.

Indications by Bach: Fear of the mind being over-strained, of reason giving way, of doing fearful and dreaded things, not wished and known wrong, yet there comes the thought and impulse to do them. *(Twelve Healers)*

Robert was prescribed Cherry Plum for his mental impulse to give in to his craving, reach for the drug, and let go of his resolve. This impulse was held in check by strong mental control and willpower. Yet, there was the mounting fear that he would give in to the dreaded impulse and that the impulse would win. The remedy Cherry Plum would ease the pressure and fear and would help him stay balanced and in free-flowing control. His resolve, which was mostly a rational choice, would keep the upper hand over the physical cravings that had threatened to dictate his conduct.

Typically, the negative Cherry Plum state is a state of extreme tension and anxiety when there is extreme polarity in the mind and the effort based on willpower to hold things in balance. Should the dreaded impulse win and reason lose, homicides, suicides and other forms of crime or violence can be committed in extreme cases. Specifically, Cherry Plum treats the fear of the dreaded impulse getting out of hand and reigning over one's conduct or thought processes, though one does not wish for it. During the initial stages of the negative Cherry Plum state, the thought processes are threatened with unwanted content. If tension progresses and cannot be checked, the internal battle may be expressed and put into action, and the dreaded impulse would reign temporarily.

Cherry Plum is a good remedy for all who are prone to be abusive and wish to be able to control the impulses of anger and violence as they arise. Generally, to prevent a negative Cherry Plum state from arising, especially in a person with strong mental control who may be prone to impulsive actions, watching and interpreting one's dreams is recommended. Dream interpretation ensures that messages from the unconscious mind can reach the conscious mind and prevent those deep-seated, unaccounted-for imbalances that have a life of their own from arising. An impending negative Cherry Plum state signals that unconscious material, usually of vital importance, has not been resolved and deserves to be looked at. Understanding one's needs and inner dynamics, plus healthy need fulfillment, if possible, dissolve the impending Cherry Plum state. Should this process be overlooked, impulses that are not wished for may threaten, and they seem to become stronger, the more forcefully they are pushed down and denied. They cannot be pushed back into the unconscious but need to be dealt with. As a negative Cherry Plum state develops, the remedy Cherry Plum will resolve fear and pressure surrounding the unwanted impulses; the person has more ease and a clearer overview. As fear and pressure cease, the impulses themselves become more understandable and benevolent in character, since the unconscious mind has less resistance opposed to it and can flow and express itself more harmoniously.

In Robert's case, the impulses to give in to his craving for the drug did not represent a need of vital importance in the overall picture of his health. His cells had become dependent on a certain stimulant which was craved on withdrawal, although its effects were basically detrimental. Nonetheless, a negative Cherry Plum state developed as his mind and body on the cellular level and as the dependency on the emotional level threatened to overrule reasonable insight and resolve.

In the spring, the Cherry Plum blossoms stand out radiantly white against a dark background of leafless branches, as if to indicate the mental clarity and healthy balancing power they bring in face of unwanted impulses that arise out of the unknown, unconscious mind, usually darkened to our view. Cherry Plum will open channels of creative communication between all parts of the mind.

ROCK WATER

Group: Overcare for Welfare of Others.

Preparation: Sun method, water from a special well is left in the sun for atleast one hour.

Indications by Bach: Those who are very strict in their way of living; they deny themselves many of the joys and pleasures of life because they consider it might interfere with their work.

They are hard masters to themselves. They wish to be well, strong and active, and will do anything which they believe will keep them so. They hope to be examples which will appeal to others who may then follow their ideas and be better as a result. *(Twelve Healers)*

Robert needed Rock Water because he was determined to forgo his drug habit and be strict with himself during the crucial transition phase and beyond. This is not of concern in itself but represents a worthwhile and inspiring effort, yet there arise feelings of denial and hardship which Rock Water helps to ease and balance. It takes great effort to be a hard master onto oneself and push down the urge to engage in habits or pleasures once enjoyed. Rock Water would help Robert to feel more relaxed, and less intense and strained, while following his resolve.

Since one feels rightfully proud and victorious after a continuous battle has been won again and again, especially during the crucial transitional phase from drug-dependency to drug-independency, one also wishes to inspire or appeal to others, which is what Robert did. Rock Water would keep intact his healthy desire to inspire others yet diminish the intensity of this urge, and he and others would be more at peace.

In general, Rock Water is usually indicated when the desire for health and perfection is high and healthful practices or spiritual aspirations are engaged in with too much force of will or unnecessary determination, this being a state which may negate the very purpose of the endeavor. Rock Water will help to be more gentle with oneself.

Rock Water symbolizes the tenderness and ceaseless flow of water that can smooth the rough edges of even the hardest stone. The remedy gently washes away hardship and struggle on the way towards perfection, and it corrects aspirations, should they be unnecessarily harsh or relatively unimportant in growth toward wholeness.

Comparative Study of Applicable Homeopathic Remedy:

Nux vomica was the homeopathic remedy indicated. In the mental/ emotional realm, it treats tension, irritability and lack of patience with others (Impatiens). Nux vomica also typically helps with impulsive behavior and outbursts of anger that are usually not wished for (Cherry Plum), since the Nux vomica personality tends to be conscientious and is interested in doing a good job. This desire to excel and the high achievement motivation may lead such a personality to overwork and denial of basic need fulfillment (Rock Water). Lack of internal satisfaction may then be compensated for by drugs and stimulants which further increase irritability, especially the "morning after." Craving for stimulants is a keynote of the Nux vomica picture. This remedy is often indicated in drug rehabilitation when cravings create tension and impatience. Before quitting his habit, Robert had shown a tendency to the Nux vomica state, which now was intensified due to increased demands on his vital force.

Some typical physical symptoms are: Frontal headache and pain in occiput with tense feeling in nape of neck; during colds, nostrils are alternately stopped up; ineffectual urging to vomit and constipation with ineffectual urging; sour risings from stomach, increased appetite and craving for meat and fat; awakening from sleep at 3 A.M., with restlessness and an inability to go back to sleep.

CASE 11. VERVAIN, VINE, HOLLY (CHAMOMILLA)

Ben is a boy of ten years with a keen interest in video games. His overenthusiasm motivates his friends also, and he invites them to share in this entertainment. Together they sit for hours, riveted and completely "into" it.

Trouble starts as taking turns does not work, since Ben, holding the powerful position in his own home, tends to usurp the situation.

Further trouble ensues as games do not yield the expected satisfaction, since certain points were not scored due to hasty play and commotion; and there is frustration and nervous excitement of a negative kind with occasional inappropriate language and yelling.

As Ben's mother walks in and demands that the television be turned off and peace be established, Ben asserts himself and boldly insists that he and his friends need to play at least one more game. Mother usually gives in, afraid that Ben would raise a turmoil of upset feelings and temper outbursts in case she would refuse him. The temper outbursts usually serve Ben so that he gets his way with friends and parents alike. Overall though, he is kindhearted and considered a good leader among his friends. Ben is aware himself that dominating and angry behavior is not commendable, and he keeps promising to work on it. He is also known for his enthusiastic way of attending to his interests and pastime activities with his friends, whom he motivates to share in his enjoyment.

His mother feels that his intense reaction to the video games has carried certain facets of his behavior to the extreme and that other parts of his life have been affected also. His overenthusiasm has turned into an almost fanatical endeavor, his willfulness is pushed to the extreme, and the upset feelings are exaggerated as the urge to engage in video games absorbs and rules him. Other activities have become secondary, such as reading or crafts, and his mother is somewhat concerned, yet she sees educational value in the games also. She decides, however, to somewhat curtail his favorite pastime activity, while she hopes that his interests will branch out into more diversified occupation again, one being sports and play in the fresh air which has been neglected as of late. She hopes that Ben calms down with time and becomes more peaceful, even during the engagement with video games.[19]

The following remedies are indicated: *Vervain* for overenthusiasm, *Vine* for assuming the leadership role, and *Holly* for outbursts of anger and easily vexed feelings.

Some physical symptoms or tendencies are: Restlessness, irritability; hot, red face during anger outbursts; sensitivity to smells; great thirst for cold drinks with aversion to warm drinks; occasional griping in region of navel, upset bowel system, greenish stool, usually loose bowel movements; and restlessness at night.

VERVAIN (Verbena officinalis)

Group: Overcare for Welfare of Others.

Preparation: Sun method, use of flowering spikes.

Flowering Period: June to September.

Indications by Bach: Those with fixed principles and ideas, which they are confident are right, and which they very rarely change.

They have a great wish to convert all around them to their own views of life.

They are strong of will and have much courage when they are convinced of those things that they wish to teach.

In illness they struggle on long after many would have given up their duties. *(Twelve Healers)*

The second paragraph above applies mostly to Ben, since he was not an adult yet with fixed principles and ideas. Yet, in essence, Ben resembled the Vervain type. Specifically, he was overenthusiastic and motivated to incite his friends to share in his video enjoyment or other activities that he liked to engage in. In addition, while engaged in his favorite pastime activity, he was also overzealously wrapped up in it and in a wound-up nervous state which is typical for the negative Vervain state. He thought and acted in an overenthusiastic way, which often resulted in tension and willfulness, especially around the intense occupation with video games, which greatly fascinated and motivated him.

Enthusiasm is healthy and propels learning and enjoyment, yet when driven too far may result in overzealous activity, fanaticism, or nervous tension. This is an unhealthy state of being out of balance within oneself and within one's behavior toward others whom one wishes to influence and convert.

Vervain would help Ben to be more relaxed in view of his video game activity and more in charge of the overzealous urge to engage himself and others in this type of entertainment. Also, during game activity, he would have a better overview and be more a master of the situation rather than being driven by it. His single focus towards this activity might ease and new diversion be found in other activities. The urge to influence and convert others, including his mother, would also be helped as Ben would develop respect for their choices and learn to grant others their freedom of choice.

In general, Vervain helps all those who are overzealously engaged in political, environmental, intellectual or personal causes, and who wish to convert others to their viewpoint so that their cause is carried further to a good end. Vervain helps calm and dispel the tense driven state and the urge to discuss and convert, while it gives tolerance for the others' viewpoints and puts the importance of one's own cause into perspective. The self-righteousness that often propels persons in need of Vervain subsides so that loving respect and tolerance can actualize more. Often, self-righteousness is based on sincere recognition of values and truths; in such cases, Vervain will help understand that overenthusiasm cannot change things more quickly and that over time and with concentrated action, plus with faith in the power of justice and goodness, change may come.

Furthermore, Vervain eases the tendency to drive one's personality to new heights of accomplishment, even though stamina and nerve power may be failing. People in need of Vervain often show great strength of will that may escalate into nervous tension, however, should inner warning signals not be heeded and physical needs be neglected, Vervain will restore balance and revitalize the nervous system. In extreme cases, a nervous breakdown may be diverted.

The plant is known for its wiry stems that point up sharply, as if to speak of the overzealous, nervy state they cure. Along the stem are knots that portray a ladder effect and may hint at the mounting tension and the escalating or enumerating of arguments that happens during the negative Vervain state. Vervain brings back peace and perspective, as expressed in the tiny whitish flowers that bud along the stem.

VINE (Vitis vinifera)

Group: Overcare for Welfare of Others.

Preparation: Sun method, use of flowering clusters.

Flowering Period: April to May.

Indications by Bach: Very capable people, certain of their own ability, confident of success.

Being so assured, they think that it would be for the benefit of others if they could be persuaded to do things as they themselves do, or as they are certain is right. Even in illness they will direct their attendants.

They may be of great value in emergency. *(Twelve Healers)*

Ben was considered a leader among his friends, known as skilled and strongly motivated towards the various activities he engaged in, as of late the video games. Being a leader is not of detriment to himself and others, as long as he is considerate of the others' needs and the others enjoy being led. However, as soon as personal interests begin to rule over the interests or personal choices of others, a negative Vine state comes on that needs to be corrected, especially since many people in the vicinity of the leading person may be adversely affected. Specifically, Ben, being the leader and in charge of the video games in his own home, consistently took turns when he was not supposed to, and he often intimidated his peers with his loud talk. He also was not open to most of his mother's suggestions and controlled her with his outbursts of temper. People often gave in to him, and he got his way.

Vine would help Ben to be more considerate of others and be less urged within himself to lead and control others. Getting his way would not appear so important any more, and he would actually enjoy seeing others lead, too. His positive leadership qualities, however, would not be lessened by the remedy but enhanced. His enthusiasm was contagious and his suggestions usually worthy of consideration by others. Vine would also help him to be more understanding of his mother's concerns and be more open to her suggestions. He would be less inclined to be demanding and controlling, and become a more cooperative youngster.

In general, Vine is a good remedy for all those in leading positions who tend to be too drastic and stern. Vine brings forth positive leadership qualities by opening eyes for the others' position and creating increased consideration, compassion and respect for others. It is indicated also for those who need to be led and cannot accept this condition, since they are leaders also. This attitude is often characterized by disobedience, moves towards independence, and behavior aimed at controlling the one in charge, as seen in Ben's treatment of his mother.

The Vine plant is a climbing plant that tends to overgrow other plants, indicating the negative Vine state of overgrowing and stifling others. Its fruits speak of the fruits of service and mutual cooperation.

HOLLY (Ilex aquifolium)

Group: Oversensitive to Influences and Ideas.

Preparation: Boiling of flowering twigs.

Flowering Period: May to June.

Indications by Bach: For those who are sometimes attacked by thoughts of such kind as jealousy, envy, revenge, suspicion.

For the different forms of vexation.

Within themselves they may suffer much, often when there is no real cause for their unhappiness. *(Twelve Healers)*

Ben was not particularly experiencing jealousy, envy, revenge or suspicion, but he needed Holly to calm his vexations and easily stimulated upset feelings that often resulted in temper outbursts. His reaction to the video games furthered this process; there was irritability when game rounds were lost, and overstimulation deveoped from the many sounds and the quick pace of the games. Furthermore, he was quickly angered when others, including his mother, did not comply with his wishes or stood in his way, and he would use temper tantrums, however involuntarily, to control the others' reaction and get his way.

Holly would give Ben inner peace and calm, so he would not be so easily annoyed and upset, and he would not feel the inner volcanic need to burst out and lose control. Holly would serve to protect him from being easily vexed and also from being overstimulated and nervously agitated, which are states that often precede angry outbursts and quick temper. He would learn to develop kindness and consideration of others and understand that angry outbursts hurt others and offend them.

In general, Holly is an excellent remedy to cure such strong emotions as jealousy, envy, revenge and suspicion that can rule people and often make them feel weak-willed in face of the intensity of such emotions. In extreme cases, these feelings can be so strong and upsetting as to carry the whole personality to the extreme and actually seduce to feel self-righteously empowered, driven by the dynamic intensity and force of such thought content. In the negative Holly state, one feels that others are in some way a threat to one's happiness, even if this is not clearly warranted, and one experiences the strong urge to fight and strike back, even though it might just be in one's thoughts. Yet, suffering is great when such thoughts take hold, affecting not only the bearer but also the receiver should these thoughts be expressed. Holly will reestablish inner harmony, friendship and peaceful feelings and actions towards others, and one does not feel threatened so easily.

The spiked leaves of the Holly tree speak of vexation and aggressiveness, whereas the red berries signal the love and cheer given by the healing power of this plant. In many countries, Holly branches are used for Christmas decorations, celebrating the spirit of Christ's peace and love.

Comparative Study of Applicable Homeopathic Remedy:

Chamomilla (Matricaria chamomilla) is a useful remedy for children, and also for adults; it is indicated in great irritability with demanding, overzealous attempts to convert others to one's own ideas and get one's way (Vervain and Vine). Following, one observes temper outbursts if wishes are not met, plus possible aggressiveness and loud language (Holly and Vine). Chamomilla also treats oversensitivity to impressions and overstimulation, resulting in great irritability, especially in regard to noise and commotion (Holly).

On the physical plane, there is the tendency to have a red, hot head, especially during temper outbursts, or when acute states of sickness come on; sometimes one cheek appears redder than the other. Chamomilla is a good remedy for earaches and teething pain in children when the indications exist. The following symptoms are presented: Sensitivity to noises and smells; smarting of eyes; thirst for cold drinks, aversion to warm drinks, sour rising from stomach, griping pains around the navel, colic from anger and vexation; greenish stool that appears like chopped spinach, diarrhea; aggravation of symptoms at 9 A.M. and 9 P.M.; restless nights.

CASE 12. WATER VIOLET, BEECH, OAK
(KALIUM CARBONICUM)

Annette, forty-one years old, is a single working mother, priding herself that she is able to provide for her two sons and raise them on her own. Her sons are teenagers who are going through difficult phases, and she tries hard to keep an eye on them and give them guidance. She is not happy with the company they are in and, within her mind, finds herself criticizing her sons' friends and their lifestyle. She considers herself a friendly person and is not happy with such feelings, yet they surface repeatedly.

She has also noticed that she tends to look down on people in the office who do not seem to work as hard or make as much an effort as she does, and she often feels special, superior and also more knowledgeable than others. She prides herself that her stamina is great and that she can push herself even though she might be exhausted and worn out. Furthermore, her house is in good order and her life well organized. She feels on top of things, despite her occasional periods of fatigue. During her free time, she enjoys being at home and retreating from the world, although from time to time she feels lonely, since her sons do not spend much time at home any more.

In regard to dating, she has had some dates with men but has felt rather reserved and aloof, experiencing also some feelings of reluctance and a subtle fear of rejection. She tends to hold back and not encourage intimate relations, preferring men to take all the necessary steps in the dating process. Her behavior signals proud reserve, yet her inmost feelings also show shyness and reluctance to go forward, due to some inner need to stay within her own sphere, where she feels special and safe. She further finds herself criticizing potential partners and finding something wrong with them, which gives her the excuse to not get involved. She has an ideal man in mind whom she has not been able to meet yet, although she believes that she deserves such a man.

Over time, she has become increasingly unhappy, lonely and despondent, since all her hard work at her job and at home has not brought her closer to real happiness, although she feels that rewards should come her way. Yet, she struggles on daily, not letting go of her resolve to keep working hard and stay on top of things, in charge of her life.

The remedies indicated are: *Water Violet* for feeling special and reserved, *Beech* for her tendency to criticize others, and *Oak* for her unceasing struggle in face of disappointment.

Some physical symptoms or characteristics are: Swelling of inner upper eyelids; nervousness felt in the stomach with intolerance for tight clothing, craving for sweets, bad effects from ice-cold drinks; bloated abdomen, constipation and hemorrhoids; nightly restlessness around 2 A.M.; great sensitivity to drafts.

WATER VIOLET (Hottonia palustris)

Group: Loneliness.

Preparation: Sun method, use of flowers.

Flowering Period: May and June.

Indications by Bach: For those who in health or illness like to be alone. Very quiet people, who move about without noise, speak little, and then gently. Very independent, capable and self-reliant. Almost free of the opinions of others. They are aloof, leave people alone and go their own way. Often clever and talented. Their peace and calmness is a blessing to those around them. *(Twelve Healers)*

Annette showed the characteristics of the Water Violet type; she felt special and independent, rather reserved at times, and content with her achievements, also in regard to raising her sons as a single mother. There was also a tendency to feel superior to her colleagues, not only in regard to her capabilities but also in regard to her stamina and perseverance despite fatigue. Feeling special, she also expected a special partner, whom she had not been able to meet, due to some extent to her aloofness and re-luctance to go forward engagingly, and also due to her easily adopted perception of the other's unsuitable state.

Typically for the Water Violet type, her reluctance to get involved is also reflecting an inner need to stay safe and unham-pered, in charge of her own life. Yet, loneliness is often burden-some, and Annette did have the healthy longing to love and devote herself to someone dear, which potentially would have cured her Water Violet state by making her more open to easy comradery and recognition that everybody is special. While she was still single, the remedy Water Violet would help her to be more outgoing and accepting of others in the work place and during dates so that her tendency to seek independence and aloofness could be overcome more easily and happiness be achieved. Even if a loving partner would not come her way, Water Violet would keep her open toward others and give her joy of encounter with other people.

In general, Water Violet also helps those on the spiritual path who are realizing the religious truths of existence and want to avoid the pitfalls of feeling too special or superior to others. Should one feel lack of motivation or interest in meeting others, the remedy gives the incentive to stay open-hearted so that true spiritual progress can continue. Water Violet helps to understand that healthy self-respect and feeling special comes from loving others.

The Water Violet plant speaks of separateness by its lonely habitat near or in the water. Furthermore, the plant shows different groups of blossoms that are arranged around the stem in a circular fashion at different intervals along the stem. This seems to indicate the negative Water Violet state of separating from others and feeling above them, while the rounded groups of beautiful white and cheerful blossoms speak of the joy found in unity and togetherness.

BEECH (Fagus sylvatica)

Group: Overcare for Welfare of Others.

Preparation: Boiling of twigs with both male and female flowers.

Flowering Period: April and May.

Indications by Bach: For those who feel the need to see more good and beauty in all that surrounds them. And, although much appears to be wrong, to have the ability to see the good growing within. So as to be able to be more tolerant, lenient and understanding of the different way each individual and all things are working to their own final perfection. *(Twelve Healers)*

Annette needed Beech to help her be more tolerant with other people and their perceived lack of perfection. Specifically, she felt critical of her sons' friends and their lifestyle, of her colleagues and their perceived lack of excellence and stamina, and of her suitors whom she found unsuitable. She easily saw flaws and shortcomings in other people, while priding herself on being special. Yet, she felt basically friendly at heart and somehow aware that her attitude was not correct. The remedy Beech would help her to focus on the others' positive and lovable traits which would reveal as she devoted herself more fully.

In general, a negative Beech state can come on after one has lost something or someone dear and special, and nothing else measures up to the standards once enjoyed. In that case, there may also be sadness, helped by Star of Bethlehem, and longing for the past, treated with Honeysuckle. Beech helps to see beauty in surrounding people and circumstances, even if earlier standards are not met with, and one develops tolerance and appreciation instead of judgment and appraisal.

A negative Beech state can also come on when one is aware of high standards, through education and knowledge, without actually having experienced them in one's own life, and when one is critical if existing conditions do not measure up, as in Annette's case. Beech will give new appreciation and gratitude.

A negative Beech state may also result from resentment (Willow) due to the perceived wrong received from another, or it may be incited by jealousy (Holly); both of these attitudes may instill the need to constantly find fault with someone, also in areas other than their perceived wrongdoing or perceived threat, as in "cognitive dissonance," this being the psychological term for this state. Cognitive dissonance describes the mental state of having formed a certain opinion about someone and bending reality and one's impressions to fit this picture, which is usually of a negative kind. Beech will bring back kindness of heart and an open frame of mind not bent on faultfinding.

The Beech tree is marked by great beauty, considering the stately growth, smooth bark, the delicately shaped leaves and the ornamental white flowers. It speaks of perfection and clarity of form, signaling its power of bringing heightened recognition of beauty and the healing of intolerance and unnecessary criticism.

OAK (Quercus robur)

Group: For Despondency or Despair.

Preparation: Sun method, use of whole stalk of red female flowers.

Flowering Period: April and May.

Indications by Bach: For those who are struggling and fighting strongly to get well, or in connection with the affairs of their daily life. They will go on trying one thing after another, though their case may seem hopeless.

They fight on. They are discontented with themselves if illness interferes with their duties or helping others.

They are brave people, fighting against great difficulties, without loss of hope or effort. *(Twelve Healers)*

Annette needed Oak for her tendency to work hard even to the point of exhaustion. It was important to her to stay on top of things, fulfill her duties, have stamina, and be a caring mother; and her efforts were unceasing. Despondency would overcome her from time to time, as disappointments in her private life made her feel heavy at heart and weary, while she had been wishing all along that the hard work would earn rewards and happiness. Specifically, in the area of partner search she felt that no results had been forthcoming, while her general workload was intense, and she longed for a breakthrough of some kind that would allow her more ease and happiness. Yet, even when disappointments would come and feelings of despondency surfaced, she would struggle on bravely, yet with a heavy heart, and this is typical for the negative Oak state.

The remedy Oak would give her strength and set joyful incentives to go on, instead of resolve of willpower, while it would uplift her occasional feelings of despondency and bring lightness of heart, even if rewards were still not forthcoming and disappointments continued to exist. She may also realize that working beyond one's reserves is unhealthy and that regular rest and recreation are her prerogatives.

To sum up, people in need of Oak are resolved, with great strength of will, to struggle on despite exhaustion and disappointments, while they try to hold their commitments in balance. Over time, they may become stoic or deeply worn out or develop a one-track mind bent on task completion. Their continued stamina is admirable and will not be reduced by the remedy but rather raised to new lightness of heart, mind and action.

The Oak tree resembles a somewhat worn or bent state, indicating the Oak mentality of working to the point of exhaustion and yet going on with willpower. The green foliage and acorns speak of renewal and sustenance, both of which the remedy Oak will instill.

Comparative Study of Applicable Homeopathic Remedy:

Kalium carbonicum was the remedy indicated. In the mental/emotional realm, this remedy is marked by strong mental control and perseverance during task completion (Oak). This state may instill pride in one's stamina and superiority over others (Water Violet), with simultaneous criticism of others who do not seem as well in charge of themselves or are lacking in other ways (Beech). In the Kalium carbonicum state, one tends to ignore emotional needs and rules with an iron fist. Yet, emotions cannot be suppressed and usually reassert at night when the Kalium carbonicum patient experiences disturbed sleep with frequent waking and restlessness. Stifled emotions also may affect inner organs and create damage, since they do not find recognition within the consciousness. Kalium carbonicum patients may carry stoically the burdens of unfulfilled dreams, which have been denied by circumstance, on top of a demanding work load which they manage with willpower and perseverance. The tendency to superiority and criticism, though not necessarily visible in each Kalium carbonicum case, roots in this valuable, to them seemingly unparalleled, effort to sustain one's demands.

Some major physical symptoms are: Swollen upper eyelids, inner angle; gums separate from teeth; nervous stomach, with feelings of anxiety experienced in stomach, sour eructation, bad effects from ice water, tight clothing is not tolerated; constipation and hemorrhoids, bloated abdomen; restless waking with frequent urination at night and inability to go back to sleep; waking at 2 A.M. and between 4 and 5 A.M. Annette had most of these symptoms.

CONCLUDING REMARKS

This presentation of the thirty-eight Bach Remedies showed the appropriate selection of Bach Remedies, based on recognition of the individual dynamic of each case. Case material, plus added general remarks about the remedies, served to bring out the unique character of each healing essence.

The homeopathic remedies presented in these twelve cases have been analyzed in their main characteristics as well, highlighted by the specific dynamic of each case. These homeopathic remedies, however, cover more possible mental/emotional states and, of course, more physical symptoms than those presented in the cases. Especially the polychrests span a wide range of mental/emotional and physical states, yet these states will remain within each remedy's typical essence or picture. Depending on the case, certain facets of these possible characteristics are being highlighted, usually not all in equal intensity. Yet, one always recognizes the main dynamic.

The next chapter will give one example of a remedy that has been analyzed as completely as possible in regard to the mental/emotional states it cures. The appropriate Bach Remedies will be listed as well, and an overview of the main physical symptoms is included.

8

LYCOPODIUM CLAVATUM: EXAMPLE OF A COMPLETE ANALYSIS OF A HOMEOPATHIC REMEDY AND ITS CORRESPONDING BACH REMEDIES

- Mental/Emotional Symptoms
- Physical Symptoms

MENTAL/EMOTIONAL SYMPTOMS

There are genetic, climatic or nutritional reasons, plus other physical and mental/emotional factors, that determine the emergence of a chronic remedy picture in the mind/emotions/body totality. Should basic physical needs be fulfilled, the predominant etiology lies in the mental/emotional realm, since imbalances in mind and emotions, if persisted in, greatly affect the overall health. Certain types of people portray different tendencies to mental/emotional and physical imbalance. These imbalances are generally stirred up when mind and emotions go astray, pulling the whole economy with them. The vital force will then express this layer of health disturbance, that may represent a genetically inherited tendency to imbalance, in this specific area of the mind/emotions/body totality. These genetic tendencies can be held at bay or be overcome by one's personal interest in developing and safeguarding one's healthy mind and emotions and maintaining physical welfare, and by using specifically indicated Bach Remedies and homeopathic remedies, should imbalances begin to assert.

The most common mental/emotional etiology leading to the *Lycopodium clavatum* picture stems from not feeling recognized or accepted and having to defend against such perceived treatment. By evaluating others too readily as not accepting, the mental perception of reality is bent and fueled by emotions. From this perception may arise a state of feeling inadequate, which is not tolerated by the self and defended against to guard one's healthy self-image. Should defenses actually involve external behavior, there may be bragging or an exaggerated outward show of courage and competence; these attempts may be based on true ability, nonetheless. Lycopodium clavatum persons are generally found to be good intellectual workers and achievement-oriented.

Internal insecurities that may threaten but are not wished for are best treated by *Larch* or *Cerato,* whereas *Mimulus* would apply to the person's need to defend against a possible negative appraisal that is feared and not wished for. Mimulus would also deal with anxieties that arise in regard to others finding out that one is in need to put on a show or has to defend against a possible unfavorable evaluation by others. Furthermore, Lycopodium clavatum is listed under anticipatory fears; there may be the need to give oneself a push before one presents oneself to the world and before a new task is tackled. Mimulus helps with this dynamic also. *Elm* for feelings of being overwhelmed and *Hornbeam* for mental clarity and for overcoming of procrastination could be of service also.

Persons prone to develop the Lycopodium clavatum state may also be affected adversely by contradiction or by condescension against them, and they are greatly offended by this treatment. Anger and hurt feelings are stirred up easily, and they may decide to vent their annoyance or keep it inside, while outwardly manifesting the posture of defiance. Should feelings of resentment not be expressed adequately and kept within, internal arguments and conversations concerning the issue stay with them, even after points of contention have been smoothed over or have dated back some time. Lycopodium clavatum people have a hard time accepting accusations and unjustified appraisal, and they often play back conversations and disputes in their mind, trying to figure out what they should have said and deciding on the best way to defend and counteract; as they need their self-image to stay intact, also for future purposes, should disputes flare up again. There is also a tendency to mental preoccupation with concerns other than arising from confrontation; and, as these concerns evade solution, a painful process of irresolution and vacillation between two solutions or possibilities could unfold. This creates internal discomfort, threatening one's internal stability and clarity of purpose, and there is the further need to defend one's self-image. There is embarrassment, should others learn of this process of vacillating, since one does not want to appear weak-willed or indecisive.

Holly would treat the state of being stirred up and annoyed; *Willow* would heal the internal resentment, while *White Chestnut* would give mental serenity and reduce mental arguments and conversations. White Chestnut would also lessen mental preoccupation, and *Scleranthus* would help with the tendency to vacillate between two options.

As a further step of defiance, people in the Lycopodium clavatum state may also raise themselves above others and condescend against them in an attempt to stay on top, feel special, and not allow the others to pull them down. There also may be impatience with others who may be slower in thought and action.

Putting oneself above the others is treated by *Water Violet,* and the remedy *Impatiens* would reduce irritability and impatience with others.

Lycopodium clavatum persons may also enjoy positions and attitudes of power which can be used as a further defense against possible threats to the self-image. Should power be misused, an imbalance occurs within the self that actually works to augment threatened feelings of inadequacy instead of improving them. True self-respect, as recognized within one's own experience, and true respect granted by others are based on one's kindness of attitude and genuine deference to the others' identity and aspirations rather than on domination.

Vine is the healing remedy for the tendency to misuse power against others.

Should impulses exist to engage in dominating or inappropriate behavior or thought patterns that are not wished for, *Cherry Plum* would help to restore balance.

In case the demands and problems of living reduce enjoyment and ease, while mental preoccupation with problems may separate from free-flowing contact with others, a state of depression and joylessness could arise which is helped by *Mustard.*

Lycopodium clavatum persons also have a bent to joking and humor that may be held in check by *Chestnut Bud,* should it be inappropriate or not in unison with the current situation.

The plant Lycopodium clavatum is a moss with upward-stretching stems carrying spores. At the top, the small stems divide into two fibres which carry the spores. According to the Doctrine of Signatures, moss symbolizes the experience of feeling low, inadequate, or threatened in one's self-image, whereas the upward-stretching stems hint at the urge to grow above, achieve and be recognized. The twofold fibres remind of the vacillation and uncertainty which often grip Lycopodium clavatum persons in their endeavors.

PHYSICAL SYMPTOMS

In an acute case, Lycopodium clavatum patients may have the characteristic tension headaches in temples with the tendency to clamp the jaws together and press down the chin. Sore throats typically develop on the right side and then move to the left. Coughs are worse lying down; they tend to be persistent, and there may be rales. Desire for warm drinks predominates; there may be inability to eat large amounts of food, and there is bloating of the abdomen. One foot may be hot, the other cold. Characteristic time of aggravation of symptoms is from 4 to 8 p.m.

In a chronic Lycopodium clavatum case, the above symptoms may be present in varying degrees of intensity and with intervals. Headaches may be common; emaciation around neck and shoulders can occur; chronic coughs, liver problems, bloating, digestive sensitivity to beans and cabbage, and restlessness may be present. Irritability and fatigue are greatly increased between 4 and 8 p.m., so are the other symptoms present. These chronic tendencies may not only arise from mental/emotional imbalance; they may be enhanced also by fatigue, increased demands of living, malnutrition, or stem from the aftereffects of acute illnesses.

In any major or minor illness, the original physical disposition, linked closely with the type of personality, decides which remedy picture the vital force will choose to express the imbalance in the totality of the person in response to a given acute or chronic stress.

⌘

CONCLUSION

Bach Remedies, by easing the strain, fatigue and overly stressed state of the mind/emotions and body, gives the vital force a chance to rest and organize into a synchronized expression of imbalance, which then can be treated most effectively by homeopathic medicines.

Hahnemann, in his later years, was also aware of the need to clear a chronic case and stimulate the vital force into clarity of expression. He routinely prescribed Sulphur to open the case and repeated this remedy until new symptoms indicative of a more precise remedy emerged. The new remedy was then given at once and the case moved forward.[20] Hahnemann chose Sulphur to activate and clear the chronic miasm psora which he had identified as a major layer of health disturbance commonly experienced by the population. Psora relates to states of impurity throughout the organism, from fears and hesitancy in the mind/emotions to skin affections and intestinal toxemia.

In this context, Bach had felt his nosodes to be of service also. He believed that they successfully removed the miasm psora, in this way clearing the organism of a major basis for chronic disease. The nosodes have also been employed in cases which did not respond to well-chosen homeopathic remedies and needed the additional benefit of the nosodes' cleansing and activating effect. Bach's unceasing efforts for finding medicines derived directly from nature, however, led him to the discovery of the Bach Remedies which replaced the nosodes and greatly surpassed them in cleansing and restoring power of the mind/emotions and body.[21]

The catalytic healing effect, stimulated by the nosodes as well as by the Bach Remedies, appears to root also in their electromagnetic polarity. Both show a negative polarity, whereas potentized homeopathic remedies present with a positive polarity. It had been Bach's goal to replace the original nosodes and their deep-reaching effects, which he believed to be caused by negative polarity, with plants from nature that would be prepared to resonate with a like polarity; and this was secured with Bach's unique method of potentization that relies on the application of heat and forgoes excessive dilution and succussion. Negative polarity appears to release the very seat or root of the disease, even beyond the power of homeopathy.[22]

In my observation, in continuation of the practice to clear and prepare a case for in-depth homeopathic treatment, I have found the Bach Remedies to release and unravel the innate layers of health disturbance in most gentle ways; the remedies work as catalysts, clear and cleanse the organism from deep within, beginning at the root of all trouble, this being the disharmony in the personality. As major layers of health disturbance clear and the defense mechanism is strengthened, increasingly the Bach Remedies alone may assist in creating harmony and overall health.

The most complete state of cure is the gift of health which comes from being in touch with one's inner light and grace, and devoting oneself to the world and its people. This state, although greatly furthered by the remedies, is a personal motivation and dedication, a personal decision for mankind's health.

NOTES

[1] Refer to Trevor M. Cook, *Samuel Hahnemann: The Founder of Homoeopathic Medicine* (Wellingborough, Eng.: Thorsons, 1981), p. 59. To study the principles of homeopathy, refer to Samuel Hahnemann, *Organon of Medicine,* trans. J. Künzli, A. Naudé, and P. Pendleton from 6th German ed. (1921; rpt. London: Victor Gollancz, 1992).

[2] See George Vithoulkas, *The Science of Homeopathy* (New York: Grove Press, 1980), pp. 273-94, for a presentation of Hahnemann's proving of the remedy Arsenicum album. This book is also recommended for further in-depth study of the theoretical and practical aspects of homeopathy.

[3] Harvey Farrington, *Homeopathy and Homeopathic Prescribing* (1955; rpt. New Delhi: B. Jain, 1987), p. 152. This ink could also have been "potentized" and given as a curative remedy, a process called "isopathy," termed and described by Lux in Switzerland in 1833 (refer to seminar by Francis Treuherz, "Materia Medica of the Nosodes," Homeopathic Educational Services, Berkeley, 13-14 Apr. 1991). In isopathy, one uses the same substance that was responsible for the illness and prepares it homeopathically, so as to clear the organism of the crude substance's negative influence. (Explanation of "potentization" follows in next paragraph of text.)

[4] Vithoulkas, *Science of Homeopathy,* pp. 161-68.

[5] The scientific Journal *Nature* published a report of a reaction in waterbase between cells and a certain antibody that continued after the antibody had been diluted and shaken inten-

tionally to a point where all molecular content was removed. These findings support the assumed existence of an innate carrier or essence that exists within the molecular structure and can be released from it without losing its effectiveness, even though the carrier is undetectable at that point. For reference, see: E. Davenas et al., "Human Basophil Degranulation Triggered by Very Dilute Antiserum against IgE," *Nature*, 333 (1988), 816-18.

The author has noted the oscillating nucleus of the hydrogen atom as being capable, due to the succussion, of absorbing and transferring the unique resonant frequency pertaining to the medicinal substance, thus storing this frequency even after Avogadro's number has been superseded. Refer to: Cornelia Richardson-Boedler, "A Potential Antidote for the Necrotic and Systemic Effects Caused by the Brown Recluse Spider (Loxosceles Reclusa): A Homeopathic Preparation from the Spider," *Journal of the American Institute of Homeopathy*, 91 (1998), 277-83.

The curative effectiveness of homeopathic remedies themselves has been tested, as seen in: J. Kleijnen, P. Knipschild, and G. ter Riet, "Clinical Trials of Homoeopathy," *British Medical Journal*, 302 (1991), 316-23.

[6] Refer to James Tyler Kent, "Lecture VIII: On Simple Substance," in *Lectures on Homoeopathic Philosophy* (1900; rpt. Berkeley: North Atlantic Books, 1979), pp. 67-76.

[7] One common repertory used in the United States is Kent's repertory: James Tyler Kent, *Repertory of the Homoeopathic Materia Medica*, 6th ed. (1957; rpt. New Delhi: B. Jain, 1991). Examples of important standard textbooks for materia medica are: James Tyler Kent, *Lectures on Homoeopathic Materia Medica* (1904; rpt. New Delhi: B. Jain, 1984); and William Boericke,

Pocket Manual of Homoeopathic Materia Medica, 9th ed. (1927; rpt. Santa Rosa, Calif.: Boericke & Tafel, n.d.).

[8] The examination of "essences" of states of illness, as identified by homeopathy, was further developed by George Vithoulkas. In his book *The Essence of Materia Medica,* 2nd ed. (New Delhi: B. Jain, 1990), he shows how the psychological essence penetrates to the physical plane and determines the expression of symptoms.

[9] Bach's life, his early thoughts, and the discovery and application of the Bach Remedies is best described in the biography by Nora Weeks, *The Medical Discoveries of Edward Bach, Physician* (London: C. W. Daniel, 1940).

[10] Refer to Treuherz "Materia Medica of the Nosodes" for a good analysis of the Bach Nosodes. Further details can be found in: John Paterson, "The Bowel Nosodes," *British Homoeopathic Journal,* 40 (1950), 153-63; and Elizabeth Paterson, "A Survey of the Nosodes," *British Homoeopathic Journal,* 49 (1960), 161-86. The latter article was based on a paper read to the Faculty of Homoeopathy in England on November 5, 1959. The Patersons were instrumental in researching the bowel nosodes and determining their affinity with homeopathic remedies.

[11] Later on, Bach discovered the plant *Scleranthus annuus* as healer for states of changeability and vacillation. This plant appears to have been the direct replacement for the Coli mutabile nosode. By then, however, Bach had abandoned all work on replacing the nosodes with plants and had concentrated on finding healers for various mental/emotional states. (The correlates - plants and nosodes [excepting Morgan] - are concluded).

[12] Weeks, p. 62.

[13] This list of four basic ways of using the remedies leans on Bach's Wallingford lecture, given on September 24, 1936, on his 50th birthday. Refer to: Edward Bach, "Wallingford Lecture," in *Collected Writings of Edward Bach,* ed. Julian Barnard (Hereford, Eng.: Flower Remedy Programme, 1987), p. 7.

[14] Edward Bach, "Some Fundamental Considerations of Disease and Cure," *Homoeopathic World,* 64 (1930), 295-99.

[15] This case, with the application of the Doctrine of Signatures in regard to the healing substance, was developed thoroughly in the following article: Cornelia Richardson-Boedler, "Uranium Nitricum: New Pointers to the Remedy," *Homoeopathy International,* 8, No. 2 (1994), 21-23.

[16] Weeks, "Results Obtained by the Thirty-Eight Herbal Remedies," pp. 124-33.

[17] Edward Bach, *The Twelve Healers and Other Remedies* (London: C. W. Daniel, 1936). All quotations by Bach in regard to the indications for each remedy are taken from this book and are annotated as *(Twelve Healers)* at the end of each quotation.

[18] For beautiful photographs, biological descriptions of plants and their natural habitat, plus some reference to the plants' expressive potential, I recommend this book: Julian and Martine Barnard, *The Healing Herbs of Edward Bach* (Hereford, Eng.: Bach Educational Programme, 1988).

[19] Video games are fun and usually educational; they may only lead to over stimulation and irritability in one's reactions if engaged in to excess. This can happen with most forms of entertainment.

[20] Close study of Hahnemann's latest case books revealed the use of Sulphur in chronic case management, as described by Rima Handley, "Classical

Hahnemannian Homoeopathy or What Hahnemann Really Did: Preliminary Observations," *The Homoeopath,* 7 (1988), 106-14.

[21] The clearing and activating use of the nosodes in homeopathic treatment has been described. Refer to: John Paterson, pp. 153-63; Edward C. Whitmont, "The Intestinal Nosodes," in *Psyche and Substance: Essays on Homeopathy in the Light of Jungian Psychology* (Berkeley: North Atlantic Books, 1991) pp. 226-29. (In recent times, homeopathic drainage remedies, prescribed to drain and cleanse specific organs, have also been postulated to clarify the remedy picture; refer to Trevor M. Cook, "Diploma Homoeopathic Course" [Staines, Eng.: British Institute of Homoeopathy, 1988].)

[22] For references, see: Weeks, p. 37; Edward Bach, "The Rediscovery of Psora," *British Homoeopathic Journal,* 19 (1929), 29-50.

This distinction between the vibrational healing pattern of homeopathic medicines ("positive polarity") versus that of Bach Flower Remedies and of the original Bach Bowel Nosodes ("negative polarity") was not addressed in the author's dissertation; hence, the paragraph ending with the note 22 was added postscript. One may view the complementary method of using homeopathy and Bach Flower Therapy combined, as well as the catalytic method of eliciting layers and miasms via Bach Remedies, on this background of polarity; as it explains why each method's contribution is unique and does not interfere, unless in a cooperative way, in the workings of the other. A further exploration of this topic can be found in Lesson 1 of the course: Cornelia Richardson-Boedler, "Bach Flower Practitioner Course" (Staines, Eng.: British Institute of Homoeopathy, 1997).

BIBLIOGRAPHY

Bach, Edward. "Some Fundamental Considerations of Disease and Cure." *Homoeopathic World,* 64 (1930), 266-68, 295-99, 327-31; 65 (1931), 13-17.

—————. "The Rediscovery of Psora." *British Homoeopathic Journal,* 19 (1929), 29-50.

—————. *The Twelve Healers and Other Remedies.* London: C. W. Daniel,1936.

Barnard, Julian, ed. *Collected Writings of Edward Bach.* Hereford, Eng.: Flower Remedy Programme, 1987.

Barnard, Julian and Martine. *The Healing Herbs of Edward Bach.* Hereford, Eng.: Bach Educational Programme, 1988.

Boericke, William. *Pocket Manual of Homoeopathic Materia Medica.* 9th ed. 1927; rpt. Santa Rosa, Calif.: Boericke & Tafel, n.d.

Cook, Trevor M. *Samuel Hahnemann: The Founder of Homoeopathic Medicine.* Wellingborough, Eng.: Thorsons, 1981.

Davenas, E., et al. "Human Basophil Degranulation Triggered by Very Dilute Antiserum against IgE." *Nature,* 333 (1988), 816-18.

Farrington, Harvey. *Homeopathy and Homeopathic Prescribing.* 1955; rpt. New Delhi: B. Jain, 1987.

Hahnemann, Samuel. *Organon of Medicine.* Trans. J. Künzli, A. Naudé, and P. Pendleton from 6th German ed. 1921; rpt. London: Victor Gollancz, 1992.

Handley, Rima. "Classical Hahnemannian Homoeopathy or What Hahnemann Really Did: Preliminary Observations." *The Homoeopath,* 7 (1988), 106-14.

Kent, James Tyler. *Lectures on Homoeopathic Philosophy.* 1900; rpt. Berkeley: North Atlantic Books, 1979.

—————. *Lectures on Homoeopathic Materia Medica.* 1904; rpt. New Delhi: B. Jain, 1984.

—————. *Repertory of the Homoeopathic Materia Medica.* 6th ed. 1957; rpt. New Delhi: B. Jain, 1991.

Kleijnen, J., P. Knipschild, and G. ter Riet. "Clinical Trials of Homoeopathy." *British Medical Journal,* 302 (1991) 316-23.

Paterson, Elizabeth. "A Survey of the Nosodes." *British Homoeopathic Journal,* 49 (1960), 161-86.

Paterson, John. "The Bowel Nosodes." *British Homoeopathic Journal,* 40 (1950), 153-63.

Richardson-Boedler, Cornelia. "A Potential Antidote for the Necrotic and Systemic Effects Caused by the Brown Recluse Spider (Loxosceles Reclusa): A Homeopathic Preparation from the Spider." *Journal of the American Institute of Homeopathy,* 91 (1998), 277-83.

—————. "Uranium Nitricum: New Pointers to the Remedy." *Homoeopathy International,* 8, No. 2 (1994), 21-23.

Vithoulkas, George. *The Essence of Materia Medica.* 2nd ed. New Delhi: B. Jain, 1990.

—————. *The Science of Homoeopathy.* New York: Grove Press, 1980.

Weeks, Nora. *The Medical Discoveries of Edward Bach, Physician.* London: C. W. Daniel, 1940.

Whitmont, Edward C. *Psyche and Substance: Essays on Homeopathy in the Light of Jungian Psychology.* Berkeley: North Atlantic Books, 1991.

SEMINAR

Treuherz, Francis. "Materia Medica of the Nosodes." Homeopathic Educational Services, Berkeley. 13-14 Apr. 1991.

COURSES

Cook, Trevor M. "Diploma Homoeopathic Course." Staines, Eng.: British Institute of Homoeopathy, 1988.

Richardson-Boedler, Cornelia. "Bach Flower Practitioner Course." Staines, Eng.: British Institute of Homoeopathy, 1997.

COMPUTER SOFTWARE

Richardson-Boedler, Cornelia. *The Richardson-Boedler Bach Repertory.* San Rafael, Calif.: Kent Homeopathic Associates, 1993.

⌘

BOOK TWO

THE PSYCHOLOGICAL/CONSTITUTIONAL ESSENCES OF THE BACH FLOWER REMEDIES

*Includes the Remedies Use in Mental and
Psychosomatic Illness with Descriptions of Plants
in Light of the Doctrine of Signatures.
Contains a Bach Remedy Repertory*

BOOK TWO

THE PSYCHOLOGICAL/CONSTITUTIONAL ESSENCES OF THE BACH FLOWER REMEDIES

INTRODUCTION

*T*his book presents thirty-eight psychological dynamics, each one of them healed by a specific Bach
Remedy, and it offers a unique Bach Remedy rep-
ertory.[1] The description and differentiation of those thirty-eight
dynamics alone, fundamental to humanity, makes this text an
insightful tool in the endeavor to understand the human personality, enhancing the careful descriptions of psychology and
psychiatry.

In his searches to unravel the intricate relationship between
mind/emotions and body, physician Edward Bach concluded
that sickness derived primarily from mental/emotional imbalances was cured best if these causative imbalances could be
healed. He was in unison with psychosomatic medicine but went
beyond in discovering specific natural medicines, grouped with
the homeopathic healers, that were to heal the states of mental/
emotional imbalances he had observed in his patients and
throughout the population. By working through the mind/emo-
tions, these remedies were found to also affect the body in exactly those areas of disturbance where the disharmonious mind/
emotions had been expressed. Yet, in view of the complexity
and individual expression of the human being, Bach did not

classify those specific sites, except for giving a few general guidelines. Over the decades, psychosomatic medicine has studied those physical correlations and come up with worthy insights and beneficial therapeutic approaches.

Bach Remedies can be applied to all health-related fields. They have a wide range of action, addressing mild tendencies to imbalance to severe states of mental illness. Specifically in this text, the remedies are applied to aid in the healing of inner psychological dynamics, in states of mental illness, and in psychosomatic illness. The key to cure is the insightful prescriber or self-prescriber who recognizes the crucial individual imbalances in the personality and begins the true process of cure.

Botanical descriptions of plants, reflecting their essence, their individual dynamic of growth, form and behavior, show parallels to the human psychological dynamics in a unique correlation between man and nature. Several disciplines merge, homeopathy, psychology, psychiatry, psychosomatic medicine and botany, to come to a synchronized approach to the healing of the human being.

1

SEVEN MODES OF CONSCIOUSNESS –
SEVEN GROUPS OF BACH REMEDIES

The English physician Edward Bach (1886-1936) observed that mind and emotions played an important role in the formation and cure of physical disease, and he devoted his life to developing gentle homeopathic medicines which were to heal the mental/emotional imbalances and subsequently benefit the body as well.

His remedies were derived from the plants of nature, from flowers, bushes and trees, as well as from one well in Britain known to carry healing properties. All remedies were thoroughly tested on himself and others and found to heal deeply without any harmful effects. The remedies work by stimulating through subtle homeopathic vibrations the innate source of wholeness and the positive potential in the mind/emotions, thus to restore equilibrium in those areas of imbalance within the personality.

Bach's work originated in close observation of people, their behavior and their internal psychological dynamics; subsequently, he would research outdoors and in the laboratory those special plants he deemed to carry healing potential specific to the mental/emotional imbalances he had identified. This process unfolded during several years of concentrated work, until he had detected thirty-eight different mental/emotional states and their respective healing remedies.[2]

The prescriber's task is to distinguish the patient's exact mental/ emotional imbalances according to Bach's classification and indications. A thorough interview will usually reveal the necessary remedies, or simply observation will guide to the correct choice. Bach organized the remedies into seven groups according to their indication, and to provide easier reference and distinction.

On examining Bach's seven groups of Bach Remedies, one realizes seven different ways of disharmonious mental/emotional behavior in relation to the world. Within the framework of consciousness imbalances, these ways can be considered basic modes of consciousness or basic existential expressions of living in and relating to the world and its people. Each group of Bach Remedies shows several remedies which treat the nuances and different facets within one mode of consciousness. The remedies aim at restoring the one healthy mode of consciousness which consists of wholehearted devotion to the world and its people, while simultaneously achieving a sound self-relatedness and preventing physical illness which may derive from long-persisted-in consciousness imbalances.

In the group of *For Those Who Have Fear,* consciousness retreats from the world in dread and does not want to go forward. It is overly impacted on by adverse forces from outside and from within the self and recoils. The different facets within this mode are represented by five remedies:

Rock Rose treats states of intense fear, terror and heightened nervousness.

Mimulus is for everyday fears of concrete objects, persons or circumstances.

Cherry Plum treats states of tension with the intense fear of losing control and engaging in unwanted dreaded acts or thoughts.

Aspen heals states of foreboding and vague, haunting fears for which no explanation can be given.

Red Chestnut is indicated in fear for the welfare of others.

The group of *For Those Who Suffer Uncertainty* shows a mode of consciousness not certain in its expression towards the world. There is wavering and lack of steadfastness of inner will and diminished decisive force, all of which stifle wholehearted active engagement in life. The six different facets of this mode of consciousness are healed by the following Bach Remedies:

Cerato heals inner uncertainty, lack of self-assurance and dependence on the advice of others.

Scleranthus is for the tendency to vacillate between options and suffer delay in decision-making.

Gentian treats discouragement and reluctance to get involved in the world.

Gorse deals with hopelessness and retreat from active engagement in the world.

Hornbeam heals mental fatigue, listlessness and procrastination in face of the duties of the world.

Wild Oat addresses a lack of motivation and incentive plus uncertainty in regard to choosing a definite career path.

The third group, titled *Not Sufficient Interest in Present Circumstances,* represents a mode of consciousness not drawn to the world, since internal dynamics divert from the beauty of the present moment. The present does not hold a strong enough appeal to engage the mind fully. Seven different remedies treat the facets of this mode of consciousness.

Clematis treats daydreaming and longing for future happiness, based on the belief that the present circumstances cannot provide such fulfillment.

Honeysuckle is for those who live in the rich memories of the past, believing that such happiness can never be repeated again in the present or future.

Wild Rose helps those withdrawn in apathy and resignation from unfavorable present circumstances.

Olive is for those too exhausted to attend to their daily business.

White Chestnut treats states of mental preoccupation and intense worry which remove from concentrated involvement in the present.

Mustard heals withdrawal into depression and gloominess.

Chestnut Bud deals with states of inattentiveness and lack of restful concentration on the present moment.

The fourth group of Bach Remedies addresses states of *Loneliness.* Inner loneliness arises from a self-centered attitude towards life. While being in this mode of consciousness, one is removed from heartfelt engagement with others for personally chosen reasons. Three remedies heal the different facets within this state.

Water Violet is for those who remove themselves in proud and reserved dignity.

Impatiens heals the tendency to force one's own fast pace of work or recreation onto others and not tuning into their natures.

Heather helps the state of being overly concerned with one's personal problems and not wanting to talk of anything else.

Oversensitive to Influences and Ideas forms the fifth of Bach's groups. This mode of consciousness is marked by a heightened sensitivity to impacts from outside. Four remedies address the different facets of this state.

Agrimony heals oversensitivity to turmoil, strife and quarrel; one suffers from disruptions in peace and tries to restore it.

Centaury helps those seeking to please and serve others, and in so doing undermine their strength. They are overly sensitive to the demands and needs of others.

Walnut treats heightened mental sensitivity to impressions from outside; one is unstable and too easily influenced in one's inner self.

Holly heals those overly distressed and easily made upset and irritated by vexing and annoying circumstances.

The sixth group of Bach Remedies or mode of consciousness is that of *For Despondency or Despair* when one's consciousness is weighed down and unable to rise above despairing conditions. In this state, one cannot give to life fully, since inner lightness and freedom from cares are absent. There are eight different facets within this mode of consciousness, healed by the following remedies:

Larch is for those suffering from low self-esteem and feeling despondent and hampered in their approach to life.

Pine brings relief from the states of guilt and self-reproach which may weigh heavily upon one's consciousness.

Elm treats states of being overwhelmed and burdened by tremendous tasks.

Sweet Chestnut heals unbearable anguish and despair with concurrent faithlessness and a sense of meaninglessness of life.

Star of Bethlehem addresses the burden of grief plus trauma and shock, and their aftereffects.

Willow is for those not favored by fate or mistreated by others and developing despair, bitterness and resentment.

Oak treats states of stoic perseverance in face of hardship and despair.

Crab Apple helps those unable to rise above shameful aspects of the self and despairing over them.

The seventh mode of consciousness is represented by group seven, titled *Overcare for Welfare of Others*. In this state, consciousness is overbearing in its expression, attempting to shape the world and its people according to its own ideas. Five different facets of this mode are healed by the following remedies:

Chicory heals an overly fussy and self-centered approach to caring for others and being cared for by others if unwell, accompanied by the need to bind others closely to oneself.

Vervain treats states of overenthusiasm for ideas, accompanied by the exaggerated attempt to convert others to one's view.

Vine is for those who consider themselves leaders and control others against their wishes.

Beech heals states of undue criticism and intolerance, as one judges others according to one's own ideals and standards.

Rock Water helps those overly motivated to inspire others with their personal path of self-mastery.

From his observation of people, Bach determined twelve major states or nuances of these modes of consciousness which represent important tendencies within the personality, whereas the remaining twenty-six are less entrenched states of consciousness and may arise more in response to concrete circumstances of life. Bach actually discovered these twelve major states before the remaining twenty-six, since they were more easily detectable and more commonly found throughout the population. These major states or types of personality imbalances, together with their respective healing remedies or type remedies, are:

For Those Who Have Fear:

Fear and shyness (Mimulus); heightened nervousness and fragile sensitivity, with easily stimulated fear and panic (Rock Rose).

For Those Who Suffer Uncertainty:

Self-distrust (Cerato); indecision (Scleranthus); doubt or discouragement (Gentian).

Not Sufficient Interest in Present Circumstances:

Indifference or boredom (Clematis).

Loneliness:

Impatience (Impatiens); pride or aloofness (Water Violet).

Oversensitive to Influences and Ideas:

Sensitivity to disquiet, mental torture or worry (Agrimony); being a too willing servitor, with weakness (Centaury).

Overcare for Welfare of Others:

Overconcern for the welfare of others, with fussiness (Chicory); with overenthusiasm (Vervain).

All modes of consciousness are represented by one, two or even three type remedies, except for the group of *For Despondency or Despair.* The remedies belonging to this group deal more with responses to hardship and insurmountable conditions rather than reflect inherent traits of personality imbalance. The special type remedies, however, are also prescribed in acute or chronic states elicited by special life circumstances and do not necessarily have to be identified as imbalances in character or personality. Vice versa, the remaining twenty-six remedies can accomplish a deep-reaching change within the personality structure. All remedies are equally important, have a broad range of application and a unique psychological essence of depth. For this reason, the type remedies, while worthy of special consideration, will not be especially highlighted in the following text.

⌘

2

THE METHOD OF PRESENTING THE ESSENCES

T his presentation by modes of consciousness serves as an introductory guideline and gives an over view to the Bach Remedies' healing system. The presentation of the essences themselves is given in alphabetical order for easy reference. Each remedy description is divided into six sections, these being MIND, EMOTIONS, PHYSICAL TENDENCIES, DOCTRINE OF SIGNATURES, METHOD OF PREPARATION and GOAL OF THERAPY.

Under MIND, each remedy is examined in its mental characteristics, these being the angles of perceiving and understanding the world, and these being the mental dynamics propelled by the psychological imbalance. Mental clarity, power of concentration, and reasoning and discerning powers fall under this rubric. The use of Bach Remedies in major forms of mental illness will be described, following the criteria in the *Diagnostic and Statistical Manual of Mental Disorders* (DSM). These disorders are listed under mind yet have emotional aspects also, those being reflected in the emotional indications of the specific Bach

Remedy. Bach Remedies do not necessarily claim to heal all forms of mental illness, yet, if applied correctly, can lead to healing of the underlying psychological dynamic. In lighter cases, the Bach Remedies alone can address the symptoms, while they are recommended as supporting treatment in more severe cases.

The EMOTIONS of the imbalance itself are examined plus those emotional tendencies deriving from and accompanying the imbalance. The mental dynamics of perceiving the world are often shaped by the emotions which portray the movement of the psyche, what motivates and repels. They represent the longings of the heart, the need to give and receive love, and the disappointments, frustrations and disillusionment. Both, the mind and emotions constitute the *essence,* the innate psychological dynamic of the remedy picture, which is also reflected in the plant's essence, in view of the Doctrine of Signatures.

The PHYSICAL TENDENCIES to imbalance and sickness derive secondarily from the imbalances in the mind/emotions and complete the overall picture of the psychophysical or constitutional state of imbalance. Certain areas in the body are known to express certain emotions, such as the stomach and intestines may suffer during fear and intense worry. Each Bach Remedy has an amazing healing potential on the physical plane. Yet, since the remedies are indicated on the mind/emotions, it is hard to predict in some cases what areas of the body or what kind of sicknesses are best affected by a certain Flower Remedy. For some Bach Remedies, more than for others, there are some general guidelines, and my personal observations and conclusions plus additional insights on mind/body relationships gained in psychosomatic medicine[3] will be given.

Each psychosomatic disease will be listed with the one specific Bach Remedy which most reflects the underlying dynamic of the disease. One, two or three supporting remedies may be necessary in a given case to address additional facets within the mental/emotional dynamic. Bach Remedies may heal or greatly alleviate psychosomatic illness but do not claim to do so in each case. Lighter cases would benefit from the single use of the remedies, while more physically ingrained cases warrant additional treatment approaches. The major psychosomatic diseases will be reflected in the text.

Except for the sudden precipitation of psychosomatic illness due to shock, only the long-standing, chronic mental/emotional imbalances with gradually developing physical concomitant symptoms lead to psychosomatic illness in predisposed individuals. In empirical studies and seen from an existential/phenomenological viewpoint, those mental/emotional states most commonly demonstrated in certain psychosomatic diseases are then recognized as being linked with the disease. This does not mean that certain Bach Remedies are automatically linked with certain diseases; and, although guidelines can be given, each case needs to be assessed individually from a fresh point of view.

The DOCTRINE OF SIGNATURES refers to an historic way of discovering and interpreting medicinal plants. It was understood, and this is equally valid today, that plants of healing express in their physical, behavioral and habitual properties the human sickness or imbalance and also often point to the plant's positive healing quality. In the case of the Bach Remedies, nature's signature reflects the essence or innate psychological indications of each remedy. For example, the plant Impatiens, which is the healer for impatience and irritability, is marked by an explosive scattering of seeds, reminding of sudden outbursts of temper and irritability.

The METHOD OF PREPARATION shortly describes how to prepare each plant's healing medicine. The main differentiation lies in the heating method, either through sunlight or through boiling, and in the parts of the plants which need to be used. The following chapter explains the general preparations and procedures necessary for making one's own remedy.

Under GOAL OF THERAPY, a succinct summary is given of the main goals and aspirations of the healing process. These can also be given to the patient as inspiring guidelines and positive affirmations to open the mind to the far-reaching possibilities of healing. Bach suggested to his patients, who often felt overwhelmed by the strength of their mental/emotional imbalances, to strive for the opposing virtue or healthy state and not battle against the wrong or painful state within. This focuses the mind on the goal and moves it along the road of transformation more powerfully. While having one's goals and aspirations in mind, the wholehearted concentration and devotion to the world and its people, with simultaneous leaving behind of worry, self-centered attitudes, or self-preoccupation, is the best way to reach a healthy mode of consciousness. This positive attitude, together with the healing power of the remedies, overcomes the hindrances between one's consciousness and the world, as described above in the seven modes of consciousness.

HOW TO MAKE YOUR OWN REMEDY

You can easily grow your favorite flowers, bushes or trees in your garden or patio. If not readily available, order the special plants through your nursery, either in the form of seeds or as young plants. When in full bloom on a sunny day, pick the flowers or flowering sprigs and get ready to prepare your own remedy.

For the sun method, fill a glass bowl with clear spring water and place the blooms on top of the water. Leave the bowl in bright sunshine for several hours until the petals show signs of fading. This can last from two to seven hours depending on the strength of the petals. Remove the flowers or strain the water imbued with healing power and add an equal amount of brandy to the water. Store this mixture as mother tincture.

To complete the boiling method, pick the flowers or flowering sprigs on a sunny day and boil for half an hour. Strain the water and add an equal amount of brandy and store as mother tincture.

From the tincture bottle, take two drops and fill into a 1 ounce (30 ml) dropper bottle filled with brandy to form the stock bottle. From this stock bottle, take again two drops and add to a 1 ounce dropper bottle filled with spring water. Add 1 teaspoon of brandy or vinegar to preserve the remedy. Label this bottle, as well as the others, with the remedy's name and add the date of preparation. From this dispensing bottle, take four drops four times a day, either in a teaspoon or added to a glass of water, juice, or any other mild drink.

The remedies can be taken singularly or in groups of two, three or four. Six at once is the official limit, but usually it is not necessary to send so many healing impulses at once. Add two drops from each chosen stock bottle to the 1 ounce dispensing bottle and shake gently. During warm times of the year, you may want to keep the bottle in refrigerator to preserve maximum freshness.

The remedies work in chronic and acute cases. As soon as healing is achieved and one senses that the remedies are no longer necessary, they should be discontinued. In some cases, it is advisable to continue treatment to safeguard the progress made and prevent a relapse from occurring.

In learning to prescribe for oneself or others, one always gains in awareness and understanding of human, psychological dynamics in general. A truly differentiated and in-depth understanding of the human psyche is offered in the Bach Remedies' healing system, which is ready to reveal its wisdom to all in search of deepened and most gentle cure.

4

THE BACH REMEDY ESSENCES

- Agrimony (Agrimonia eupatoria)
- Aspen (Populus tremula)
- Beech (Fagus sylvatica)
- Centaury (Centaurium umbellatum)
- Cerato (Ceratostigma willmottiana)
- Cherry Plum (Prunus cerasifera)
- Chestnut Bud (Aesculus hippocastanum)
- Chicory (Cichorium intybus)
- Clematis (Clematis vitalba)
- Crab Apple (Malus sylvestris/pumila)
- Elm (Ulmus procera)
- Gentian (Gentiana amarella)
- Gorse (Ulex europaeus)
- Heather (Calluna vulgaris)
- Holly (Ilex aquifolium)
- Honeysuckle (Lonicera caprifolium)
- Hornbeam (Carpinus betulus)
- Impatiens (Impatiens glandulifera)
- Larch (Larix decidua)
- Mimulus (Mimulus guttatus)
- Mustard (Sinapis arvensis)
- Oak (Quercus robur)
- Olive (Olea europaea)
- Pine (Pinus sylvestris)
- Red Chestnut (Aesculus carnea)
- Rock Rose (Helianthemum nummularium)
- Rock Water (Aqua petra)
- Scleranthus (Scleranthus annuus)
- Star of Bethlehem (Ornithogalum umbellatum)
- Sweet Chestnut (Castanea sativa)
- Vervain (Verbena officinalis)
- Vine (Vitis vinifera)
- Walnut (Juglans regia)
- Water Violet (Hottonia palustris)
- White Chestnut (Aesculus hippocastanum)
- Wild Oat (Bromus ramosus)
- Wild Rose (Rosa canina)
- Willow (Salix vitellina)
- Rescue Remedy

AGRIMONY (AGRIMONIA EUPATORIA)

Agrimony, along with Centaury, Walnut and Holly, belongs to the group of *Oversensitive to Influences and Ideas,* as classified by Bach. These four remedies help those who are unduly distressed or overly influenced by disturbing factors or powerful impressions in their environment. Specifically, Agrimony treats a heightened sensitivity to the environment that is caused by the tendency to ignore worries or hide them within.

MIND: The mind is unsettled and restless, prone to be distracted. There is avoidance instead of facing disturbing thoughts or dealing with problems. The tendency exists to glide over difficulties, with an attempt to stay cheerful, find diversion, or reach for stimulants (alcoholism and other forms of drug abuse are frequent). Since inner disharmony is not attended to with insight and care, and kept in vicarious balance, outside disturbances of peace are hardly tolerated and threaten to disrupt the inner stability, however tentative.

Inner cares and worries, instead of leaving when not attended to, as is the intention, reassert continually and work to undermine mental peace and restful devotion to the present moment. Anxieties build up; restlessness and a sense of dissatisfaction perpetuate inner disquiet.

EMOTIONS: An Agrimony state may develop after or while living through experiences of grief or other forms of disappointment, severity, resentment or guilt which are not being worked through and cannot find healing from deep within. On the surface, the mind works to achieve balance through cheerfulness and diversion, but true release needs deepened attention to unresolved conflicts or trauma.

There often is a deep sense of longing for fulfillment or adventure, for love and personal growth. Inner restlessness, a sense of boredom in face of present circumstances and unfulfilled needs propel forward. This urge may be without a concrete, feasible or wholesome structure and often finds some relief in drugs, entertainment or other forms of diversion.

Love of peace and longing for harmony are dominant emotional traits. Quarrels distress and bring unhappiness; there is an effort to restore peace, among people, with one's friends or family, within oneself. Often, people in need of Agrimony show the desire to not let others down and burden them with their personal problems, instead they intend to spread cheer and uplift others. In this way, their own emotional needs may not be attended to and continue to disrupt inner peace. Typically in the Agrimony state, one tends to not acknowledge and express strong emotions which could bring disharmony or strife to oneself or others. Resentment and antagonism nonetheless build up within and may find release unexpectedly in spiteful remarks or in masked aggressive behavior.

PHYSICAL TENDENCIES: There is restlessness in mind and body, internal disquiet, nervousness and the urge to hurry. Anxieties and worries stifle physical ease and well-being. Craving for stimulants is a frequent indication. Liver disturbances may exist. (Traditionally, Agrimony has been used as an herbal remedy for liver troubles.)

Since internal imbalances are often not expressed on the surface, the body may convey internal messages through pain, illness or physical discomfort. Suppression, overcompliance and denial of emotions has been seen as a major contributing factor in psychosomatic illness, even though suppression in some cases is truly worthwhile, coming from ethical standards and benefiting social and individual peace.

Agrimony will greatly ease pain in a patient who is smiling and cheering others despite pain and internal torture.

DOCTRINE OF SIGNATURES: The Agrimony plant grows upward in a single spike resembling a steeple and demonstrating peace and awe, these being qualities this plant instills. "Church Steeples" actually is one of the colloquial names for this plant. This may convey the message of bringing one's worries onto God, of releasing them to the heavens.

Five-petalled yellow flowers grow directly on the stalk and bloom progressively toward the top, leaving below the faded blossoms. These change into rough burs which are caught by passers-by and adhere to their clothes. This progression of blooming points at the cheerfulness and positive attitude on top, while "burs" and troubles remain unresolved underneath. Although one wants to avoid facing worries, they catch up with oneself and adhere wherever one goes. The burs' vicinity to the stem symbolizes the incessant pressure and closeness of worries and minor anxieties. Interpreted positively, one could see the upper blossoms as healing or radiating wholeness over troubling "burs" and disquiet.

The plant has deep roots with tentacles suggesting to "dig deep" to come to the bottom of internal imbalances, instead of staying on the surface of things and ignoring the messages from deep within. It prefers to grow on mild, chalky grounds, parallel to a person's need for peaceful and mild surroundings, and avoids acid grounds, hinting at the typical Agrimony intolerance for acridity and strife.

METHOD OF PREPARATION: The flowering stalks are floated onto a bowl of water and left in the sun for several hours. The water imbued with healing power is strained and used as medicine.

GOAL OF THERAPY: To free the mind of disquiet and worry and allow for enjoyment and full appreciation of the present moment and its treasures. To yield restless need and desire for adventure to feelings of peaceful happiness. To unify the internal will and fully integrate troubling and unresolved content into consciousness.

ASPEN (POPULUS TREMULA)

The remedy Aspen belongs to the group of *For Those Who Have Fear,* as determined by Bach. The other fear remedies are Rock Rose, Mimulus, Cherry Plum and Red Chestnut. The specific indications for Aspen point to vague, hovering fears and forebodings.

MIND: In the Aspen state, the mind is overly receptive and too easily impressed with the great "unknown," the dark and sinister side of life. The balancing and protecting functions of reason and faith lose their hold, and primordial fears and threatening dark forces of doom may penetrate to the depth of one's being.

There is preoccupation with delusions, superstitions, omens, fateful encounters, prophesies and ghost stories. Belief in higher powers exists, yet these are not seen as protective but as uncanny and dangerous. Some people develop personal rituals to establish a sense of protection; still, there may be the continued lure of the unknown, evoking a mixed response of sensationalism and fear.

Fears usually do not have a concrete content; they are not based on the world of facts and science. Sensations of foreboding are vague and may be solely imaginary; some people, however, are truly intuitive and may accurately sense future disasters or present threats, this being a talent of perception which may burden them and bring eerie feelings and fear. Intuitive, spiritual or psychic paths of personal development may lead people into the Aspen state.

Aspen is indicated in states of fearful delusions and paranoia when fears are based on imaginary content with haunting features. Aspen also helps to protect the boundaries of consciousness when disturbed by haunting impact from outside or from within the psyche (cf. Walnut). In panic disorders, when no apparent reason can be given for the attacks, Aspen can be of service (cf. Cherry Plum, Rock Rose).

EMOTIONS: Eerie sentiments are experienced with great dread in extreme cases, while the anxiety is more hovering in less intense cases. Emotions may be ambiguous; there is recoiling in face of foreboding and darkness with a simultaneous sensation of fascination and lure. Underneath these impressions lies the longing for light, safety and grace.

Oftentimes, as a person decides to enter the world of service and goodness, especially in terms of tuning into others and their needs, an Aspen state may develop. The inner life of despair, loss, grief and the reality of death may open up in a new dimension of depth and overwhelm and frighten the service-oriented explorer, as he grows in compassion and understanding. The remedy Aspen helps to answer the longing for mercy and shelter; it gives protection and fortifies the "trembling heart" in patient and helper alike.

PHYSICAL TENDENCIES: Anxiety attacks marked by the typical vague Aspen fear, episodes of trembling, sleeping disorders and insomnia due to nightmares of an eerie, haunting kind can be helped by this remedy. In some cases, Aspen can greatly benefit those unable to fall asleep due to their fears of letting go, of not knowing what awaits them in the land of sleep and dreams, and this same dynamic is also helped in someone envisioning death with foreboding and anxious disquiet in mind and body.

An Aspen patient can show symptoms of mental/emotional withdrawal and, under extreme circumstances, become dejected or haunted in appearance.

DOCTRINE OF SIGNATURES: The Aspen tree is known to tremble and quiver even in a light breeze, reminding of a fearful, foreboding state. This receptivity to wind is caused not only by the rounded and easily swayed shape of the leaf but also by the flattened stalks of the leaves which vibrate and "flutter" the leave when stirred by breezes.

Pale-green leaves, a silvery-gray smooth trunk with a green sheen, predominantly dark-gray catkins speak of a ghostly or eerie quality. The tree grows best in sandy or even poor soil, adapts well to high altitudes, and is frequently found in damp woodland, reminding of haunted or ghost-stirred places. It is considered a pioneer species, growing readily after fire and logging and on abandoned fields. Its also blooms earlier in the year than most trees, as early as cold February, symbolizing the healing mind in search of new life which grows out of cold and abandoned territory, disaster and alienation. The outgrowing fuzzy catkins portray a sense of warmth and fertility in the midst of adversity, while their dark-gray color still blends in with gloom and shadows.

On a sunny day, the leaves swirl with gold and lightness, reminding of grace and playfulness.

The Aspen tree with its foliage, bark and buds is unusually attractive to all kinds of wildlife, providing nourishment throughout all seasons. This shows the Aspen state of being readily impacted on by forces beyond one's control. And yet, the healing attitude is implied also: As the tree stands calmly, one also thinks of openness, trust, ability to share and give, and fearlessness in face of nature's destructive forces. Nourishment and sustenance growing out of the tree speak of its healing quality.

METHOD OF PREPARATION: Small twigs with leaf buds and clusters of flowers, which are the catkins, are boiled for half an hour. Both, the male catkins, being gray with tinges of red anthers or yellow pollen, and the smaller gray female catkins are selected. Subsequently, the water is strained and used as medicine.

GOAL OF THERAPY: To heal fear and instill a sense of protection, a growing above preoccupation with the invisible world. To foster faith in the loving care of a friendly universe. To strengthen reasonable insight and being centered in one's tangible reality.

BEECH (FAGUS SYLVATICA)

Together with the remedies of Rock Water, Vine, Vervain and Chicory, this remedy belongs to Bach's group of *Overcare for Welfare of Others*. These five remedies deal with attitudes of control and overcare toward others. Specifically, Beech treats the tendency to criticism and intolerance.

MIND: In the Beech state, the mind raises itself above others with the self-appointed right to assume critical judgment on another person's expression of life. It is a state of arrogance, an attempt to impress upon others one's own standards of assessment considered special or perfect. Faultfinding, criticism and intolerance are predominant traits.

Judging others creates superiority, and those criticized are held low, condescended against. Oftentimes, one actually does not want them to measure up to one's own perfect style so that one may continue to consider oneself as special. To keep the critical opinion against another, even though the other might have changed, is considered a state of "cognitive dissonance" which is the psychological term for this phenomenon. The mind does not want others to move up in standard, and it gives more personal satisfaction to keep them in their place. Dissonant impressions are rejected, and a "double bind" is created for the criticized person who may try to measure up to the other's standards and finds a no-win situation.

The Beech attitude may also be less condescending, more nagging and dissatisfied.

The mind is narrowed in perception, tolerance and judgment, although one believes oneself to have the right attitude and capacity for assessment. This results in self-deception.

In the treatment of persecutory delusions or paranoid personality disorders, Beech lessens the tendency to overly criticize others and fit them into a specific image with threatening features (cf. Holly, Willow).

EMOTIONS: Although the Beech state may seem arrogant or exasperating, there is often an underlying sadness, a personal loss of a more perfect reality that is mourned. To have personal perfect standards and finding reality wanting implies a loss, a sense of being let down. This may not be in regard to "cognitive dissonance," since the other's lack gives satisfaction, but in regard to life's essentials, including loved ones. For example, the perfect husband was never found or has died; the present one is criticized, with a tinge of buried sadness.

In many cases, if grief was not allowed to be fully experienced or worked through, if there was denial, shock or lack of understanding, there may develop a Beech state. The event or person is criticized or rejected instead of mourned. A Beech block surrounds the heart, sheltering the heart from unbearable or inexplicable sadness.

PHYSICAL TENDENCIES: People in need of Beech may appear haughty and rigid in body posture; in some cases, frequently raised eyebrows can be observed.

DOCTRINE OF SIGNATURES: Beech trees prefer to grow together and do not readily allow other species to enter their domain, due to their thick foliage that filters out sunshine and rain. This suggests the elitist thinking of people in the Beech state. The Beech tree is marked by beauty and perfection; the bark is smooth and elegant, the leaves refined, the flowers delicate. All details are pointing to the high standard of beauty and perfection characteristic of the Beech state.

It is almost impossible to climb up on a Beech tree, due to its smooth bark and the long distance from the ground to the first branches. It is equally hard to "climb up" in another person's opinion, once criticized or condescended against.

METHOD OF PREPARATION: The remedy is prepared by the boiling method. Small twigs and male and female flowers - they are found on the same tree - are boiled for half an hour. The boiled water is strained and used as medicine.

GOAL OF THERAPY: To open the mind to the realization that there is present and potential beauty in people and surroundings. To give tolerance and loving acceptance. To get in touch with hidden sadness and experiences of loss that have not been released or dealt with.

CENTAURY (CENTAURIUM UMBELLATUM)

The remedy Centaury belongs to Bach's group of *Oversensitive to Influences and Ideas,* along with the remedies of Agrimony, Walnut and Holly. The Centaury sensitivity is described as a heightened serviceability that is marked by the inclination to please and accommodate others.

MIND: In the mental realm, the balance of perception is tilted overly in favor of others. In the Centaury state, the mind is easily impressed with the needs and demands of others, to the point of wishing to do good and be of service. One gives others priority over oneself, seeing their needs first and de-emphasizing one's own.

This attitude is truly enriching for oneself and others, except under certain circumstances. As a person's life unfolds, there comes a moment when a decision of destiny has to be made. Old ties are meant to be loosened or broken at such a point and new commitments envisioned. The Centaury mentality might be so strong, the habit of serving so encompassing, as to impede one's view of fresh horizons leading to deepened self-realization. Feelings of guilt and loyalty may further bind and narrow one's way. Hidden talents may not be furthered; life may seem more as drudgery than adventure.

The other mistake the service-oriented person may make is to overlook growing personal weakness and exhaustion. As needs of others seem predominant, one's own assume less importance, and one's health and strength may be undermined slowly. Change of perception is important at such a point, shifting from the overemphasis on the value of others to one's own value as a person with needs and wishes, from unceasing helpfulness to still reserve, recreating one's strength.

In mental illness, if excessive submission and attempts to please others are part of the underlying dynamic, Centaury is of service, as in dependent personality disorder (cf. Cerato).

EMOTIONS: In the Centaury state, emotional involvement and relationship issues may be strong.

Serving others may be a refuge for some, a binding up of one's identity with a positive attitude, a way to build self-esteem and find approval by others. Usually, however, Centaury people feel true love and sympathy for others which motivates them to be helpful and kind. They find joy in service and often do not understand why others are not equally giving and unassuming.

If give and take is unequal between two people, however, there may easily develop the attitude of servant and master, one humbling himself, the other augmenting himself. From this may grow resentment or frustration in the helpful person as opposed to insensitivity and neglect in the demanding person.

Joy of service may change into duty over time, as parts of the personality become too enmeshed with the needs of others and personal creativity and satisfaction are hampered.

The helpful person may also lack courage to make his needs known, or his ethical principles may forbid to entertain resentful impulses and assert over the needs of others.

There may be sadness within, due to unfulfilled potential or unanswered needs. There may also be disappointment in people and an inner sense that one has not been recognized for one's output. Yet, the unceasing and reliable satisfaction of service is experienced, healing the soul continually and impeding negative emotions from sinking in.

PHYSICAL TENDENCIES: Weakness in mind/emotions and body, lack of stamina may be apparent; people may not seem fully invigorated or empowered.

Overcompliance and disregard of one's own needs (cf. Oak) may lead to psychosomatic diseases when the body expresses the unvoiced psychological need in symbolic form or simply shows signs of continued engagement in overly demanding service. The psychosomatic diseases of hypertension (cf. Willow), hyperthyroidism (cf. Vervain), insulin-dependent diabetes, soft tissue rheumatism and rheumatoid arthritis (cf. Chicory and Willow for the last two) have been linked with an exaggerated sense of service and suppression of self-centered impulses.[3]

DOCTRINE OF SIGNATURES: The Centaury plant is very delicate; small five-petalled blossoms grow in clusters, found in grass and among the weeds. The plant is unassuming as are service-oriented people, yet beautiful and refined as one looks more closely. It can easily be overlooked or stepped upon, as there may be the tendency to disregard the humble attitude of the servitor.

Alpha Centauri is the star nearest to our earth, just as the positive Centaury quality inspires most brightly.

METHOD OF PREPARATION: Pick the flowers, put them in a bowl of water, and let them sit in the sun for several hours. The water imbued with healing power is strained and used as medicine.

GOAL OF THERAPY: To give strength of self-realization. To recreate energy and stamina. To help free from wrong obligations and stifling commitments, while upholding genuine desire to serve.

CERATO (CERATOSTIGMA WILLMOTTIANA)

The remedy Cerato, along with Scleranthus, Gentian, Gorse, Hornbeam and Wild Oat, belongs to Bach's group of *For Those Who Suffer Uncertainty.* Cerato has the indication of uncertainty of self in regard to formulating judgments and decisions and in regard to personal self-expression.

MIND: In the Cerato state, the mind is lacking the connection to inner wisdom and intuitive guidance. The perceptive power of the mind is not supported by inner certainty and truthful interpretation from deep within. Consequently, there is continued doubting, uncertainty, and lack of personal decisiveness and self-assurance.

Since inner guidance has not been tapped into, persons in the Cerato state rely heavily on the advice of others, often admiring their decisive move through life and feeling less adequate themselves. They are overly impressed with outward shows and trends, people in charge of themselves and the situation, while they feel hampered in regard to their own creative self-expression, often blaming themselves for this uncomfortable lot.

Internal social agony, preoccupation with oneself, hampering self-observation and shyness are common (cf. Mimulus, Larch). In extreme cases, there may be speech problems and other distortions of expression of personality, fixed ideas, irrational anxieties, inappropriate laughing and immature behavior.

Indecisiveness and uncertainty, while hampering one's social and personal expression, may also extend to all concrete situations of life where decisions are called for. There is mistrust in one's capacity to judge correctly and make the appropriate decision. One feels that oneself and others cannot rely fully on one's inner state of wavering and uncertainty.

Cerato is indicated in speech problems arising from inner uncertainty; it is also of service during language development when inner certainty and dynamic of word use need to be improved. Furthermore, it could assist in developmental disorders by helping the mind gain certainty and enhancing learning potential (cf. Chestnut Bud).

In mental illness, this remedy can be of service in gender identity disorders, anxiety disorders, delusions, elimination disorders and sexual disorders (cf. Cherry Plum, especially for the last two), or whenever there is an underlying dynamic of uncertainty of consciousness expression. In avoidance personality disorder, Cerato can successfully treat the timid reliance on the favorable evaluation by others and help overcome avoidance of social situations (cf. Mimulus). In dependent personality disorder, Cerato addresses the excessive dependence on the approval and advice of others (cf. Centaury). In regard to anxiety disorders and delusions, Cerato can help those lost in their own reality so that new certainty can grow in their remaining healthful aspects and the wrongly based certainty of their illusions and imaginings fade.

EMOTIONS: Consequently, the person in the Cerato state has to balance a continued array of emotions.

There is lack of self-esteem and easily stimulated feelings of inferiority. One is impressed by the others' decisive demeanor, wants to measure up, wishes for recognition and approval by others. Unfortunately, others often sense the person's discomfort and may turn away in disregard, increasing the person's uncertainty.

Uncertainty and frequent feelings of inferiority undermine one's enjoyment of life, and one may feel trampled by the force of others.

Usually, however, one attributes the fault for one's distress to oneself; one feels caught within one's own stifled and hampered expression of personality.

Oftentimes, in the Cerato state, there develops a deep longing for truth, personal clarity and independence. One knows what is missing yet does not understand how to reach this special elixir of life. For many, the way of service and love, of tuning into others rather than preoccupying with oneself and being in the way of oneself, is the road to healing.

PHYSICAL TENDENCIES: Lack of forcefulness of appearance may exist; the person is rather retreating and allows others to lead. In regard to uncertain, unsteady gait or posture, especially if caused by reluctance and inhibition, Cerato will give physical assurance.

In diseases of the immune system, when the inner intelligence which operates automatically does not know how to achieve health, Cerato may aid in reviving inner certainty and help the organism decide on a strategy of defense.

DOCTRINE OF SIGNATURES: As the positive Cerato state seems elusive and hard to find, so the plant itself is rare and was long hidden from view in distant Tibet, its place of nativity. Tibet, the land of wisdom and meditation, grew this special flower which brings insight, inner balance and truth perception. Although it has been imported to the Western World, it still is considered a specialty plant and rarely found.

The riveting blue-purple color gives clarity just by looking at it.

The flowers grow in clusters; they open successively, each flower lasting only one day. Here again is the elusive quality of wisdom and inner certainty, so craved and seen as unattainable by the person in the Cerato state. This short-lasting blooming may also speak of the spurts of wisdom and insight that guide the healthy person, since the viewpoints of clarity must be achieved anew in each particular situation. Yet, the positive Cerato state, once achieved, gives consistent strength and decisiveness, making life more meaningful.

METHOD OF PREPARATION: Fresh flowers are put in a bowl of water and allowed to sit in the sun for several hours. The water imbued with healing power is strained and used as medicine.

GOAL OF THERAPY: To transform excessive and hampering self-consciousness into healthy tuning into others and objective problem- centering. To increase intuition, truth perception, self-assurance and trust in one's judgment.

CHERRY PLUM (PRUNUS CERASIFERA)

The remedy Cherry Plum belongs to the group of *For Those Who Have Fear,* as classified by Bach. Further remedies in this group are Rock Rose, Mimulus, Aspen and Red Chestnut. Specifically, Cherry Plum treats the fear of losing reason and mental control in face of unwanted impulses, dreaded urges, or strong mental pressures.

MIND: In the Cherry Plum state, the mind is overstrained and out of balance. This state may come on after prolonged mental effort, especially when achieved with great strength of will and forceful concentration despite failing nerve power and exhaustion. Or it may be the result of unanswered vital needs and pressures, either consciously experienced or active in the unconscious, that cannot be satisfied but nonetheless send impulses of thought to the mind, as if crying for recognition.

In both cases, the result is a flooding of the mind with unwanted thought content that is strongly resisted, since it is shocking in nature, considered antisocial, dangerous to oneself or others, or bizarre. The person in this state tries desperately to stay normal within, to balance continually the reasonable faculties in face of these unusual mental pressures. As these forces are opposed vehemently, they respond with heightened intensity, mental strain is escalating, and there arises the fear that all balance will be lost and the impulsive, unwanted thoughts will win. This is the typical Cherry Plum fear.

There are varying degrees of the Cherry Plum state. In lighter cases, the person may just do thought control, trying to purify the mind or reasserting reason and self-esteem over embarrassing, unwanted, or unnerving, agitating thought content or imaginings. Cherry Plum can be of service in nervousness, shyness and stage fright, these being unwanted mental states which one tries to fight within oneself. In a more intensified state, not only the world of thought is threatened but the world of active doing as well. Impulses dictating to carry out certain acts, dangerous to oneself or others, or socially unfit, may demand attention and threaten to dictate conduct. Many crimes and suicides are committed while being in the Cherry Plum state. All problems in regard to impulse control fall under the healing action of this remedy (cf. Impatiens, Holly, Vervain, Vine).

Cherry Plum, should the indications exist, treats phobias of all kind (cf. Mimulus, Rock Rose) and fear of sudden physical/mental failure, as in stammering or in diseases such as epilepsy or repeated fainting. It is indicated whenever there is fear of losing control over one's mental/ emotional faculties or physical happenings; one feels helpless in face of overwhelming dynamics which, though resisted to, seem to have a life of their own. During drug rehabilitation or during attempts to heal addictive imaginings, Cherry Plum treats the fear of losing one's resolve and succumbing to former habitual satisfaction.

Within the Cherry Plum dynamic, one also finds obsessive-compulsive, perfection-oriented, or ritualistic behavior or thought processes engaged in with the intention to avoid succumbing to the dreaded impulse (cf. Crab Apple, Pine).

The remedy is invaluable in treatment of delusional and psychotic states when the boundaries of consciousness are disintegrating and the mind becomes subjected to unconscious and primordial forces.

EMOTIONS: Great anguish and distress are experienced in the Cherry Plum state, along with the intense fear of losing control. Milder cases may feel more exasperated or nervous in face of unwanted thoughts, rather than experiencing anguish.

While the mind is out of balance, the emotions are too. Oftentimes, there are unfulfilled emotional needs at the bottom of the mental pressures. Some vital part is not heard properly, becomes suppressed, only to reassert through bizarre or inappropriate expression.

In some cases of willful abuse or crime, one can observe a fascination with the Cherry Plum state which is engaged in for the sake of thrill or excitement. To contemplate forbidden things may arouse in some a taste of adventure, and the dangers are played with in one's mind, the tension savored, until the negative balance is won. One will do the forbidden deed and one feels empowered; newly balanced certainty grows out of the temporary Cherry Plum state, but at the wrong end. Moral consciousness, in such instances, is not powerful enough to offer sufficient deterrence in face of these antisocial impulses. Cherry Plum will help these people to be less drawn to forbidden, tension-provoking content and reduce the fascination found in danger and unusual thrill, while moral insights would have to be strengthened concurrently.

Oftentimes, the opposite effect is encountered, as a standard of high morals and a strong sense of propriety impel an upright person into a Cherry Plum state. Thoughts have to be proper, and one feels responsible to guard them constantly.

Ethical principles and love for one's neighbor, however, which are often at the bottom of the true Cherry Plum fear and which enhance the need to balance, self-observe and protect others, also offer a way to find peace by de-emphasizing preoccupation with internal dynamics and concentrating one's focus on caring for others.

PHYSICAL TENDENCIES: Extreme nervousness, threatened nervous breakdown (cf. Impatiens, Rock Rose, Vervain), nervous twitches, grimaces, gestures are common in severe cases. The body expresses the mental struggle taking place within. The remedy is of service in tic disorders, elimination disorders and sexual disorders (cf. Cerato). Mounting tension can release suddenly in unpredictable outbursts of violence. Cherry Plum can help people suffering from diseases of the nervous system to find added peace in mind and body (cf. Rock Rose). The physical concomitant symptoms and affected nerve paths related to speech problems can benefit from the calming influence of this remedy.

During drug rehabilitation, physical and mental/emotional cravings can be reduced and the organism rebalanced.

In severe pain, when one feels almost unable to bear the strain and torture, when the mind is at the verge of breaking down, Cherry Plum brings relief. In some cases, unbearable pain can lead to homicide or suicide.

DOCTRINE OF SIGNATURES: The Cherry Plum tree stems originally from the Balkan, a land known for intensity in the mind/emotions and overenthusiasm.

Cherry Plum blossoms are the first white blossoms to appear at the end of winter. They effectively stand out from leafless, dark branches, symbolizing healing lights on the background of shadowed unconscious forces. The blossoms are pristine, pure, radiating peace and clarity, these being qualities the plant instills in a mind tortured by shocking thoughts and internal ·battles.

METHOD OF PREPARATION: Twigs of flowers are picked and boiled for half an hour. The boiled water is strained and used as medicine.

GOAL OF THERAPY: To reduce mental preoccupation and direct the viewpoint to people and content outside of oneself, with emphasis on love and service. To reduce pressure from the unconscious, allowing for peaceful communication between the varying needs of the self, for example by analyzing one's dreams. To give mental peace and relaxation.

CHESTNUT BUD (AESCULUS HIPPOCASTANUM)

The remedy Chestnut Bud, together with Clematis, Honeysuckle, Wild Rose, Olive and White Chestnut, belongs to Bach's group of *Not Sufficient Interest in Present Circumstances*. These remedies help those not fully engaged in the here and now. Specifically, Chestnut Bud treats a young and impulsive mind not prone to integrate the lessons of daily life.

MIND: In the Chestnut Bud state, the mind is restless and impulsive, easily distracted, absent-minded, and not set on learning in the factual and moral sense. Chestnut Bud treats a mind with a bent to immaturity; there is still a potential for growth and deepening of learning, especially in regard to one's reflective and reasoning powers.

In learning environments, the mind in need of Chestnut Bud is marked by skipping from topic to topic, or superficially through a text, or rushing ahead impatiently. Deepened concentration, savoring and reflecting on learned material are not fully present. Consequently, learned material is not contained very well, although capacity for memory is usually present. It is the manner of addressing the learning material which prevents deepened learning from taking place. Distractions are welcomed; things are not taken seriously enough, or one may jump at conclusions prematurely. There may be inappropriate laughing or gliding over reprimands. These observations not only apply to learning environments but actually extend into parts of life where understanding and achieving are called for.

This includes the moral arena, where the same dynamic can be observed. Life's experiences, even if they contained lessons and painful consequences, are not integrated in such a way as to further character growth and inner wisdom. One glides through life rather superficially, living according to one's spontaneity and emotional motivations rather than balancing with reason, clarity and meaningful reflection.

In developmental disorders, hyperactivity (attention-deficit hyperactivity disorder) and disruptive behavior disorders, Chestnut Bud helps the mind to settle into restful concentration and retain the learning material. In the treatment of disruptive, antisocial or criminal behavior, factitious disorders, and malingering, when learning and growth in moral insight are not forthcoming, Chestnut Bud is of service.[4] In personality disorders marked by a refusal to change and acquire empathy for others, such as in antisocial personality disorder, Chestnut Bud can spur moral growth (cf. Vine).

EMOTIONS: Since the mind is not very trained in constructive self-observation and the resolute fostering of positive aspirations, emotions rule much of the conduct. One is easily carried by positive as well as negative emotional content and may appear unreasonable, easily swayed, naive, emotionally unstable, impulsive, defiant and somewhat lacking in integrity or depth.

People not willing to obey laws and adjust to a normal socialization process often are in need of this remedy. They do not learn readily from experience, are often heedless or careless, even after having been reprimanded or curtailed in their freedom. There is also a bent to easy comradery, hilarity and joking.

Besides affecting the whole character, the Chestnut Bud state can also be experienced by a person usually strong in integrity and insight. A repeated tendency may exist, or there might be moments in life when one feels unsettled, easily distracted, more superficial in certain aspects of life, or one temporarily avoids to draw lessons from one's experiences.

PHYSICAL TENDENCIES: Impulsiveness of physical conduct and some degree of hyperactivity or restlessness can be concomitant physical features.

One may bring the self and others in danger through recklessness or disregard important physical needs.

DOCTRINE OF SIGNATURES: The remedy is prepared from the opening buds of the Horse Chestnut tree. Apparently, these buds are known as very powerful shoots, almost visibly growing on observation. This symbolizes the impulsive dynamic and spontaneity of expression of the mind still young in its reflective and reasoning powers.

METHOD OF PREPARATION: The young twigs with shoots are boiled for half an hour. The water is strained and used as medicine.

GOAL OF THERAPY: To help the mind find calm focus and become receptive to reason, clarity, reflection and development of inner wisdom.

CHICORY (CICHORIUM INTYBUS)

Chicory belongs to the group of *Overcare for Welfare of Others,* as classified by Bach. The other remedies in this group are Rock Water, Beech, Vine, Vervain. This group deals with mental/emotional imbalances in regard to caring for or controlling others. Specifically, Chicory treats a heightened care for others that is marked by possessiveness.

MIND: In the Chicory state, the mind is bent on taking care of others according to one's own design or idea. It is a self-centered approach to caring, since the true needs of the care recipient may not be noticed or found unimportant by the care-taker. The care received may be interpreted as too forceful or unnecessary, and, as soon as this message is conveyed, there develop sentiments of self-pity in the care-giving person, a sense of not being appreciated for one's efforts. This is the double-sided dynamic of the Chicory state.

The Chicory mind sets up fairly rigid opinions and ways of working with others. There is the conviction that one's perceptions and opinions are correct, and one assumes the right to force them on others. This usually happens with good intentions of passing on the right way but may be experienced by others as too controlling or interfering. There is also the tendency to be overly careful with details, one's daily duties, and with cleanliness. Possessiveness of people, as well as of goods, is another indication for this remedy.

There also exists an inactive Chicory state when attention is desired through retreat, manipulations and pretense, and one waits for others to connect and provide security and love, rather than actively going out towards them. In both cases, the goal is to bind others closely to the self. The active Chicory type may experience the inactive Chicory state during times of illness when self-pity and demands for attention are forthcoming.

This remedy is indicated in the treatment of feigning of sickness in order to gain attention, called factitious disorder (cf. Chestnut Bud, Heather), in eating disorders (cf. Crab Apple,

Mustard), should the inactive Chicory dynamic be present. In conversion disorders, also called hysterical neurosis of the conversion type, when the body expresses through illness the unvoiced psychological need for attention and love, Chicory can help heal the underlying dynamic.[5] Hypochondriasis (cf. Heather, Mimulus), somatoform pain disorder, which is a preoccupation with pain without physical findings, and somatization disorder, this being based on long-standing medical complaints without actual illness, can also rest on a Chicory need for attention gain. In histrionic personality disorder, based on attention-seeking within the sexual sphere, Chicory can remove the underlying dynamic (cf. Cherry Plum).

EMOTIONS: The Chicory state, although seemingly overbearing to others, does root in a heartfelt desire to love and serve, and find closeness. Devotion and caring are undermined, however, by the Chicory persons' insistence on their own style and their self-centered idea of how to convey their care for and interest in others.

Furthermore, there is the underlying motive of binding others closely to oneself for the sake of power, influence, or to escape loneliness. In the Chicory state, one has a very hard time letting go of others and relinquishing one's rights as caretaker.

Another personal reason, sidetracking with true love and devotion, is the need for attention and appreciation. One serves others with the intention to find recognition and be seen as valuable or indispensable. The typical Chicory self-pity comes in as appreciation is not expressed, efforts overlooked or even resented. Self-pity, hurt feelings and retreat are also common in courtship when a partner is rebuffed or treated unfairly.

Next to the active Chicory attitude, there is also the inactive attitude of expecting attention and caring, simply for being in the world. There is the need to be the center of attention and be appreciated, even though special efforts have not been forthcoming. Self-pity, sulkiness and pouting are common, if affectionate attention is not offered. If consoled, there may be annoyance and persisted-in self-pity, as if intended to arouse even more sympathy in the other. This state is commonly experienced in children, although seen in adults as well, except that the adults' mannerisms or ways of expressing the emotional message may be less childlike and differ more from person to person. People may resort to manipulation, power play, pretense, threat, possessiveness, or feigning of sickness in order to convey that they feel hurt, offended, or overlooked. If attended to, they may reject being consoled which increases their self-pity and may create further alienation in others rather than bring the desired appreciation. In case attention is accepted, there may be fussiness and capriciousness, and nothing may please. Overcoming a self-centered attitude and self-pity, while tuning in to the needs of others, helps to break this fruitless cycle.

PHYSICAL TENDENCIES: Fussy mannerism may be noticeable in some people. A face prone to pout or look hurt and withdrawn may portray the Chicory state of self-pity.

The inactive Chicory type may show conversion disorders, these being the involuntary, physical symptomatic expression of an unvoiced love need (cf. Scleranthus). Hypochondriasis, somatization disorder, and somatoform pain disorder can be further expressions of the inactive Chicory type. Others resort to anorexia, vomiting, nausea, bulimia and overeating in an effort to draw attention and love to the self. Bronchial asthma, characterized by difficulty in expiring, can rest on a basis of emotional hurt, self-pity and a refusal to give, hence the inability to expire, to give of oneself; this refusal to give can also grow out of the self-protective, anxious attempt to hold in emotions, since they were not responded to properly.[6] All these conflicts rest on unconscious dynamics that the patients are not aware of.

In addition, some types of patients with gastroduodenal ulcers, if prone to tyrannical outbursts and yet falling ill whenever affection is withdrawn, portray the manipulative tendency to call for attention through nonverbal means.[7]

In the diseases of soft tissue rheumatism and rheumatoid arthritis, should they be of psychosomatic origin, the active Chicory state may be one factor in the formation of disease. Patients have been found to be overly controlling and service-oriented, while suppressing hostile emotions and demanding attention when sick.[3] Chronic constipation (cf. Mustard, Willow) has been interpreted as inability to part with something.[8]

DOCTRINE OF SIGNATURES: The Chicory plant grows by the wayside in the form of a small bush. Numerous blue flowers grow right out of the stem or branch which is rigid and appears unyielding. This symbolizes the exaggerated attempt to bind others closely to oneself, as in overcare and overly close bonding with one's children or loved ones. In passive cases, when self-pity and need for attention dominate, the binding closely, the need to be together, is the underlying motive as well.

The plant, usually growing along dusty, dry roads, needs a long root to obtain water. Likewise, insects need to spend more time during pollination on this plant than on most others, since the stamens have to allow pollen and nectar to be released. This symbolizes that "give," releasing the pollen and nectar, and "take," absorbing water, do not come easily in the Chicory state. Affectionate interchange may be overshadowed by effort and delay. The flower, however, containing the healing power, speaks of the desired union by its circle of sky-blue petals.

METHOD OF PREPARATION: The flowers are picked, floated in a bowl of water, and let sit in the sun for several hours. The strained water is used as medicine.

GOAL OF THERAPY: To instill love that seeks not to acquire for personal gain but is selfless and self-forgetful in service and true understanding of another person's individuality, potential and needs.

CLEMATIS (CLEMATIS VITALBA)

This remedy belongs to the group of *Not Sufficient Interest in Present Circumstances,* as classified by Bach. The additional remedies of this group are Honeysuckle, Wild Rose, Olive, White Chestnut, Mustard and Chestnut Bud. This group of remedies helps those not fully engaged in the here and now. Specifically, Clematis has the indication of longing for a future state while experiencing indifference or disinterest towards the present.

MIND: The mind is set on dreams of future fulfillment rather than seeing the present as promising and trying to find happiness therein. Reality may actually appear hazy, as if veiled, and there may be the tendency to suddenly lose touch and become drowsy or sleepy. Or one may feel lightheaded or vacant in one's mind, as if the mind is removed and not fully centered or concentrated.

These states can come on not only from daydreaming about future happiness but also from fatigue, from a strenuous or saddening daily routine that one removes oneself from internally, as if it is too painful to experience fully or look too closely.

In school settings, one may notice the unmotivated, day-dreaming student whose absent-mindedness is prevalent, although interrupted here and there by spurts of interest.

In delusional states with ecstatic content (cf. Vervain), with pleasant visions and reveries, Clematis removes the lure and brings the mind back to reality.

EMOTIONS: Although reality is wanting and does not promise happiness, the person in the Clematis state is hopeful. The view directs to a bright future when longing ceases and completeness, fulfillment and rewards are forthcoming. As one dwells on these dreams and reveries, one is most happy. Reality, seems harsh in comparison, void of meaning, lonely or sad. Yet, these are the present circumstances, and, every time one wakes up to them, disillusionment sets in. The mind cannot bear this state for very long and is drawn again and again to happy imaginings, as if addicted.

If longing is expressed in art, which means a grounding of this inner dynamic, the Clematis state may be alleviated or cured, just as direct devotion to people and helping them realize their dreams will defocus the awareness of one's own dilemma and bring enjoyment of the present moment. Usually, however, one feels more passive, awaiting changes to come and staying out of touch with people and present circumstance.

PHYSICAL TENDENCIES: The body may seem as if not "inhabited," as the mind draws to future dream castles or removes due to exhaustion or emotional hardship. One is shocked by sudden noise and startles easily when touched. Sleepiness, drowsiness, fainting and vertigo are common. In some comatose states, Clematis can restore consciousness. Some people may have out-of-body experiences.

DOCTRINE OF SIGNATURES: The Clematis plant gives an ethereal impression, and, being a climbing shrub, it overgrows, intertwines, proliferates, ranks and weaves much like reveries weave through the Clematis consciousness. The plant needs to attach to other bushes or trees to find support for growth; it ranks above other plants, just as the Clematis mind ranks over and above reality.

The white flowers have wispy, tufted seed heads that are seen floating in autumn, reminding of clouds and dreams. Autumn is a time when reality becomes stark and wanting in color, and the mind may be prone to revert to dreaming or imagining, to "floating in the clouds."

METHOD OF PREPARATION: Flowers are picked with the stalk, placed in a bowl of water, and allowed to sit in the sun for several hours. The water is strained and used as medicine.

GOAL OF THERAPY: To ground in reality and find meaningful occupation, to appreciate the present moment and become receptive to all its joys with clarity of mind and perception.

CRAB APPLE (MALUS SYLVESTRIS/PUMILA)

The remedy Crab Apple, together with Oak, Willow, Star of Bethlehem, Sweet Chestnut, Elm, Pine, Larch, belongs to the group of *For Despondency or Despair,* as classified by Bach. These remedies deal with mental states of severity when a condition burdens and one does not have sufficient power or possibility to grow above. Specifically, Crab Apple treats persistent feelings of shame in face of unwanted personal attributes or failings.

MIND: In the Crab Apple state, the mind is overly concentrating on one aspect of the self considered unclean, shameful, bothering and burdensome. Other aspects of the self, such as positive character traits, are not equally important or regarded. The one displeasing state assumes inappropriate dimensions, and one loses perspective of what is most important in life or about oneself. This attitude is enhanced by underlying feelings of helplessness one feels in regard to the problem. One feels unable to shake off or overcome the disturbing condition, and feelings of despair may develop.

In some cases, the shameful aspect experienced or engaged in is fostered by addictive perpetuation and hidden from others so that a personal prison of shame and self-disgust develops.

In other cases, the Crab Apple state is marked by obsessive preoccupation with beauty flaws or states of sickness considered unclean and unbecoming. Here the problem may be openly shared with others.

In yet another situation, contamination is feared through a source outside of the self, such as by germs or unclean surroundings, and a strong reaction of dislike or disgust may be aroused in some people. This strong stance reflects their inner sensitivity in regard to personal hidden shame, or it reflects fear of and possibly temptation to uncleanness in thought or action which has not been dealt with properly.

In cases of abuse or molestation, a Crab Apple state may come about in the victim who feels soiled or abased, even though there is no personal guilt or wrong. The indication for this remedy is the perception that something unclean or base has touched the self, either from within the personality sphere or from without, and one wishes to be cleansed of it.

In treatment of obsessive-compulsive behavior with personally shameful content, this remedy brings release (cf. Cherry Plum, Pine). In body dysmorphic disorder, which entails obsessive, exaggerated preoccupation with imagined or hardly noticeable physical defects, Crab Apple is the indicated remedy.

EMOTIONS: Feelings of uncleanness and shame may weigh heavily upon the heart and stifle personal enjoyment of life. True despair and despondency may develop, as one feels unable to free or cleanse oneself. This holds true especially when repeatedly engaging in sinful or shameful behavior and regretting it later on.

Another emotion of intensity is the obsessive or hysterical undertone that can develop while being in the Crab Apple state. Minor problems assume disproportionate importance, and, since there is usually no ready cure, obsessive despair may escalate.

The Crab Apple view is too self-centered; one's own self is overly dealt with and the view lost to others and their special needs or place in life. Oftentimes, it is shame about one's appearance or inner guilt and uncleanness which prevents one from enjoying direct eye contact, and much opportunity for personal enrichment through careful tuning into others and concentrating away from oneself is lost.

Some people feel an intense craving or desire to be cleansed and purified from within. This may be part of a moral or spiritual awakening, or it may be a purist's attitude of striving for perfection and ultimate health in body and consciousness. Crab Apple would help in both cases.

PHYSICAL TENDENCIES: This remedy can be of service in unclean skin, acne, accumulated wastes in the blood stream, cleansing of digestive tract, long-lasting viral infections and chronic poisoning due to environmental hazards.

It also helps to draw out impurities from a wound if applied to the bandage.

In psychosomatic medicine, chronic diarrhea, among other causes, has been linked with the psyche's effort to get rid of something, to cleanse and free the self. Feelings of disgust or repulsion have been interpreted to be at the bottom of anorexia, vomiting, nausea and emaciation (cf. Chicory, Mustard).[8] Bulimia can also be motivated by strong repulsion towards the food consumed, with the urge to vomit. Basically, both anorexia and bulimia rest on the Crab Apple tendency to obsess with weight problems and put too much emphasis on a slim figure with abhorrence of any unnecessary fat. Body dysmorphic disorder can grow out of this dynamic (see definition above).

DOCTRINE OF SIGNATURES: The very name "Crab Apple" refers to this remedy's property of cleansing from "crab" and impurities. Apples are generally recognized as cleansers for our bodies. The fruit of this tree is bitter, however, and may speak of the "forbidden fruit" that leads to shame and personal decline. Often, the tempting situations of life lead, if engaged in, to the Crab Apple state.

The blossoms, however, growing before the fruit ripens, restore healing or safeguard inner purity, should it be threatened. Endowed with a beautiful scent, the radiantly white petals with a touch of light-pink around the edges speak of pristine beauty and clarity, standing off effectively from dark-green foliage.

This tree grows in the wild, unfettered by pruning or domestication, just as Crab Apple liberates from the curtailing impact and the narrowing walls of negative self-appraisal.

METHOD OF PREPARATION: Small twigs with whole clusters of flowers are boiled for half an hour. The water is strained and used as medicine.

GOAL OF THERAPY: To bring a sense of self-acceptance and forgiveness of one's shameful aspects. To direct the mind to positive attributes of oneself, as well as to reestablish priorities such as love and kindness over self-preoccupation and despair. Directing the view to the care of others and finding the joy of service, with simultaneous raising of one's self-worth, brings deepened healing.

ELM (ULMUS PROCERA)

The remedy Elm belongs to Bach's group of *For Despondency or Despair,* along with the remedies of Crab Apple, Oak, Willow, Star of Bethlehem, Sweet Chestnut, Pine and Larch. These remedies deal with states of hardship of the oppressive, burdening kind. Specifically, Elm treats a state of feeling overwhelmed and subdued in face of tasks and responsibilities.

MIND: In the Elm state, the mind feels unable to rise above challenges or duties that are being presented or still lie ahead. One actually perceives the task as insurmountable, as if it had literally grown above one's capacities, looming ahead, while one feels weak and small in front of it.

One also makes the mistake to view the many steps of present and future tasks as one whole mass of overwhelming duty, instead of concentrating on one step at a time and letting the rest be.

"Duty" is another aspect of the Elm state. Whereas, previously, the tasks may have been enjoyable and within one's strength of achievement, they now look somewhat threatening, intimidating, like a burdensome or dreaded duty.

Elm is also indicated for the mind busy at work on details, while not having an appropriate overview of the various tasks and not being able to plan the best approach to completing the job. One may get lost in details and feel that progress has not really been made.

During emotional hardship, Elm may help a mind unable to sort through the intensity of feelings and may aid the person to come to a place of calm within, where an overview can be reached and the balancing strength of reason and clarity be regained. In case life's problems burden, evade solution and fixate the mind into preoccupation, this remedy helps to regain mastery within this mental dynamic (cf. White Chestnut).

EMOTIONS: In the Elm state, one experiences the emotions of being overwhelmed, of dread, anxiety, internal exhaustion, intimidation by the amount of duties, inadequacy, disillusionment, despondency and despair. It is a state of not feeling empowered, of losing one's wings of joyful progress. Whereas before there was hopeful looking ahead into the future, there now is dread in face of enormous tasks. There can be feelings of sadness, especially when ideals were high and the service attitude strong and one suddenly realizes that one's goals were unrealistic and not within one's reach. Helpers in the arena of human suffering may frequently experience this state.

Some people, while being in the Elm state, do not want to give up but try to struggle on. Personal high expectations and a strong sense of duty will still give some incentive, although the message may be to rest and take care of oneself. Other people avoid facing the particular insurmountable situation and busy themselves with other duties in their lives, those being more easily within their range of present capacity.

PHYSICAL TENDENCIES: There is a tendency to exhaustion in mind, emotions and body, to listlessness and lethargy.

Unresolved, overwhelming conflicts and work loads can lead to the formation of psychosomatic diseases, if healthful recreation and diversion are not balancing the impact (see White Chestnut).

DOCTRINE OF SIGNATURES: The Elm tree is characterized by a large billowing crown which extends over the lower branches, reminding of the mind feeling overwhelmed by insurmountable tasks. The leaves themselves are shaped specifically to indicate a leaning back or overwhelmed state.

Elm trees are susceptible to overwhelming influence from outside; they are sensitive to diseases such as the widely spread Dutch Elm Disease. An Elm tree, hit by a car and suffering what seems to be minor damage, may suddenly decide to die. The tree's vital force seems easily distraught, much as a person in the Elm state seems to have less vitality and strength in face of overwhelming challenges.

METHOD OF PREPARATION: Boil twigs and blossoms for half an hour, strain the water and use as medicine.

GOAL OF THERAPY: To uplift the mind to a position where tasks can be perceived calmly and their completion be planned most efficiently. During task completion, to concentrate on one step at a time, while envisioning the whole in its progress. To overcome despondency and despair and rekindle joy of taking on challenges.

GENTIAN (GENTIANA AMARELLA)

The remedy Gentian, together with Cerato, Scleranthus, Gorse, Hornbeam and Wild Oat, belongs to the group of *For Those Who Suffer Uncertainty,* as classified by Bach. These remedies help those suffering from doubts and uncertainty in the daily affairs of their lives. Specifically, Gentian treats discouragement, a lack of faith and diminished optimism.

MIND: The Gentian mind is easily discouraged. As one moves through one's tasks and life's challenges, one may feel disheartened and ready to give up as soon as hindrances arise. One retreats from the situation at hand, thinking circumstances to be wrong or believing fate is not on one's side, or simply doubting that one is capable to persevere and be successful. There is lack of inner stamina and faith, weakened capacity for perseverance and lack of courage to give one's all to a task or challenge.

Forcefulness of personality is lacking; the self-assured grip that tackles life's problems without delay or doubt needs to be brought forth.

The mind has the tendency to exaggerate, to build minor hindrances into major ones, to view small setbacks with disheartenment, to draw the wrong conclusions and foster self-undermining beliefs. As belief in one's capacities wavers frequently, one also does not readily trust the care of a higher power or God.

EMOTIONS: In the Gentian state, the easily stimulated doubting and disheartenment weaken enjoyment of life and personal self-assurance. Lack of faith in oneself and the tendency to give up, even during projects that may be enjoyable, possibly lead to a diminished fullness of life, to a lack of interest and stimulation with withdrawal from challenges and from involvement in the world. Sadness or depression often accompany this state.

Lack of faith in a higher power can further reduce the safety feeling and undermine the assurance of having a handle on one's tasks and life's vicissitudes.

In the Gentian state, one also does not feel grounded or centered enough, more like superficially touching at things and not fully sinking into vigorous crafting of one's goals.

PHYSICAL TENDENCIES: Lack of physical stamina may be common. This remedy helps to accelerate physical healing in a patient plagued by doubts and discouragement about the slow process of cure.

DOCTRINE OF SIGNATURES: The Gentian plant, showing multiple blossoms, is marked by a sturdy appearance, growing in a pyramid. There are more flowers and leaves on the bottom, narrowing towards the top. This suggests a grounding of the self, a binding with the earth, and sturdy footage within one's tasks and challenges. The multiple pink-purple blossoms remind of warmth and bounty, hinting at the fruitfulness of a steady, persevering heart which grows into manifestation without reluctance.

This plant readily grows on the hillside, where one finds inspiration and gains an overview, as the remedy will give faith and empowerment.

METHOD OF PREPARATION: Flowers are picked, floated onto a bowl of water, and left standing in the sun for several hours. The strained water is used as medicine.

GOAL OF THERAPY: To give faith and encouragement, to invigorate personal trust in one's capacities and instill perseverance. To ground the self in a more complete union with accomplishments and daily tasks.

GORSE (ULEX EUROPAEUS)

This remedy belongs to Bach's group of *For Those Who Suffer Uncertainty,* together with the remedies of Cerato, Scleranthus, Gentian, Hornbeam, and Wild Oat. These remedies help those suffering from states of doubt, hopelessness, uncertainty, and lack of clarity of purpose in their daily affairs. Specifically, Gorse treats a deep hopelessness that may affect the vitality of the person.

MIND: In the Gorse state, the mind cannot perceive a way out of a difficult situation, and all incentive to give oneself to new ideas and hopes is gone. It is a state of deep-reaching hopelessness and resignation.

With giving up the belief that anything can be done to find lasting improvement, there comes the cessation of uncertain hopes, of denial and recurring disappointment, of struggle and rebellion against one's fate. One accepts one's lot, succumbing to adverse forces. It is a state of lowered vitality, dangerous for those in sickness; the life spark itself is losing its incentive to live and fight on. Although there is certainty that all hopes are lost, uncertainty still remains in regard to what exactly lies ahead.

EMOTIONS: After an initial turmoil of emotions, as occurs in situations of great severity, one now becomes calmer, as inevitability of events is accepted. As people make suggestions for improvement, one might go along with them, knowing full well that there is no way out.

Although one may appear calm, there is also underlying sadness and a sense of misfortune and suffering. In cases of true hopelessness, such as terminal illness, Gorse will help to raise spirits while in the here and now and give a new, inspiring outlook into the beyond. The certainty grows that all will be well and one is taken care of.

The Gorse state is not confined to sickness but can be experienced during various situations of life, in business and family life, whenever a situation seems hopeless and one succumbs to it.

PHYSICAL TENDENCIES: Lowered vitality, sinking of strength and loss of the incentive to live may accompany the Gorse state.

DOCTRINE OF SIGNATURES: The Gorse bush is characterized by multiple small yellow-golden blossoms which radiate light and healing power. The branches have long thorny spikes, reminding of the state of severity which brings forth great hopelessness. Amidst the threatening spikes grow the flowers of healing, in profusion, signaling new life and vitality.

Gorse is an evergreen plant, and blossoms can be found throughout the year. This conveys the message of the plant's special blooming and healing power which asserts itself despite unfavorable weather conditions, despite adversity and hardship.

METHOD OF PREPARATION: Flowers from the bush are placed in a bowl of water and allowed to stand in the sun for several hours. The strained water is used as medicine.

GOAL OF THERAPY: To raise the heart and mind to new hope and give incentive and will to live and move forward. To raise vitality and positive expectancy.

HEATHER (CALLUNA VULGARIS)

The remedy Heather, together with Water Violet and Impatiens, belongs to Bach's group of *Loneliness*. These remedies help those suffering from inner loneliness as a result of being too centered within their own selves and losing the connection with others. Heather treats an increased urge to talk about oneself, stemming from the need for attention and care.

MIND: In the Heather state, the mind is overly concentrating on personal affairs and attaches much importance to experienced hardship and dilemma. One believes the own concerns to be so paramount as to have to be shared at all cost with others who then, so it is expected, will give understanding and caring insight. There exists a self-centered view of life, and one holds the assumption that one deserves sympathy and regard.

There is great inner urging to share through words; talkativeness is an important characteristic of the Heather state. Inner pressure of loneliness and self-related worry needs to be expressed; the craving for attention and sympathy needs to be stilled.

Should words alone not have the desired effect, other attention-getting behavior is added to this dynamic, either consciously (factitious) or unconsciously (somatoform), such as feigning sickness, hypochondriasis (cf. Chicory, Mimulus), or other expressions classified under factitious and somatoform disorders (see Chicory, Chestnut Bud); or verbal flow centers increasingly around obsessively fixated themes (cf. White Chestnut).

EMOTIONS: Oftentimes, the cause of the Heather state is true emotional need, coupled with the inability to find an appropriate partner or avenue of expressing the internal suffering. In case of injustice received or if one was undermined in one's honest efforts, there is an even greater need and internal pressure to find sympathetic listeners who give support. In the Heather state, one craves to find understanding of one's inmost self. One needs the connection with others. This Heather state can show itself even when talkativeness has not come forth yet; the internal pressure to share oneself and find a sympathetic listener is enough indication to prescribe this remedy.

As compared to cases of deeper emotional hardship, there appears the emotionally lighter case of Heather, where talkativeness over seemingly unimportant details is prevalent. Here the talking serves to gain attention, feel special and vent self-pity. In case words alone do not get the desired effect, these people more readily resort to pretense and other manipulative ways of expressing their needs for attention, such as by feigning sickness. The true underlying emotional challenge, however, is not so much to find sympathy for hardship but to open the view to the needs of others and de-emphasize preoccupation with personal affairs. This new experience would fill the inner isolation more deeply than the misleading attempt to bind others' attention and sympathy to one's own self.

PHYSICAL TENDENCIES: The person can appear overbearing and agitated in demeanor.

Factitious and somatoform disorders, centering around feigning or unconscious production of sickness with concurrent urge to talk about symptoms, can occur.

DOCTRINE OF SIGNATURES: Heather grows profusely throughout meadows, spreading like words or channels of sharing. It grows in small bushes and shows numerous delicate blossoms of a soothing purple color. To look at a field covered with this generous sweep of color gives peace of mind and expands the inner self.

This remedy widens the inner center of individuality to the welcome of others.

METHOD OF PREPARATION: The flowering stems are placed in a bowl of water and allowed to sit in the sun for several hours. The water is strained and used as medicine.

GOAL OF THERAPY: To open the mind to the needs of others and reduce preoccupation with self. Specifically, in regard to talkativeness, to learn to be a good listener.

HOLLY (ILEX AQUIFOLIUM)

The remedy Holly belongs to the group of *Oversensitive to Influences and Ideas,* as classified by Bach. Additional remedies in this group are Agrimony, Centaury and Walnut, all helping those suffering from vulnerability to disturbances from outside. Specifically, Holly treats negative or aggressive feelings or thoughts that are often marked by anger or agitation in response to a perceived threat.

MIND: In the Holly state, one easily perceives disturbances in the form of circumstances or other people as threats to one's peace and well-being. One reacts with oversensitivity to often minor occurrences which would leave many others undisturbed. The irritated mind is set on rejection in such a state, on being free of the annoyance, even to the point of inflicting harm, as happens in extreme cases. The Holly state is a fighter's mentality, an agitated, aggressive state, either expressed through words or gestures or simply held within, as stirred-up emotions grip the self.

The mind, being too quick to perceive others as threatening, is prone to be swayed and become unreasonable due to suspicion, envy, jealousy, revenge, anger and wounded pride.

In regard to mental disorders, this remedy is of value in treatment of antisocial personality disorder, conduct disorder (cf. Chestnut Bud, Vine), paranoid personality disorder and delusional or any other disorder with aggressive or jealous features. In persecutory or paranoid delusions, there can be heightened accusation and antagonism against the imagined threat of others (cf. Beech, Willow). In problems with impulse control, when rage is not bridled, Holly can restore the necessary inner control (cf. Cherry Plum, Impatiens, Vervain, Vine).

EMOTIONS: Emotions experienced in the Holly state can be very strong and rule the self. Oftentimes, they are invested in with much personal force, as one relishes and stirs up the negative. One may even feel empowered or invigorated by such sentiments, since the fighter's charge runs through the self. Then again, as the initial thrust cools off, one may find oneself plotting calmly or quietly engaging in devious thought.

The more one loses perspective and augments the negative sentiment, the more difficult it is to find the heart-centered balance that is called for.

This remedy is also of help to a person with good intentions who is irritable and easily annoyed without necessarily investing in negative thinking or doing. The Holly state can be a state of exhaustion, frazzled nerves and of being overstimulated by environmental impact. Excessive noise and turmoil, as may be caused by children, can spoil the mood and create the urge to "fight" oneself free. If held within, there is much internal suffering and agony; if expressed, others suffer as well, while there might be the illusion of having helped the self to feel less stifled. Much violence and abuse originate in this agitated Holly state, and uncontrolled behavior may happen even if not wished for (cf. Cherry Plum).

To be prone to vexation and upset is a painful experience, creating much internal suffering. Often, these people long for quiet repose and peaceful surroundings. There is the tendency to seek the cause of disturbance in the outside world, although it is the internal balance between impact and reaction that needs to be restored, ideally by avoiding unnecessary turmoil or vexing situations, while seeking tolerance of response and a loving attitude within.

PHYSICAL TENDENCIES: Nervousness, physical irritability, tension headaches or migraines may occur; headaches may come on after annoying experiences or reflect the force of suppressed anger.[3] Persons may be prone to outbursts of anger, rage, or violence which are not only detrimental to their own psyche and organism but can also lead to injuries for oneself and others.

The suppressed Holly state can result in psychosomatic illness over time (see Willow).

DOCTRINE OF SIGNATURES: The Holly tree is marked by spiked leaves, signaling defense to an outside threat. These leaves exist mostly towards the bottom of the tree to deter the animals from eating them, whereas the spikes almost disappear towards the top of the tree. In the Holly state, one likewise reacts with "sharp pricks" to a perceived threat or invasion from outside.

During the flowering period, tiny white flowers appear along the twigs, seemingly hiding behind the much larger leaves. This symbolizes the dominance and strength of the negative emotions, once engaged in, in comparison to kindness and inner beauty which hide behind the aggressive facade. The flowers, carrying healing essence, have a very powerful, sweet scent, however; as if to remind the heart of its lost bliss. If these subtle inspirations are obeyed, the fruits of service, symbolically expressed in form of the red berries, are then forthcoming, aglow with the bright-red color of love and warmth.

No wonder, this tree has been chosen as an ornament during the Christmas season.

METHOD OF PREPARATION: Flowering twigs are boiled for half an hour, the water strained and used as medicine.

GOAL OF THERAPY: To reduce oversensitivity and force of negative emotions by calming the inner, easily agitated self and allowing for feelings of kindness to come forth more readily. To instill the desire to give love.

HONEYSUCKLE (LONICERA CAPRIFOLIUM)

The remedy Honeysuckle belongs to Bach's group of *Not Sufficient Interest in Present Circumstances,* along with the remedies of Clematis, Wild Rose, Olive, White Chestnut, Mustard and Chestnut Bud. These remedies are for those not fully engaged in the here and now and consequently not living to the fullest. Specifically, Honeysuckle treats the undue longing for the happiness of the past.

MIND: In the Honeysuckle state, the mind dwells overly on past memories; its viewpoint directs to former experiences, instead of guiding its full focus to the present moment. Usually, the mind seeks those happy, fulfilled moments of the past and replays scenes and sentiments over and over again, as if to derive nourishment from them. Reminiscences and nostalgia carry more fascination than the colorless present. In fact, in the Honeysuckle state, one sadly believes that the happiness of the past can never be repeated in the present or future, and one hangs on to it.

In mental illness, when sentimental visions of the past grip the self repeatedly, or when one experiences delusions, visions or voices of lost loved ones in reaction to unresolved trauma or severe grief (cf. Star of Bethlehem), Honeysuckle will bring relief.

EMOTIONS: Sadness is the predominant emotion, yet it is tinged with the sweet pain of cherishing something lost, of longing to relive former happiness, if only in one's memories. There is also hopelessness and resignation in regard to present and future potential for happiness, and there is certainty that nothing can replace the lost fulfillment.

Oftentimes, these feelings are based on facts, as in old age when the losses cannot be replaced in this life. The children have moved on; one's health is fading; the partner may be dying. Honeysuckle will help even then to ease the sadness and direct the view to the remaining joys of the present moment.

Honeysuckle may apply to many different situations of life, whenever a lost preferred state calls from the past and diverts from fully exploring the present. Homesickness, a lost love, even loss of beauty or position in life can lead to the Honeysuckle state.

PHYSICAL TENDENCIES: Lethargy, sleepiness and diminished vitality can be concomitant symptoms.

DOCTRINE OF SIGNATURES: Honeysuckle is a climbing plant, overgrowing hedges and small trees, reminding of the memories of the past as they overgrow and weave through consciousness. The flowers grow in a cluster of red "tendrils" which point upward, as if to clasp at the mind or draw into states of yesterday.

As soon as the "tendrils" open, yellow-white flowers unfold, shooting upward in a lively swing and pointing at new prospects of regained happiness. They omit a heavy, laden scent, and, while it may stimulate reminiscences, it also directs longing to the future, to new dimensions, to the new growing out of the old.

METHOD OF PREPARATION: The flowering heads are picked with a few leaves and boiled for half an hour. The water is strained and used as medicine.

GOAL OF THERAPY: To give hope and incentive that happiness can be regained, to direct the mind from overindulgence in memories to enjoyment of the present moment, to soothe sadness.

HORNBEAM (CARPINUS BETULUS)

The remedy Hornbeam, together with Cerato, Scleranthus, Gentian, Gorse and Wild Oat, belongs to Bach's group of *For Those Who Suffer Uncertainty.* These remedies help those suffering from lack of certainty or strength of purpose in their daily affairs. Specifically, Hornbeam treats a mind not fully invigorated and lacking clarity of focus.

MIND: The mind in need of Hornbeam is fatigued and listless, and the body may feel this lethargy as well. One has to use willpower and push oneself to work, and still the mind may feel dull or lacking in power of concentration.

Due to fatigue, avoidance of work and procrastination may occur. Work does not appeal; one feels lax in fiber, thinking that one needs strengthening before duties can be fulfilled joyfully and with ease. It is as if the mind is not fully connecting with or seizing the tasks at hand. Brightness of concentration and devotion are diminished.

There is no deep-seated exhaustion, however; and one usually manages well, once one has mustered strength and willpower.

This remedy is of value in study and school settings, or whenever prolonged mental work is called for. It will revitalize mental powers of clarity and concentration and give perseverance. It is of service in developmental disorders, learning disabilities, and retardation (cf. Chestnut Bud, Mustard, Wild Oat).

EMOTIONS: Emotions center around the fatigue, and one copes with listlessness, frustration, temporary feelings of being overwhelmed, lack of interest, boredom, mild depression, occasional resentment and unkindness. One is more prone to be irritable and may be less inclined to be of assistance or do extra work for others, mostly because one needs the extra strength for oneself.

There are lighter Hornbeam cases, when one feels fairly well but lacks some invigoration or internal strengthening so that tasks are tackled more joyfully.

PHYSICAL TENDENCIES: Lethargy in mind and body, which may seem like a mild depression in some cases, often accompanies the Hornbeam state. The remedy can be of service after head injuries when power of concentration is diminished and fatigue sets in readily (cf. Scleranthus, Mustard, Wild Oat).

In brain dysfunction due to physical causation, as in organic mental syndromes and disorders, and in retardation, Hornbeam can help restore maximum clarity of consciousness within the physical limitations.

A chronic Hornbeam state may lead not only to physical fatigue but also to reduced interest in living a healthful life, with subsequent loss of overall vitality (see Wild Oat).

DOCTRINE OF SIGNATURES: As the remedy invigorates and strengthens mind and body, so does the tree have exceptionally durable and tough wood, akin to a "horn"; the wood actually has a whitish appearance and resembles a horn when polished. It lends itself to the manufacture of tool handles and other durable wooden articles. In comparison, the remedy Hornbeam enables one to use one's "tools" more efficiently; it enlivens and brings forth the best physical fibre and most invigorated consciousness to apply to one's tasks. Despite being tough, however, this wood can be bent into sturdy arches and frames, suggesting the flexibility and lack of harshness of a clear mind and toned-up body.

On looking closely at the foliage, catkins and flowers, one notices their droopy or relaxed nature, their apparent lack of fibre, hinting at the fatigued mind and body in need of this remedy.

Hornbeam helps to take life by the "horns," to move forward into accomplishment. It sends a "beam" of light into the mind.

METHOD OF PREPARATION: Collect twigs with both male and female flowers; the males are the catkins, whereas the females are smaller and actually look more like flowers and grow at the end of the twig. Boil for half an hour, strain the water and use as medicine.

GOAL OF THERAPY: To give alertness, brightness of consciousness, help with learning and task fulfillment. To invigorate mind and body.

IMPATIENS (IMPATIENS GLANDULIFERA)

Together with Heather and Water Violet, this remedy belongs to the group of *Loneliness,* as classified by Bach. All three remedies bring healing to those suffering from inner loneliness mostly due to self-centered reasons. Specifically, Impatiens treats a lack of patience and a tendency to tension and restlessness.

MIND: The mind is in a tense, wound-up state, and there is the urgency to work and move fast. Speeding in mind leads to speeding in one's movements, propelled by internal agitation and restlessness. Efficiency is a desirable goal in this state. One works fast and counts one's progress; one gets the job done. This inner dynamic, usually coupled with ability and skill, gives the personal perspective of being a leader or role model whom the others should follow or keep up with. Impatient people may be ruthless or self-centered, short of temper and intimidating.

In a less apparent case, there may be internal agitation and impatience but less urging on of others or ruthlessness. Still, this inner intense state is expressed through signs of mental and physical tension and occasional outbursts that are kept in check as much as possible. Here, the suffering may be great, since outlets of inner tension are blocked out of consideration for others, and inner tension may mount to an advanced stage of nervousness. In extreme cases, a nervous breakdown is threatened (cf. Cherry Plum, Rock Rose, Vervain).

Impatiens is indicated in all situations of life calling for increased patience and forbearance, or when one's lifestyle has become tense and driven.

In problems with impulse control and during drug rehabilitation, this remedy can help restore balance in mind/emotions and body, and increase self-mastery (cf. Cherry Plum, Holly, Vervain, Vine).

EMOTIONS: While being in the more expressed Impatiens state, one usually feels less inclined to linger with others and pay thoughtful attention but drives oneself and others from one activity to the next. Commonly, there are experiences of anger, frustration, dissatisfaction and irritability. A self-centered attitude may persist, and the feeling may exist that others should pay attention and revolve around the impatient person's idiosyncrasies.

The less expressed impatient type, since stifling the pressure within, may experience despair more easily, or feelings of being overwhelmed by high situational demands coupled with inner lack of nerve power and calm control.

For both types, inner peace is not easily achieved, and one can rarely rest calmly within oneself. Inner speed and tension constantly seek an outlet through engagement in activity and restless motion.

PHYSICAL TENDENCIES: Concomitant symptoms are nervous tension, strain, problems with high blood pressure, heart trouble and threatened nervous breakdown in extreme cases;

internal and external agitation and sudden explosions of temper with possible violence are common.

Since life and other people often do not move as fast as the impatient person, the impatient urges and the tendency to high-speed performance have to be held within, there creating nervous tension and cardiovascular strain.

DOCTRINE OF SIGNATURES: The Impatiens plant is marked by beautiful mauve flowers, emanating healing and calming by their special, soothing color. In resemblance of sudden temper outbursts, the plant's pods suddenly explode when ripe and scatter the seeds in all directions.

The plant's leaves have a tight appearance, standing rigidly from the stalk without the least sign of drooping. They have serrated edges, reminding of a saw or of the nerve strain and pain experienced in the Impatiens state.

METHOD OF PREPARATION: The mauve flowers are picked and floated onto a bowl of water which is left in the sun for several hours. The water is strained and preserved as medicine.

GOAL OF THERAPY: To give inner peace and freedom from restless pressure and agitation. To calm the nervous system. To concentrate on others and their needs; to grow in patience which is enjoyed rather than perceived as a burden.

LARCH (LARIX DECIDUA)

Bach grouped the remedy Larch under *For Despondency or Despair,* together with the remedies of Crab Apple, Oak, Willow, Star of Bethlehem, Sweet Chestnut, Elm and Pine. Specifically, Larch treats states of low self-confidence.

MIND: In the Larch state, one does not perceive oneself as capable or successful. One anticipates failure and feels that one cannot quite measure up to the challenges of life. For this reason, one may avoid new opportunities for growth and advancement, and this neglect further instills the wrong thinking pattern of not being in command and deserving failure.

Next to the perceptual mistake that one is not capable, one also compares oneself with others, believing everybody else to be more in charge of themselves and their lives. This further error of perception undermines the self-image, and the free-flowing expression of creativity and achievement is hampered. Basically, in the Larch state, the view into life is refracted and too much directed within the confines of oneself and one's perceived difficulties, rather than focused towards the people and tasks in one's environment (cf. Cerato, Mimulus). Worry about oneself detracts from the true duty of giving oneself in self-forgetfulness to the service and advancement of others. Once the importance of the other is understood, the hampered self is able to flow freely, and the feeling of success is experienced. Self-confidence is supported further as positive feedback lifts the self-image and gives joy of accomplishment.

EMOTIONS: While being within the confines of the self and not feeling empowered to rise to life's challenges, one may experience internal sadness, regret, despondency and even despair. In the Larch state, one feels suppressed within oneself, and it may seem impossible to rise above these limitations, despite one's despairing wish to do so. Feelings of inferiority, fear of failure, shyness and lack of personal strength may hurt deeply and gnaw at the root of life's happiness. There may also be a sense of loneliness and alienation from others, since one retreats easily, not feeling indispensable or as a valuable group asset. This may be interpreted as not tuning in to people or not paying them deference.

Larch is also a good helper for those undergoing demanding tasks and finding themselves intimidated or without confidence only occasionally. In the Larch state, one may feel lax and dampened, without energy or incentive. This experience may resemble the state of depression when there is no real courage or joy of going forward, of tackling life.

PHYSICAL TENDENCIES: Lack of energy, drooping sensation, weary limbs and reluctant posture may be concomitant features. One may appear withdrawn or not animated.

DOCTRINE OF SIGNATURES: The Larch tree has drooping branches, reminding of low energy or of a lack of feeling empowered. The flowers, however, point upward and are red and vibrant, speaking of new growth and creative expression.

Larch is a native tree of the European tundra which is known for long, cold winters with solidly frozen grounds. It is also found in cold mountainous regions. Here, only those trees survive that are able to live without water for an extended period of time. The Larch tree is one of them. In order to survive, the leaves are shed early, and tree life comes to a standstill, as it is unable to draw water from the frozen ground. For many months of the year, the tree is only seen with dark cones. This state reminds of the person's state of being hampered or of lacking energy, of coming to a standstill within the process of growth and renewal.

In spring, as frost declines, water is again raised through the trunk, and leaves and flowers have a chance to grow. This refreshing rebirth resembles the new surge of energy and confidence that flows through the person activated by joyful service and concentration on the duties of the moment, outgrowing the state of being stifled within oneself. New sap brings forth fruits in nature and person alike and ends the state of being "sapped."

METHOD OF PREPARATION: Twigs with young leaves and flowers are picked and boiled for half an hour. The water is strained and used as medicine.

GOAL OF THERAPY: To instill confidence and raise self-esteem by activating the joy of service. To connect with the world, to ground the self, instead of being confined within it.

MIMULUS (MIMULUS GUTTATUS)

Mimulus belongs to Bach's group *For Those Who Have Fear*, along with the remedies of Rock Rose, Cherry Plum, Aspen and Red Chestnut. Specifically, Mimulus treats concrete fears of a known origin.

MIND: In the Mimulus state, the mind envisions concrete fearful events, objects, or persons and shrinks away from them with a sense of dread. Or one lives in a constant state of fear, shyness and nervousness, due to immediate unfavorable circumstances plus chronic engagement in faulty thinking patterns.

Usually, Mimulus treats anticipatory fears which may even subside as the dreaded situation is encountered. This would apply to concrete events such as exams, surgery, a public appearance. Or one carries phobias of a chronic nature which reassert occasionally. These are fixations or obsessions of the mind, usually generated by a coupling of fearful experiences with a certain object, symbol or event. Mimulus also treats deep-seated existential fears such as fear of death, of poverty, of accidents, of loneliness and of other kinds of misfortunes. Hypochondriasis (cf. Chicory, Heather), excessive self-observation (cf. Cerato, Larch) and carefulness in one's endeavors are further signs of the Mimulus state.

The main differentiation from other remedies covering fears is the concrete nature of the content feared. In the Mimulus state, the mind always knows exactly what is feared, what is the object of dread. Dreaded things, persons or events are seen as a hurdle or as a dangerous deterrence that one seeks to avoid and retreats from. The remedy heals by lessening the impact of fearful content; dreaded events, objects or persons become just one usual occurrence in the continuum of life, instead of looming ahead and overshadowing one's consciousness. The remedy instills courage, a sense of being in charge.

This remedy is invaluable in all forms of anxiety disorders and phobias when there are concrete objects, persons or situations of fear (cf. Cherry Plum, Rock Rose).

EMOTIONS: Fearfulness, shyness or nervousness undermine the self-image, and one may feel inferior to others and embarrassed about one's lack of courage, tendency to fearful worry, and fear of appraisal. For this reason, fears are often not shared with others. On the contrary, one may try to conceal inner insecurities from others with an outward show of bravado, this state being defined in the Webster's dictionary as "pretended courage or defiant confidence, where there is really little or none." Depending on the case, this could grow into a potentially dangerous state of recklessness or demoralization of behavior. Usually, under milder circumstances, people secretly bear their dread.

Mimulus treats chronically shy people. A common emotion accompanying this state is regret or sadness about such internal hindrances which they often feel powerless to rise above. Shyness may also manifest physically and lead to easily aroused nervousness, usually responded to by the individual with attempts to hide this state from others; Mimulus successfully treats this state as well.

In severe states of dread, there can be a sense of internal agony or a slumping of personal vitality.

PHYSICAL TENDENCIES: Nervousness, not of a severe nature, lowered stamina and decrease in vitality are possible side effects of the Mimulus state. Fear lodges in the stomach region and creates disturbance; there are frequent loose bowels and intestinal griping pains during acute states of anxiety; in long-standing states of fearfulness, chronic diarrhea may develop. Hypochondriacal, obsessive anxieties can develop in regard to the manifestations of minor symptoms and intensify them. During physical rehabilitation after accidents or surgery, or during sickness or old-age infirmities, when every move frightens and small pains intimidate, Mimulus gives new courage and a more carefree attitude in mind and body.

In psychosomatic medicine, cardiac neurosis, duodenal ulcers in the passive-dependent patient, "emotional diarrhea," urticaria and atopic dermatitis have been closely linked with anxiety, excessive self-observation and fear of rejection.[3]

DOCTRINE OF SIGNATURES: The Mimulus plant is found throughout the land, preferring wet places, from sea marshes to mountain streams. This plant actually grows half in the water, lowering its roots deep into the gravel along streams. This nearness to sparkling and soothing streams indicates the plant's power to wash away hampering fears and free the mind. It also speaks of the plant's fearlessness; it is risky to grow near water, also in terms of fertility; the seeds often fall into the water and are washed away.

The bright yellow flowers, instead of pointing upward, are growing sideways along the stem, their position reminding of a dejected or tugged-in state. They appear to be retreating, as the Mimulus person retreats from dreaded events or imaginings.

Interestingly, the plant's common name is "Monkey Flower," reminding us of age-old myths and tales featuring the monkey as a symbol of fear. The botanists chose this name due to the arrangement of the petals which resemble a gaping mouth.

METHOD OF PREPARATION: Flowers are picked, placed in a bowl of water, and left to the sun's action for several hours. The water imbued with healing power is then strained and prepared as medicine.

GOAL OF THERAPY: To give freedom from internal stumbling blocks of a fearful kind, lessen preoccupation with fears, keep the mind in the here-and-now, and create feelings of safety and trust.

MUSTARD (SINAPIS ARVENSIS)

The remedy Mustard belongs to Bach's group *Not Sufficient Interest in Present Circumstances,* along with the remedies of Clematis, Honeysuckle, Wild Rose, Olive, White Chestnut and Chestnut Bud. Specifically, Mustard treats states of depression and gloom.

MIND: While being in the Mustard state, the mind is overshadowed by darkness and gloom, and there may be the sensation of a weight or downward-pull that depresses the person as a whole. The mind actually appears to receive less light, and the person cheers up in the warm, bright rays of the sun. People who crave light and sunshine are often in need of this remedy. Bach describes this state as a sensation of a dark cloud which descends, sometimes for inexplicable reasons.

The depressive character of this state makes the person turn inward, as if locked within, and the connection to the outside world is weakened. It takes effort to perk up and lift oneself out of this state; one may appear as absent-minded, introverted or disinterested in present circumstances. Cheerfulness or light-ness of being are not easily achieved under these circumstances. Life does not appeal; tasks and interaction with people seem to give no incentive or joy.

In depressive disorders, this remedy helps to bring about cure. In retardation, Mustard can help alleviate withdrawal and joylessness (cf. Hornbeam, Wild Oat).

EMOTIONS: Depression and gloom may bring the emo-tions of sadness, regret, boredom, self-pity and a sense of mean-inglessness. Or one may be morose and ill-tempered, seeking to retreat from involvement with others, while succumbing to gloom.

In severe cases, there may also be despair and a sense of desolation, of loneliness. One may feel as an island; life holds no incentive, while other people seem busy and cheered. The purpose of existence is veiled in the Mustard state; life seems to stagnate, and aspirations lie dormant.

In lighter cases, depression does not seem so overbearing but rather like a passing mood that reasserts from time to time. Some experiences, such as failure, sadness or regret, may bring on the Mustard state. At other times, the dark cloud descends unannounced, without apparent reason, to stifle the joy of the day. Here too, a lack of meaningful occupation, based on dormant potentials and unrecognized soul purpose in work and human relations, may lie at the root of the problem.

PHYSICAL TENDENCIES: Depression may lead to lowered vitality, lethargy, chronic fatigue; appetite disturbances (cf. Chicory, Crab Apple, Wild Oat), resulting in either weight loss or, should solace be found in eating, in weight gain; and constipation (cf. Chicory, Willow). There may also be sleep disturbances (cf. Pine, White Chestnut), disinterest in physical recreation, and a general decline in healthful interests and habits (see Wild Oat).

A head injury can be a mechanical reason for the appearance of the Mustard state. Nerve damage or faulty alignment of skull plates along fissures may dampen consciousness which may not be able to receive as much brightness and light as before the accident (cf. Hornbeam, Scleranthus, Wild Oat).

DOCTRINE OF SIGNATURES: The yellow Mustard plant spreads across the land profusely, reminding of the cheer-bringing rays of the sun. The plant usually grows above other grasses and weeds in the field, reminding of its healing quality to uplift and raise the mind above gloom. It also gives the idea of lightness and joy, not only by its color but also by its light dance in the breeze.

Mustard seeds have the tendency to lie dormant in the ground for many years; they suddenly spring up when the conditions for growth are right, and this is usually after the ground has been freshly plowed. Similarly, human potentials and talents may lie buried at the bottom of the inner self, preventing the soul's sparks of joy and meaningfulness from germinating. Plowing the inner self in the process of self-discovery, usually brought forth through the experience of the self in and through the world and its people, will help to air one's inner treasures. In biblical terms, the Mustard seed is used as a symbol of the inner kingdom of grace which grows to bring joy and fulfillment to the soul.

METHOD OF PREPARATION: The flowers are picked above any seed pods and boiled for half an hour. The water is strained and prepared as medicine.

GOAL OF THERAPY: To uplift the mind/emotions so that life appeals again and brings new adventure. To turn self-hampering, depressive introversion into fruitful relatedness, thus releasing sparks of self-actualizing creativity.

OAK (QUERCUS ROBUR)

The remedy Oak belongs to the group of *For Despondency or Despair,* as classified by Bach. The other remedies in this group are Crab Apple, Willow, Star of Bethlehem, Sweet Chestnut, Elm, Pine and Larch.

Specifically, Oak treats states of stoic perseverance and re-solve of willpower in the face of hardship.

MIND: In the Oak state, the mind is bent on perseverance in life's duties, even though strength and vitality may be failing. Or there may be unceasing disappointments or lack of rewards despite efforts made, and still the Oak person does not give up but resolves to struggle on with great strength of will and ever renewed hope.

In the Oak state, one may develop "tunnel vision," ever

focused on task completion and on upholding of life's commitments. Recreational activities and diversion of routine are not readily engaged in, since one stoically has in mind specific goals of accomplishment, while attempting to uphold strength and willpower. Inner weariness and lack of motivation may surface repeatedly, yet the battle is won again and again, and new incentive is raised when others would have given up a long time ago. Self-discipline, seriousness of intention, a tendency to overwork and loyalty are characteristic of the Oak mentality.

EMOTIONS: In the Oak state, emotions may be held at bay, as one struggles to uphold one's duties and loyalty. Emotions, if engaged in, are considered as disturbing to the routine and resolve of willpower, especially if they are related to self-pity, discouragement, selfishness, or longing for amusement and rest. This lack of pampering of the self leads to the typical Oak stoicism, as one rules oneself with an iron fist. Although there is satisfaction and personal pride obtained from self-discipline, vital emotional and physical needs are not met, and despondency and despair may grow from such suppression, especially if there is additional lack of progress or failure to achieve satisfying rewards in one's work.

Oftentimes, however, other people may benefit from such strength of will, as the Oak person works with loyalty, determined to never let anybody down. This in turn also gives new incentive to the hard-working person who finds rewards, if only temporarily, in offering such reliability. There are times, however, when work-oriented loyalty, typical for the Oak state, threatens to take precedence over family duties, and careful balancing is called for.

PHYSICAL TENDENCIES: Mental/emotional and physical weariness are common in the Oak state. Overwork and strength of will may lead to physical strain and undue stress. Older people may become bent from overexertion and one-sided activity.

In sickness, the Oak person struggles unceasingly with great determination to not succumb to invalidity. There is the urge to avoid necessary rest and restful recreation, even though both may be of vital need. Over time, psychosomatic diseases may express the continued rule of willpower over the need for healthful diversion and renewal (see Centaury).

DOCTRINE OF SIGNATURES: The sturdy English Oak, which is used for this remedy, is known for its stately growth and beautiful, durable wood which has been used extensively for building and paneling. This wood, as the person in the Oak state, is reliable and strong but also somewhat rigid and hardened. The tree has the tendency to grow tall and wide and reach a very advanced age; even when the first decay appears, leaves will struggle to form and renew the life cycle, just as the Oak mentality endeavors to never give up.

Oak trees are rich in nourishment and shelter; they sustain many life forms in their vicinity and, through one of their species, even give "food" and sustenance to the work-oriented human mentality. The tree's richness also expresses the human reliability and loyal tendency to support others, as portrayed in the Oak mentality.

METHOD OF PREPARATION: Red female flowers are gathered and put in a bowl of sunlit water for several hours. The water is strained and prepared as medicine.

GOAL OF THERAPY: To open the mind to new balanced options of work and recreation. To instill playfulness and lightness of will, even when working.

OLIVE (OLEA EUROPAEA)

The remedy Olive, together with the remedies of Clematis, Honeysuckle, Wild Rose, White Chestnut, Mustard and Chestnut Bud, belongs to the group of *Not Sufficient Interest in Present Circumstances*, as classified by Bach. Specifically, Olive treats states of exhaustion in mind/emotions, body and spirit.

MIND: In the Olive state, the mind is too weary to carry on, and one knows that a certain limit has been reached and reserves are depleting. It is a state of exhaustion reaching deep into the self, undermining the very spirit or inner core of existence.

As one tries to struggle on with life's duties, may they be mainly in the mental, emotional or physical realm, one realizes that they grow above one's head and are hardly within one's power to accomplish. One begins a certain task and cannot complete it; the urge to slow down and rest is simply too strong. Consequently, one may appear absent-minded, disinterested or lethargic.

In the field of social service, as burn-out syndrome develops, during or after prolonged sickness, during any demanding times asking for extra effort, Olive comes to the rescue, bringing the healing spark to carry on.

EMOTIONS: In the Olive state, emotional life is weary as well. One is unable, as in the burn-out syndrome, to care as much about others as one used to. One cannot get worked up or excited over people and issues which previously gave incentive and joy. Due to having depleted inner reserves, one now finds oneself retreating to an inner core, harboring strength and trying to protect those remaining powers necessary to get through the day.

Sadness, depression, discouragement, a sense of meaninglessness and apathy may accompany the exhaustion. The inner spiritual core may falter in faith and be devoid of seeing purpose and beauty in life.

PHYSICAL TENDENCIES: Weariness and exhaustion permeate all physical structures and call for rest and recuperation.

DOCTRINE OF SIGNATURES: The Olive tree, native to the Mediterranean, gives the appearance of weariness and lack of vibrancy by its grayish color; the bark is gray-brown and the leaves have a gray-green sheen. In addition, this tree does not reach a great height and its fruits are bitter, becoming edible only after having been soaked in salt or lye solution, hinting at the bitterness and discomfort experienced in the Olive state.

On the other hand, the evergreen tree portrays the life-giving quality of the remedy. It reaches a great age, ceaselessly bringing forth flowers and fruits. Even if cut to a stump, it will regenerate shoots, soon bearing fruit. These are rich and wholesome, once treated, and provide energy to a depleted metabolism, as well as offering a well-balanced oil, ideal for consumption. The creamy-white flowers are abundant, carrying the plant's hidden healing power of regenerating the body, mind/emotions and inner spirit.

METHOD OF PREPARATION: The flowering clusters are placed in sunlit water for several hours. The remedy is prepared from the strained water.

GOAL OF THERAPY: To revitalize the person as a whole, recharge one's reserves, give new incentive to engage in life.

PINE (PINUS SYLVESTRIS)

The remedy Pine belongs to Bach's group of *For Despondency or Despair,* together with the remedies of Crab Apple, Oak, Willow, Star of Bethlehem, Sweet Chestnut, Elm and Larch. Specifically, Pine treats states of guilt, regret and self-reproach.

MIND: In the Pine state, one is introverted, subdued by the burdens of guilt and regret. Or one may experience the Pine state more superficially, since a bad conscience has been suppressed and not heeded, only to reassert as inner uncertainty and lack of integrity. In this case, the remedy will bring to one's moral consciousness the true content of guilt, to be worked through and understood. In the introverted, reflective Pine state, however, the person usually responds to a very finely tuned conscience which does not allow for ease and pressures the conscientious mind, even though there may be little real guilt. Here the remedy will reduce self-blame and set the self free.

These are the two extremes of the Pine state, the middle ground being occupied by the normal Pine mentality, asserting itself after true wrong doing which is regretted subsequently and wished to be undone. The remedy will lighten this burden and give the feeling of having a new chance.

In the Pine state, one may preoccupy or obsess with guilt and self-reproach, and some burdens may not be released for years, creating a sense of unworthiness from deep within. In some severe cases, the mind may be drawn to the act of guilt again and again, either replaying it or actually carrying it out, as if to overcome the internal sense of failure, or as if to make sure that maybe the degree of wrong doing was not as severe as thought. These exercises seemingly deaden the conscience, if only temporarily, and are to help the self integrate those unwholesome experiences which do not readily fit into the desired self-image. Actually, they serve to perpetuate the problem by adding continued focus and denial rather than releasing the guilt content through moral resolve and reconciliation with those offended. In other cases, ritualistic cleansing acts may be repeated over and over again to calm one's conscience. This also detracts from true soul release which is best achieved in active conversion and social reconciliation.

In the treatment of mental illness, Pine is indicated in obsessive-compulsive, self-punitive, and perfection-oriented or ritualistic behavior and thinking, as in obsessive-compulsive personality disorder (cf. Crab Apple, Rock Water, Vervain). The remedy is of service in delusional disorders and paranoid personality disorder with fear of being punished or persecuted (cf. Aspen). In these cases, inner unresolved guilt calls for release through punishment by higher persons or powers. It is not the "others," however, but the persons' own conscience or exaggerated conscientiousness haunting them.

EMOTIONS: In the usual Pine state, as well as in the overly conscientious Pine state, emotions center around shame, regret and self-blame in regard to not having fulfilled one's high ideals. One may also experience true despondency and despair, as one feels unable to rise above the burdens of guilt and failure to forgive oneself. Conscientious people may even assume responsibility and blame for failure when in reality other persons have caused the wrong doing or neglect.

In the fleeting Pine state, the emotional side is colored by gliding over the dictates of conscience, taking the issues lightly, growing in carelessness and insensitivity, while inner guilt feelings stifle soul peace and leave a sense of unresolved regret.

Should repeated guilt feelings grow into obsessive or ritualistic preoccupation, one actually sees a decline in emotional content, as the mind tries to establish balance by a rather monotonous, mechanical way. Secondary emotions, such as frustration, anger, rigidity and alienation from oneself and others, may arise from such fixation.

PHYSICAL TENDENCIES: The body may show signs of becoming burdened, depressive or rigid, due to excessive introversion and self-blame.

In psychosomatic medicine, obsessive-compulsive states and exaggerated conscientiousness have been found, in extreme cases, to lead to gastric and duodenal ulcers, irritable colon, pruritis (skin disorder with itching), nervous breathing syndrome and insomnia (cf. Mustard, White Chestnut).[3] These illnesses represent examples of expressing deep-seated conflict through the body and show possible physical side effects of obsessive guilt.

DOCTRINE OF SIGNATURES: This specific pine tree, also called Scots Pine, is native to the Scottish Highlands, a land known for high morals and introversion, the latter due mainly to its thin population. From these highlands, the tree grew to be the most widely distributed pine in the world, providing Europe with a major source of timber. It is also grown as an evergreen ornament and Christmas trees, reminding of its healing quality of reconciliation and rebirth.

The tree's crown has a tendency to grow in irregular branches and may appear somewhat crooked or out of line, although the entire tree is beautiful and stately. In the Pine state, the personal "crown" of pride in oneself is damaged or out of line, and one bows one's "crown" in regret and apology.

The pine oil carries medicinal properties by relaxing and also toning muscles, if applied topically; it works against rigidity which may grow out of exaggerated conscientiousness and obsessive guilt. Furthermore, the plant shows tolerance to city smoke and helps to keep the air clean; actually, extracts from this plant are used for cleansing purposes, to cut through dirt and add a pleasant scent, these properties being symbolic expressions of the plant's power to release the burdens of guilt and bring renewed freshness to the soul.

The longevity of pines and their evergreen needles may hint at the length of some of our unresolved guilt feelings which may root in childhood experiences, sending repeated "needle pricks" of conscience throughout life.

METHOD OF PREPARATION: Twigs with male and female flowers are picked and boiled for half an hour. The boiled water is strained and prepared as medicine.

GOAL OF THERAPY: To let go of the past, while making amends. To experience self-forgiveness and regain lightness of the inner self, akin to feelings of rebirth. To forgive others their faults.

RED CHESTNUT (AESCULUS CARNEA)

The remedy Red Chestnut belongs to Bach's group *For Those Who Have Fear,* together with the remedies of Rock Rose, Mimulus, Cherry Plum and Aspen. Specifically, Red Chestnut treats fear for the welfare of others.

MIND: In the Red Chestnut state, the mind reaches out to a loved one, who is usually not within one's reach or within one's power to be helped, and one worries fearfully about the other's welfare. The idea that someone loved and cherished whom one enjoys caring for is out of reach, unassisted and threatened, undermines one's strength and nerve power. One wants to help yet cannot, and the nervous energy finds no outlet, simply "eating" away at one's reserves.

An active imagination, anticipation of something dreadful, plus loss of faith in the benevolence of the other's destiny compound the problem and may propel the mind to irrational heights of anxiety. In this state, one cannot let go; although physical distance, old age, sickness or dangers have severed the safety of the love bond, one's mind and heart are still with the other who is most precious and unbearable to lose.

EMOTIONS: Usually, grief and worry surround the Red Chestnut state; the trauma of grief may account for the sense of danger; the loss of safe vicinity and togetherness may explain the fears for the other's life and limb, any separation resembling death.

Feelings of helplessness and self-blame for inability to assist may further weaken emotional stability.

PHYSICAL TENDENCIES: Physical nervousness and anxious weakness can be extreme, with tightening from fear in the stomach and abdominal region. This internal tightening is a psychosomatic attempt to hold on to the other and give protection from dangers.

DOCTRINE OF SIGNATURES: Originally, the Red Chestnut tree stems from a chance crossing between the American Red Buckeye, *Aesculus pavia,* and the Horse Chestnut tree, *Aesculus hippocastanum,* which is native to Europe. This new tree was first discovered around 1820. It is unusual for any Bach

Remedy to have grown out of two different plants, yet in this case, there may be a symbolic message. The Red Chestnut state grows out of a bond between two poles which were once unified and then severed by distance, though still connected through mutual love and fearful worry. The trees, springing up in two different continents and forming a new tree with healing power, may express the two poles of people, the dividing Europeans, as they set out to conquer the American land. The pioneers and their relatives of the home land, which stayed behind in the safety and affection of family life, were connected by a Red Chestnut bond which spanned an unusual distance and reached into uncharted territory. The tree carrying the healing remedy formed shortly after the North American continent reached self-determination and independence from the mother continent in 1776, just as the remedy brings independence and mutual trust in the other's strength to those closely linked by a Red Chestnut bond.

The Red Chestnut tree shows beautiful raised clusters of red flowers, effectively contrasting with a background of dark-green leaves. This vibrant impression signals danger, the red color speaking of alarm or nervousness. The tree is also known to be undermined by sickness or decay more readily than other trees, portraying the nervous weakness and loss of power experienced in the Red Chestnut state. Yet, the overall impression of the tree is beauty and clarity of color and form, these resembling the assets of clarity and reason it brings to a mind torn by fear for another.

METHOD OF PREPARATION: The flowering clusters are boiled for half an hour. The boiled water is strained and used as medicine.

GOAL OF THERAPY: To release others to their destiny with faith. To balance fear, irrational worry, and exaggerated imagination with trust and reasonable insight. To give stamina and increase nerve power.

ROCK ROSE (HELIANTHEMUM NUMMULARIUM)

This remedy belongs to Bach's group *For Those Who Have Fear,* together with the remedies of Mimulus, Cherry Plum, Aspen and Red Chestnut. Specifically, Rock Rose treats states of intense fear and panic, plus a chronically weakened nervous system.

MIND: This is the state of fright and heightened anxiety when threats and dangers propel to run or speed, even though it may just happen in one's internal self. The Rock Rose response is a typical "fight or flight" response, as the whole organism prepares to either fight and defend or escape from a perceived threat. Inner agitation and nervousness can be extreme and undermine health and inner peace, if surfacing repeatedly.

Usually, the Rock Rose state originates in frightening circumstances such as the nearness of one's own or another person's death, or one is overly exposed to specific dangers or work-related hazards. Frequent nightmares are an indication for this remedy, as well as fixations and obsessions of a fearful nature, as in phobias or panic disorders. Here, repeated fearful experiences or one-time traumas of fright have become linked with a certain person, object or circumstance which will trigger renewed fear on contact even when the real danger has passed (cf. Cherry Plum, Mimulus).

In a chronic state of advanced nervousness, especially if there is frequent starting and inner trembling, this remedy is the predominant healer. Prolonged fearful worry, chronic loss of sleep, a hectic, demanding life can bring on a chronic Rock Rose state, basically this being an exhaustion of nerve power. Rock Rose is of service in all anxiety disorders, in post-traumatic stress disorder and in adjustment disorder which, in comparison to post-traumatic stress disorder, is a milder response to a less severe trauma related to fear or terror (cf. Star of Bethlehem).

EMOTIONS: While being in this fearful state, further emotions arising from fear are very intense, carried by the inner force and speed of the "fight or flight" response. In regard to fighting, we observe the additional emotions of anger, hatred, irrational resentment, impatience, whereas the flight response triggers feelings of helplessness, despair or of being caught.

In a chronic case of nervousness, in addition to chronic anxiety, there may be easily aroused tears, longing for help, desire for peace and rest, these emotions being characteristic for those predominantly engaging in the flight response. The fight reaction will elicit chronic impatience and aggressiveness towards people; or one may vacillate between the two poles. Usually, irrationality due to fear and sudden precipitation of emotions are present in both cases.

PHYSICAL TENDENCIES: Acute anxiety states cause accelerated heart beat and breathing, shortness of breath, choking sensation, dry mouth, indigestion with possible nausea, vomiting and diarrhea, dizziness and fainting, and internal and external trembling. Chronic advanced nervousness is characterized by nervous weakness, insomnia, lack of physical and mental/emotional endurance, shaking, digestive problems including lack of appetite, heightened sensitivity to noise and touch, first signs of a nervous breakdown, and other typical symptoms of an exhausted nervous system. Rock Rose can prevent a nervous breakdown from developing, and, once a nervous breakdown has occurred, this remedy restores equilibrium (cf. Cherry Plum, Impatiens, Vervain). It is also indicated in muscular rigidity due to manic or catatonic states when terror is an underlying factor (cf. Cherry Plum).

DOCTRINE OF SIGNATURES: Rock Rose is a small, delicate yellow flower with trailing branches which grow sideways before they raise their yellow flowers. This can be viewed as a shrinking away from dangers or not standing up to them in fear and terror. In addition, the soft yellow petals look slightly wilted or ruffled, reminding of a shaky, trembling or sensitive state. The flowers bloom shortly, soon fade and wilt away, speaking of nervous weakness and the nearness to death which some people experience in the Rock Rose state.

This sensitive plant also speaks of courage and stamina; in the English language, it is named after its common habitat, namely rocky soil, this being difficult terrain for any plant to take lasting hold in. Its vibrant yellow color transmits peace and calm; the bright flowers shine like warming suns on the rocky grounds. Actually, the petals themselves only open in the sun, therefore its Greek name "helios" for "sun" and "anthemon" for "flower." The sun draws out the full flower, while unfavorable cloudy skies cause it to stay closed, just as a person does not open up in face of threats and is unable to "bloom." During medicinal preparation as well, the sun's rays activate the flower's healing potential in a sunlit bowl of water.

To draw a parallel to the body, the human solar plexus, being the "sun" center of the nervous system from where important sympathetic nerve fibers pass to the visceral organs, is agitated and weakened during fright and nervousness and greatly benefits from the healing "rays" of this flower.

METHOD OF PREPARATION: Rock Rose flowers are gathered and put in a sunlit bowl of water for several hours. The water imbued with healing power is strained and prepared as medicine.

GOAL OF THERAPY: To reduce terror in an emergency, give inner peace and calm, instill courage. To heal chronic anxiety and remove the bad effects of trauma from fright and shock, to raise health of the nervous system and subsequently of the whole organism.

ROCK WATER (AQUA PETRA)

This remedy belongs to Bach's group *Overcare for Welfare of Others,* along with the remedies of Beech, Vine, Vervain and Chicory. These remedies heal the tendency to overly influence and control others. Specifically, Rock Water heals the urge to inspire others with one's example of self-mastery.

MIND: The Rock Water state comes about from having chosen a special path of personal advancement and self-discipline and adhering strictly to its rules. Though difficult at times and usually involving denial of pleasurable pursuits, this regiment instills personal pride and one feels inspired to teach others the way of perfection. The perceptual mistake is made in regard to each person's individual way of growth and self-determination in terms of choosing a particular path or simply choosing to flow through life, without regiments and denial of pleasure. One needs to recognize that one's own ways of advancement are not necessarily suited to the needs of others and may even be detrimental to oneself and others.

A differentiation needs to be made between the self-chosen path of denial and an imposed Rock Water state, propelled by circumstance and not wished for. The self-chosen path usually involves a spiritual quest, coupled with a health regiment for mind and body, which can actually undermine the very goals of spiritual awakening, those being based on release from self-preoccupation and kindling of joy on all levels of being. The imposed Rock Water state, entailing a sacrifice or loss of pleasure, actually grows out of an initial state of disappointment, severity or despair. Yet, one rises to the occasion, controls oneself and finds incentive in living without the usual ease or enjoyment. Out of this self-control and mastery of a difficult readjustment comes personal pride and the desire to inspire others to be equally strong.

Here again, though aspirations are worthwhile, one needs to take into consideration the other's individual way of growth and actually take an inventory of all possible avenues of finding joy, before the path of self-denial is consciously entered. This step is of importance to all seeking healing from the Rock Water dilemma. In addition, life's circumstances may change and offer new opportunities for satisfaction and personal fulfillment. The Rock Water mentality tends to adhere to routines and one-sided acceptance of limitations when life has moved on to new challenges. The mind overly focuses on the limitations, battles them repeatedly with willpower until one feels in charge again, instead of releasing the burdens and putting mental emphasis elsewhere.

In the rehabilitation of addictive drug use or addictive behavioral patterns, to name one example, a Rock Water state is likely to come on, as one consciously chooses the path of self-denial and self-improvement and battles the newly emerging urge of engaging in the habitual pattern. Here, sheer physical need makes this a battle of self-control, and a Rock Water state is almost unavoidable, if only temporarily.

Any time, self-martyrdom and unnecessary heroism in regard to suppression of one's gratification and desire are exhibited, Rock Water is indicated, especially so if there is additional incentive to convert others. Within this dynamic, one can also observe ritualistic, perfection-oriented, obsessive-compulsive and self-punitive behavior (cf. Cherry Plum, Crab Apple, Pine, Vervain).

EMOTIONS: In the freely chosen Rock Water state, as one suppresses desires considered unwholesome, one may block off important parts of the personality and stifle vital avenues of joy. These overriding states of willpower, rigidity and self-centered toughness may create underlying emotions of frustration, sadness, depression or anger. These "warning signals" are usually suppressed further and not permitted to deter one's self from the chosen path. A hardening of the inner personality occurs; life's ease and balanced flow are stopped, and, oftentimes, others are supposed to participate in this regiment. The idea of "misery seeks company" could apply as additional underlying motive to some cases, although the converter sees his own efforts and inspirations as only worthwhile and benefiting the other. This state of self-deception further deters from unraveling in self-analysis this self-undermining dynamic of unnecessary denial, harshness, personal pride in having achieved self-mastery, and the urge to convert others.

In the imposed Rock Water state, the emotions of sadness, depression, frustration are permitted into consciousness, yet have to be battled to some extent so as not to be too overwhelming and forceful. Simultaneously, the suppression itself of vital needs and desires takes its toll, as self-mastery, resolve and willpower are necessary to find a balance. Rock Water will help defray the intensity of the inner conflict, lessen the severity of the loss, while reducing preoccupation and the necessity of intensified willpower and allowing for gentleness and spontaneity to flow from the inner self.

PHYSICAL TENDENCIES: Rigidity and hardening of physical structures may occur. Excessive willpower may result in inner tension and strain.

DOCTRINE OF SIGNATURES: The water used for this remedy is gained from pure streams, especially from those renown to carry healing power. In England, a special well is used for the worldwide distribution of this remedy, yet other sources of healing wells may apply also.

Water is a symbol for the balanced, gentle flow of consciousness, for ease and rejuvenation. Yet, it also is persistent, timeless, and all-pervading, and even rocks are gently smoothed with time, as the water finds its path of undeterred flow. These are the healing qualities of Rock Water; it restores the gentle flow of consciousness, helps to overcome internal harshness, and washes away the rocks of denial and resolve of willpower.

On preparing the remedy, one notices the "empty" bowl in comparison to the abundance of precious flowers used in the other preparations of Bach Remedies. The Rock Water state itself is barren, without the flowers of fulfillment.

METHOD OF PREPARATION: Water from any special well known to carry healing power is placed in a sunlit bowl for only one hour and used as medicine.

GOAL OF THERAPY: To allow for gentleness toward oneself to emerge. To see perfection and self-mastery as obtainable within interpersonal relations, as one endeavors to bring true kindness to all, rather than preoccupying with personal perfectionism and denial which do not really benefit others and oneself.

SCLERANTHUS (SCLERANTHUS ANNUUS)

The remedy Scleranthus belongs to the group of *For Those Who Suffer Uncertainty,* as classified by Bach. The other remedies in this group are Cerato, Gentian, Gorse, Hornbeam and Wild Oat. Specifically, Scleranthus treats states of indecisiveness and vacillation between options.

MIND: In the Scleranthus state, the mind is swinging back and forth between two or sometimes several options and is unable to come to a satisfying decision which deems right and originates from inner certainty. As one vacillates between two options, one may continually reiterate the pros and contras of one option and then of the other, trying to find the best solution. A tentative decision is then made; one option is dropped and the other embraced shortly. Here, the Scleranthus mind cannot stay, as the other option reasserts with appealing content and the idea of losing it creates dread and regret. The tentative decision is discarded again, and one swings back to the other side to repeat the whole process.

As vacillating continues, the mind becomes increasingly preoccupied, overstimulated with internal arguments, disoriented and exasperated, while dread about possibly making the wrong choice paralyzes the inner center of decisiveness further. In this state of being overcome by inner uncertainty, by a lack of intuitive guidance, and by the disorienting flooding of the mind with details, the mind is unable to raise consciousness to a higher vantage point from where a calm overview can be achieved and a decision be made. Yet, while wrestling with the options, the person in the Scleranthus state usually is determined to solve the problem independently of others, since the decisions often are personal and of magnitude. One is aware of the importance of one's individual inner center of meaning, clarity and purpose which needs to be heard so that certainty and guidance can be conveyed to the mind.

Scleranthus is also the indicated remedy for those over-stimulated by details and cares, as they are torn back and forth between various demands and too frazzled to find peace of mind. The remedy also helps those unable to decide on a certain occupation or form of play, as in child's play; as they move from one possibility to the next without savoring any one option to the fullest. The remedy is not necessarily indicated in a decision-making process only but treats states of mental overstimulation, confusion, inability to calm the mind in response to impressions, and lack of power to come to a meditative or contemplative state.

It is of use also in the treatment of bipolar disorders, as in manic-depressive states; in dissociative personality disorders such as multiple personality disorder; and in conversion disorder (cf. Chicory, Heather), also called hysterical neurosis of the conversion type, when symptoms vacillate between extremes.

EMOTIONS: Emotional instability, capriciousness and mood swings are common in the Scleranthus state. As the mind vacillates, the emotions as well are easily swung from one extreme to the next. One minute, there is weeping, the next brings laughter; or there is incentive and enthusiasm in regard to a certain idea, when suddenly disinterest asserts itself. Capriciousness may be intense and exasperate those helpful people trying to accommodate to the various, changing demands or wishes.

Emotionally, as well as mentally, one becomes too easily impressed and overreacts, while the inner center of stability is not fortified; and decisive power and, in some cases, willpower are lacking.

The emotional state of those caught in a serious decision-making process is one of dread at the thought of making the wrong choice, of being overwhelmed, of feeling inadequate, and there may be the rising feeling of despair and futility. Even after one has settled on a decision, one may feel uneasy and weak within, anticipating some unfortunate event, believing things not to be quite right, and still lacking inner certainty and peace.

PHYSICAL TENDENCIES: The body is marked by changeability of symptoms as well. Symptoms may alternate between mental/emotional and physical expression, as in conversion disorder when the body expresses a psychological need. There may be quick fluctuations in weight. Scleranthus can help alleviate travel sickness due to disturbance in equilibrium.

After head injuries (cf. Hornbeam, Mustard, Wild Oat), when the mind seems out of balance, overstimulated, with a sense of chaos, Scleranthus can help give mental calm and restore the mind's ability to be in charge, to regain an overview (cf. Elm).

In psychosomatic studies determining the susceptibility to pulmonary tuberculosis, a state of prolonged indecisiveness, usually in regard to a vital decision, has been found to precede the onset of illness. Unable to decide, the organism resorts to illness which then subsides as the decision is made.[9] Here, indecisiveness resembles a deadlock with possible impairment of breathing, which could lay the ground for a lung infection. The free flow of breath also has been found to be deterred in a person receiving ambiguous attention and vacillating between feeling loved and rejected. The inspiratory disease Singultus, originally meaning "hiccup," has been linked with this dynamic. The person cannot receive or take in kindness regularly, and inspiration becomes disturbed.[10]

DOCTRINE OF SIGNATURES: The Scleranthus plant grows in tangled formation close to the ground, speaking of the confused mind which cannot easily rise above various impressions and gain an overview. The stems tend to split into two side stems at the end and may hint at the vacillating process between two options. This plant forms unobtrusive flowers; actually, they could be considered additional leaves, since they blend in with the rest of the plant and are without distinct petals or color. This characteristic of the plant symbolically conveys the inability to express with distinction and come to a clear decision, as experienced in the Scleranthus state.

The plant's common name "knawel" derives from the German "Knäuel," meaning a tangled knot. The plant's habitat is made on dry, sandy soil, as if to speak of a house built on shifting grounds. The remedy will help to untangle mental knots, give stability and anchoring in certainty.

METHOD OF PREPARATION: The flowering sprigs are placed in a bowl of water and left in the sun for several hours. The water is strained subsequently and used as medicine.

GOAL OF THERAPY: To give mental, emotional, physical equilibrium. To reduce the impact and distortion of vacillation and uplift the mind to a point of true insight. To strengthen intuitive perception.

STAR OF BETHLEHEM (ORNITHOGALUM UMBELLATUM)

Star of Bethlehem is listed in the group of *For Despondency or Despair,* as classified by Bach. The additional remedies of this group are Crab Apple, Oak, Willow, Sweet Chestnut, Elm, Pine and Larch. Specifically, Star of Bethlehem treats states of grief and shock.

MIND: In the Star of Bethlehem state, the mind is closed down and has retreated into a state of shock and grief. The bad news received can be so severe, as to not find full acceptance by the conscious mind which may not be able to cope with the inevitability of the grief-causing circumstances.

The mind uses several ways to defend against the integration of such shocking news. Other remedies, in addition to Star of Bethlehem, may be asked for, these being indicated in brackets in the following text. Initially, we usually encounter outcry and protest against such misfortune. Subsequently, there can be denial and a desperate hope that the news is not true, plus internal numbing or standstill which does not allow for the experience of grief to surface fully. This postponement of affects may last for years, and one usually notices signs of mental/emotional deadening, as if parts of the personality had gone to sleep or had closed down in shock (Wild Rose).

Another reaction to grief, while there may be some internal numbing as well, is the gliding over or taking lightly those things that cannot be changed, and one may actually show cheer and lift up others in their grief. Here, internal agony is present but hidden from others (Agrimony).

Another coping mechanism is undue anger and prolonged outrage which help the suffering person to overcome helplessness and reassert personal force which had been unable to prevent the saddening events (Holly). On the other hand, if helplessness and resignation are succumbed to (Wild Rose), the grieving person may retreat into introversion and depression and hide inner feelings from others, not allowing the matter to be touched or worked through with the help of others (Mustard).

Lifting the mind to a possible reunion in the future, should a loved one have died (Clematis), or dwelling on beloved memories of the past (Honeysuckle), are two other ways to lessen the severity of grief and help the mind to accept the inevitability of events. Usually, these states arise after the initial shock subsides.

Resenting one's fate and rejecting the experience is another avenue of shunning the full experience of grief (Willow), or the whole event is criticized, not fully integrated into one's heart and not allowed to create pain (Beech). One may also resort to exaggerated thoughts of nihilism and meaninglessness and discount the value of life and its treasures in general (Sweet Chestnut).

In post-traumatic stress disorder, when psychological disturbances due to the traumatic impact prevail, Star of Bethlehem brings about healing (cf. Rock Rose). The remedy is also indicated in adjustment disorder which represents a milder reaction to a less severe trauma.

EMOTIONS: If emotions are allowed to be expressed fully, there is the complete experience of sadness with heart-wrenching impact, deepest pain and despair. Despondency and hopelessness settle over the heart like a heavy blanket. In this stage of intrusiveness, meaning the full experience of emotions, additional feelings such as fear, shame, frustration and guilt can surface.

After the initial outcry that may be accompanied by denial, the stage of intrusiveness prepares the personality to integrate and work through the shocking experience and move into the stage of acknowledgment of limitations and possibilities. From here, as healing happens and emotions balance with reason and clarity, moving forward and proceeding with life is possible again.

PHYSICAL TENDENCIES: Lack of appetite, digestive problems, shock and collapse, and other symptoms of grief and shock may be present. The diaphragm is known to tighten during grief and impair breathing, leading to frequent sighing.

Ulcerative colitis and Crohn's disease have been found to be related to states of grief which have not been worked through.[3] One may interpret that the body expresses the traumatic loss by shedding parts of the bowel lining, by losing vital parts on the physical plane as well.

After accidents, as physical cells and mind/emotions carry the memory of the trauma, Star of Bethlehem acts as releasing agent.

DOCTRINE OF SIGNATURES: Star of Bethlehem belongs to the lily family and shows beautiful, pristine-white six-petalled flowers. The buds are egg-shaped and are actually formed by the petals themselves which show a green stripe on the back. This bud resembles the closed-down heart or the egg concealing life. As the petals open, this happens only in bright sunshine, a star seems to unfold in perfect symmetry of six pointed petals. This symbolizes the healing of the heart, as balance, open-ness and receptivity to experience take hold again.

The leaves are long and narrow, with straight edges and pointed at the tip, resembling a blade or a sword. Their rather aggressive appearance reminds of adversity or hardship. Out of this bed of swords grow the stars of healing, the heralds of comfort and inner light. As the Star of Bethlehem announced the coming of Christ and his healing message to all mankind, this plant brings rescue to those overcome by grief and sorrow.

METHOD OF PREPARATION: The flowering parts are boiled for half an hour. Subsequently, the water is strained and used as medicine.

GOAL OF THERAPY: To comfort the heart. To release the trauma of grief and prevent states of shock from imprinting on the mental/emotional and physical, cellular level.

SWEET CHESTNUT (CASTANEA SATIVA)

Sweet Chestnut belongs to the group of *For Despondency or Despair,* as classified by Bach. The other remedies in this group are Crab Apple, Oak, Willow, Star of Bethlehem, Elm, Pine and Larch. Specifically, Sweet Chestnut treats states of mean-inglessness and anguish beyond endurance.

MIND: In the Sweet Chestnut state, the mind is stretched to its utmost limits of endurance and seems to be unable to experience further anguish. The torture reaches deep into the self, creating meaninglessness, faithlessness, nihilism and despair. Not being able to rely on faith and not seeing meaning in one's suffering, the person experiences this severe state with intensi-fied impact; the inner reserves of soul strength have been drained.

Any severe existential crisis or religious despair with loss of faith, the "dark night of the soul," or any unwholesome, morbid preoccupation with death calls for this remedy. After a loved one has died, some people are in need of this remedy, as they do not understand where the other has gone, and they cannot accept nothingness where once was life.

Severe and prolonged physical suffering can undermine inner fortitude and create a Sweet Chestnut state. From this agony, as well as from other severe hardship which has created deep existential doubt and despair, can arise the suicidal wish, the ultimate wish to escape the unbearable state.

This remedy can also be indicated in a person free of acute anguish but nonetheless suffering from lack of aspirations and meaningful purpose to the point of nihilism and negation of life's value.

The perceptive focus in the Sweet Chestnut state is narrowed and imprisoned in the dark, nihilistic side of life.

This remedy is of service in the treatment of depressive disorders (cf. Mustard), especially when suicide is threatened and there is deep-seated despair.

EMOTIONS: The drained inner self is rather void of emotional life but feels as in a deadlock or as in darkness. Despair and despondency weigh heavily and leave no room for the forces of emotional joy and healing to operate. For this reason, death may seem the only way out of a hopeless, barren situation.

In a lighter Sweet Chestnut case, when atheism, nihilism and lack of positive aspirations have undermined soul peace, the emotional life is hampered as well. Emotions, such as love and devotion, loyalty toward higher values, and gratitude to-

wards the miracle of creation, may not be experienced sufficiently. Many times, the person has made a conscious decision
not to worship God in faith, not to believe in survival of the
soul after death, and not to strive for humility and service. Negation of these values cuts off important channels of soul joy
and impedes union with the wholesome forces of life, within
oneself and within the social context. A sense of meaninglessness of life may lead to carelessness of attitude, while deep inside despair finds a soil for growth.

PHYSICAL TENDENCIES: This remedy can be of service during physical agony when suffering seems to be unbearable and gnaws at the will to live. Physical side effects, arising
from the depression and morbid preoccupation, may resemble
those ascribed to depression (see Mustard).

DOCTRINE OF SIGNATURES: The Sweet Chestnut
tree is a stately Mediterranean tree, fairing well in hot, dry cli-
mates. Its trunk is marked by dark, deeply furrowed bark; the
furrows do not grow straight along the tree but form curves
and writing lines, reminding of a state of heavily burdened
agony or of the slow, furrowed process of writhing in unbearable pain and ceaseless, dark despair.

The outgrowth of flowers in July brings a burst of life and
color. Yellow, tufted plumes of the male flowers, along with the
small female flowers, seem to thrust into all directions, giving
the idea of abundance and new creation. These powerful and
uplifting expressions of fertility point to the sky, leaving behind
the furrowed darkness of the trunk below. Similarly, the remedy, made from the flowering sprigs, raises the sufferer out of
darkness, depth and despair to a new place of hope, regained
creativity and revival of the inner wellsprings of joy.

In autumn, the tree produces edible nuts, contained within a harsh, prickly shell, speaking of renewed sustenance given to a soul after "prickly" circumstances and a prolonged struggle.

METHOD OF PREPARATION: Flowering sprigs with both male and female flowers are boiled for half an hour. The water is strained and used as medicine.

GOAL OF THERAPY: To rekindle the inner light, raise potential for the experiences of faith and new meaning in life. To lighten states of extreme agony.

VERVAIN (VERBENA OFFICINALIS)

Vervain belongs to the group of *Overcare for Welfare of Others,* as classified by Bach. The additional remedies of this group are Rock Water, Beech, Vine and Chicory. Specifically, Vervain treats states of overenthusiasm which lead to exaggerated attempts to convert others to one's own views.

MIND: In the Vervain state, the mind is convinced enthusiastically of certain ideals or ideas and attempts to live up to them, follow through, and convert others to them. This heightened incentive may be carried by great strength of will even in face of stumbling blocks, and internal tension and drive may escalate, especially when resistance needs to be overcome. This resistance may be within oneself, as desire to rest or other attempts at diversion assert themselves, or it may stem from people who do not readily cooperate, or it may be part of the difficulty of the endeavor itself.

While everybody has the right to fight for ideals and ideas, others should not be overly influenced if they do not share equal interest. In the Vervain state, while being carried by fervency and fanaticism, one loses sight of this truth. The person is convinced of the correctness and effectiveness of the pursued ideas and may be blinded to other opinions and choices.

This remedy is indicated in the treatment of manic aspects within mental illness. For example, it is of service in bipolar disorders; in problems with impulse control (cf. Cherry Plum, Holly, Impatiens, Vine); in delusions and psychosis with excessive fervency, ecstasy (cf. Clematis) and mania; and in obsessive-compulsive personality disorder, if there is the tendency to vigorously convert others to one's perfection-oriented standards (cf. Chicory). Vervain treats the underlying élan and fervor which give many states of mental/emotional imbalance the additional impact and force and carry the psychological dynamic to renewed heights.

EMOTIONS: Not only mental concepts and ideas but emotions as well may be carried to great height, fueled by inner drive and the relentless strength of the center of will. Excitability, impressionability, quickly aroused motivation and fondness for others may stimulate and enrich. For some recipients, however, excessive joy, exaggerated and unbalanced emotions of love and friendship may be found overbearing or inappropriate; or the negative emotions of disgust and rejection may assume fanatical character. Hysterical mood swings can be carried to extremes by an underlying Vervain state.

Political fanaticism and outbursts of violence, arising from inner fervency and attempts to influence others, originate in the Vervain tendency of the personality. Self-righteousness is usually high, since one affirms one's goals fully, those often serving the needs of mankind.

PHYSICAL TENDENCIES: Escalating tension and excessive drive of willpower may take a toll on the nervous system or even lead to a nervous breakdown (cf. Cherry Plum, Impatiens, Rock Rose). In the Vervain state, one may overlook the gradual depletion of reserves and disregard warning signals. Hyperthyroidism can be helped by Vervain.

In manic and catatonic states, this remedy not only releases mental/emotional tension but also helps to relax tightened muscles (cf. Cherry Plum, Impatiens, Rock Rose).

DOCTRINE OF SIGNATURES: The Vervain plant has a wiry appearance; several rigidly upright branches grow out of a sturdy, straight stem. This speaks of a goal-oriented mind, driven by intensity. Along the branches grow tiny mauve flowers which open progressively towards the top and leave behind small knots of fruit. These tight knots symbolize the escalating of arguments and mounting of tension in this state of fervency and overenthusiasm.

The tiny flowers and fruits may also hint at the small rewards gained by hurried overenthusiasm, since foresight and calm planning are often neglected. In the Vervain state, one expends great energy and may be disappointed when results are not forthcoming more vigorously. On the other hand, great feats can be accomplished when enthusiasm and motivation are grounded and integrated into sound reality. To move upward towards one's goals in small steps, like the progressively blooming flowers, brings more solid progress and results than the overextended urge to accomplish great deeds. The remedy will help to achieve such release of calm integration, while upholding healthy enthusiasm. The mauve color of the petals speaks of calmness and relaxation, and the healing essence itself is stored in these delicate blossoms.

METHOD OF PREPARATION: The flowering branches are put in a bowl of sunlit water and left to the sun's action for several hours. Subsequently, the water is strained and used as medicine.

GOAL OF THERAPY: Step by step achievement of goals, rather than striving for too much at once. Harnessing of energy and revitalizing of inner calm and nerve power. Tolerance towards the opinion of others.

VINE (VITIS VINIFERA)

The remedy Vine belongs to Bach's group of *Overcare for Welfare of Others,* with the further remedies of Rock Water, Beech, Vervain and Chicory. Specifically, Vine treats the tendency to engage in dominant behavior.

MIND: In the Vine state, one is convinced of one's leadership qualities and assumes control over others, even if they disagree with such overbearing, inflexible treatment. The opinions and wishes of other people are disregarded, should they not fit the personal plan or desire. In an extreme case of outright controlling behavior, or overt case, dominance may lead to ruthlessness and violent abuse. In a hardly noticeable Vine case, or covert case, there may be manipulations, schemes and tricks, or flattery which help to achieve one's ends.

Usually, the degree of power held decides if overt or covert controlling behavior is used. The charging leader, invested with might, hardly has to resort to manipulations but simply has his way. His opponent or inferior, having less power to yield, has to use his wit or even deception to extricate himself and achieve a counter-position of dominance.

In both cases, personally important ends need to be achieved, and the goals assume major proportions, ruling one's behavior and blocking out perceptions of other more significant considerations regarding morals.

This remedy is of use in the treatment of mental disorders and other mental/emotional imbalances when strong resistance is shown in regard to cooperation with treatment plans, and when there is no desire to work for change (cf. Chestnut Bud). Typical Vine patients repeatedly take matters into their own hands, knowing best what is right for themselves. Vine can treat the tendency to abusive behavior and stubbornness, apparent, for example, in passive aggressive personality disorder, antisocial personality disorder, borderline personality disorder and conduct disorder. In impulse control disorders, when impulses are not resisted to but carried out readily to the detriment of others, this remedy is indicated (cf. Cherry Plum, Impatiens, Vervain).

EMOTIONS: In either the overt or covert case, the emotional life may be subjected to the goal-oriented attitude, reducing the power of compassion and active consideration of the needs of others. These are the most far-reaching and severe failures of consideration in the Vine state. One may also forget to tend to one's own needs for diversion and emotional joy and, because of exaggerated ambitiousness, become overly ruled by goals and plans.

In overt Vine cases, when power raises self-worth inappropriately, one may find the emotional states of haughtiness, egoism and self-aggrandizement, with pretentious display of one's might. Simultaneously, there may be condescension against others and absolute expectancy of obedience. Tyranny and a tendency to exploit may grow out of this state; or the senseless, arbitrary abuse of might occurs to the detriment of others, simply to satisfy the leader's need for sensationalism and self-aggrandizement. If there is resistance to orders, the emotions of anger, impatience and exasperation may surface; or the leader, in contrast to the self-aggrandizing type, is coolly calculating, in charge of his emotions and is reserved. In tendency, these dynamics can be observed in a parent or school teacher, in an industrial leader or head of state, to name some examples.

In covert cases, there is usually a deep-seated frustration, a sense of injustice, self-pity, rebelliousness and stubbornness in face of the stifling influence. Covert dominance may be preceded by overt attempts to fight back, or one may vacillate between the two behaviors, with subsequent or recurrent realization of futility and resort to manipulations. This dynamic is often visible in families, as one mate and the children manipulate and undermine the dominating parent to get their individual needs met. Covert Vine behavior may also exist in cases of no opposition, when one person quietly pulls all the strings while seemingly respecting the others' freedom, often under the pretense to help the others to their "own good."

Natural talent for leadership, however, needs recognition and a ground for operating. Vine will help to keep the heart activated and channel one's talents for best fruitfulness.

PHYSICAL TENDENCIES: In extreme cases, exaggerated ambitiousness with pushing oneself and others may give rise to coronary heart disease.[11] Exaggerated ambitiousness accompanied by envy, frustration and worry can lead to the formation of gastric and duodenal ulcers.[12]

DOCTRINE OF SIGNATURES: Vine is a climbing bush with tendrils reaching out ceaselessly into all directions without respect for the host. Other plants are used for taking hold, for proliferation and finding stature. These plants actually may be overgrown to a point of becoming weak or stifled. This shows the Vine mentality of exploiting others for one's personal ends.

The stamens are not encircled by soft, yielding petals but are closed in by a green cap which is pushed off as the stamens have ripened fully. This forceful way of growth also speaks of the "pushiness" and forcefulness of the Vine state.

The positive Vine abilities, however, are highlighted in the fruits which bring forth juice and wine. Symbolically, grapes are seen as fruits of service, based on inner wisdom and grace. The remedy helps to achieve such fruitfulness; it enables those with much personal power to do much good.

METHOD OF PREPARATION: The flowering clusters, shortly after the stamens have grown out, are put in a sunlit bowl of water and left to the sun's action for several hours. Subsequently, the water is strained and used as medicine. Only the wild vine is used.

GOAL OF THERAPY: To open eyes to the consideration of others and find joy in serving them in their quest for happiness and personal advancement. In rebelliousness against authority, to reduce stubborn preoccupation and channel one's leadership energies to more satisfying ends.

WALNUT (JUGLANS REGIA)

The remedy Walnut belongs to the group of *Oversensitive to Influences and Ideas,* as classified by Bach. The other remedies in this group are Agrimony, Centaury and Holly. Specifically, Walnut gives protection from heightened impressionability.

MIND: In the Walnut state, the mind is overly influenced by impressions from the outside world. These impressions may be in the form of trends, fads, other people and their influences and ideas, films, or other current attractions, or even mental manipulations. The person in need of Walnut is too easily impressed and swayed to the point of integrating the impression in the psyche and being led and influenced by it in daily choices, or even in important life choices.

In this state of openness, impressions sink in before discerning and evaluating power can come through and sift out unnecessary or detrimental influence. Inner stability and firmness of purpose and resolve, rational power, plus recognition of one's individual values, preferences and style, have not yet been fully formulated and established in one's mind.

In some cases, though inner firmness exists, the Walnut state is present as a heightened sensitivity, not so much to being misled morally or socially but simply to being overly impacted on by striking content. This may be in the category of true or invented stories of suffering and crime, which arouse empathy and deeply disturb one's imagination, often transmitted with visual impact through films; or even beauty may captivate unduly and overly impress the mind. Exaggerated attraction to sexual matters, even though it may just be mental preoccupation, often roots in oversensitivity to visual or imaginary impact.

During times of transitions, as one leaves behind one's usual structure of reference, and, as one gropes for new guiding posts in the new environment, the mind is overly exposed to possible harmful influence which could detract from the core identity of the inner self. These transitions may be in the form of a move or mark major stepping stones in one's life, such as beginning or ending of school, leaving one's parents, marriage, the empty nest experience, or death of a loved one. Walnut, also called the "link breaker," helps to let go of former existential structures, while safeguarding the stability of the inner self and moving it across to the next "existential link."

This remedy is indicated during the process of psychological growth when the newly found self-image is not firmly established yet and needs to be sheltered from outside deterrents.

In delusional disorders, when one feels obsessed or influenced by forces beyond one's control, Walnut can help to build a protective shield within the realms of consciousness and bring stability of boundaries (cf. Aspen).

EMOTIONS: As the mind is not invested in evaluating and protecting sufficiently and reasonably, emotions may get swayed by heightened impressionability. Impressions sink in and may create emotional disturbance from deep within.

Teenagers, for example, are easily influenced by peers, trends and fads, while they are still in the process of developing their self-identity, independence and heightened discerning powers. Much emotional suffering comes from attempting to impress those, by whom one had been impressed, and, somehow, not measuring up. Openness to biased political persuasion and fanaticism may also root in heightened impressionability. This coupling of possible harmful mental content with emotional fervor may lead to further weakening of mental judging and discerning power.

Children often need protection from outside influences, since their minds have not yet developed adequate reasoning and discerning capacity. The parents' negative evaluation of the child, for example, is communicated to the child and sinks into the self-image, undermining self-esteem and self-concept. Walnut would help this young mind to find balance and self-appreciation from deep within, and the parents' appraisal would make less of an impact.

PHYSICAL TENDENCIES: People in need of Walnut may show heightened sensitivity to radiation such as coming from neon lights or computers. They may also overreact to smells and become nauseated easily; even seemingly harmless substances such as perfumes may give a headache or nausea. In the treatment of allergies, this remedy gives the organism additional protection from being invaded and is recommended as adjunct treatment.

During spinal manipulations, should the correction not hold, Walnut may add increased physical stability.

Heightened impressionability in face of the success and prestige of others may create overambitiousness, envy and frustration and can lead to psychosomatic diseases such as observed in gastric and duodenal ulcers (see Vine).

DOCTRINE OF SIGNATURES: The Walnut tree is marked by a special fragrance, strongest during blooming times, which acts to keep insects, parasites, and even birds and other plants out of its area of growth. This indicates the protection the remedy gives to those overly influenced by outside deterrents and distracted from their personal path of growth.

As one opens a nut, one is reminded of the two halves of the human brain which, as the organ of the mind, is protected by this remedy from heightened impressionability. Even the walnut shell carries practical and symbolic properties. Crushed walnut shells have recently been used by pet merchants as cage litter. Apparently, the refuse does not combine with the crushed shell material and simply has to be sifted out. The remaining shells stay clean and free of odor.

Of all the Walnut trees, this one is "regia," endowed with queenly properties and powerful healing potential.

METHOD OF PREPARATION: Female flowers are collected and boiled for half an hour. The female flower resembles a green bud with two fuzzy stigmas growing out of the top. After boiling, the water is strained and used as medicine.

GOAL OF THERAPY: To help the mind integrate wholesome impressions and sift out those detrimental to the self. To give constancy and stability in one's inner spiritual core, in mind, emotions and body.

WATER VIOLET (HOTTONIA PALUSTRIS)

The remedy Water Violet belongs to the group of *Loneliness,* as classified by Bach. This group consists of only three remedies, the other two being Impatiens and Heather. Specifically, Water Violet treats states of aloofness and haughtiness.

MIND: In the Water Violet state, one raises the self above others and, with the attitude of a reserved dignity, removes from lively involvement with people. Due to deepened life experiences with subsequent understanding of life's truths and an intensified process of spiritual growth, one perceives oneself as special, advanced, refined and perceptive, and believes others to be less aware or matured. In case life's experiences involved grief or being hurt by others, one finds more reason to retreat from people and isolate oneself behind a wall of self-protection and feelings of superiority.

This is the twofold character of the Water Violet state; one feels superior and special, yet deep down is vulnerable and lonely. The perceptive error in this state lies in trying to establish independence and preserve one's mature and refined self-concept by shunning involvement with others, while true greatness and genuine self-respect are earned best in loving, self-forgetful service and comradery with others.

The reasons for feeling superior may also lie in one's special talents, achievements or one's heritage, as one feels uniquely endowed, accomplished or favored. In most cases, this advantage is quietly savored within, just occasionally presented and talked about. In some other cases, however, superiority is expressed more vigorously through haughty behavior, eccentricity and condescension.

In treatment of delusional disorder (grandiose type) and narcissistic personality disorder, when there is the tendency to feel haughty and eccentric, this remedy can be of service. In these disorders, usually an underlying insecurity, desire for attention and admiration, and envy fuel the grandiose perceptions and aspirations, and other remedies may be asked for.

EMOTIONS: In the quiet type, the emotional life may be subdued and stagnating, since active engagement with others is avoided or even considered as disturbing to the inner peace. This lack of involvement may be interpreted as disinterest, lack of spontaneity, or even apathy in face of social stimulation and amusement. In actuality, the Water Violet person longs for genuine human encounter but may not be fully aware of such a quest. Isolation and removal stifle from deep within and leave the inner self empty and sad. From the position of self-protection, the Water Violet person may not easily venture forth, as soon as the inner need for social interaction is coming to the fore; but may rather wait, experiencing mixed feelings of pride and sensitivity, and let the other take the initiative. This rather passive state may lead to further disappointment and work the person deeper into aloofness and seclusion.

The more expressive Water Violet type shows superiority and condescension more openly and offensively. Pride and eccentricity may alienate others unduly and keep them at bay. This more spontaneous type may not be as vulnerable inside as the quiet type but still lacks the genuine bridge of mutual appreciation and heartfelt venture towards others.

A temporary Water Violet state may come on in those who have been offended or humiliated, as they try to protect their self-image. One may choose to raise oneself above the offender, instead of accepting the negative appraisal or affront and being crushed by it. Oftentimes, the expressive Water Violet type himself may push others into this state of self-defense, as one Water Violet mentality creates another, even if just temporarily. This remedy will restore friendship and comradery where once were alienation and affront.

PHYSICAL TENDENCIES: Lack of spontaneity and of lively involvement may lead to physical stiffness and rigidity. An internal retreat or the raising of oneself above others may be reflected in a posture of haughtiness and aloofness.

DOCTRINE OF SIGNATURES: The Water Violet plant grows along brooks and streams with its roots and leaves in the shallow waters. This expresses the psychological state of being isolated, of being an island removed from people; one roots oneself in waters foreign to others. Leaves, while in other plants usually reaching out and making contact with neighboring plants, are submerged, as if to refuse contact. The leaves are feathery and needed to extract nutrients from the water, just as the Water Violet person nourishes the self in seclusion.

A single erect stem grows out of the water, presenting beautiful mauve-white flowers which emanate from the stem in a circle at various intervals along the stem. One is reminded of stages or of a hierarchy, of one group being higher than the other. This speaks of the Water Violet tendency to raise the self above others and engage in elitist or hierarchical thinking.

The circles of flowers themselves, however, portray sociableness, equality and unity. A "social circle" or a "circle of friends" commonly refers to enjoyable and affectionate friendships and encounters. The remedy Water Violet will bring new appeal to social life and teach the beauty of meeting others in equality, the beauty of circles of unity over hierarchies of separateness.

METHOD OF PREPARATION: Several flowers are picked by the stalk and left floating in a bowl of sunlit water for several hours. The water is then strained and prepared as medicine.

GOAL OF THERAPY: To meet and serve others in spontaneous kindness and self-forgetfulness, putting their desire for happiness, self-worth and personal recognition above one's own. To see and appreciate each person as special and unique.

WHITE CHESTNUT (AESCULUS HIPPOCASTANUM)

The remedy White Chestnut belongs to Bach's group of *Not Sufficient Interest in Present Circumstances,* together with the remedies of Clematis, Honeysuckle, Wild Rose, Olive, Mustard and Chestnut Bud. Specifically, White Chestnut treats states of preoccupation and intense worry.

MIND: In the White Chestnut state, the mind is preoccupied with worrisome, returning thoughts which cannot be ruled out and disturb mental peace and clarity. Usually, these thoughts circle around unresolved and deeply disconcerting content which evades solution, yet still grips the mind incessantly. One cannot leave alone those things which worry, even if one wishes to, and the mental torture continues, fueled by anxiety, helplessness and even despair. The present moment loses the power to fascinate the mind sufficiently to interrupt this pattern; one is caught within oneself and is distracted from involving spontaneously with life.

Obsessions, fixations, persistent thought patterns or persistent delusions and chronic introspection fall under the healing action of this remedy. In some of these conditions, the mind has resorted to automatic thought loops and recurrent compulsive thinking (cf. Cherry Plum, Crab Apple, Pine).

EMOTIONS: From the inability to shake off disturbing worries and preoccupation, the person experiences anxiety, exasperation, frustration and exhaustion on top of the emotional impact of the worrisome content itself. One can get worked up and desperately fixated onto disturbing content matter which is beyond one's power to solve, at least for the present moment. One has a difficult time letting go in faith and trust, giving oneself to immediate tasks, and allowing for serenity and clarity to return.

There is awareness that enjoyment and spontaneous devotion to the present moment are curtailed, and one longs for peace, for freedom from cares, and for wholehearted focus on others. While in the White Chestnut state, one may find one-self preoccupied and introverted as others are trying to communicate. The attention is diverted, the majority of the focus being turned inward. Disappointment and annoyance may grow in others and leave the worried person in regret or self-reproach.

PHYSICAL TENDENCIES: Mental preoccupation and worry often lodge in the forehead, where muscles tighten and worrisome lines begin to show. Eyes may have a lack of clarity and serenity, and some premature failures in eyesight may be compounded by a chronic White Chestnut state.

Continued thinking and worrying can last into the night and create insomnia. Both, initial mental preoccupation which prevents falling asleep (initial insomnia), as well as repeated waking up and not being able to go to sleep due to worrisome thought content (intermittent insomnia), can be helped by this remedy.

In psychosomatic medicine, irritable colon has been related to patients with a tendency to obsessive-compulsive working over of emotional experience.[13] Seen from an existential/phenomenological viewpoint, gastrointestinal symptoms such as gastralgia, hypermotility, pylorospasm and ulcers, have been related to chronic "indigestion" in the mind and difficulty in mastering something; and chronic inability to successfully work through emotional experiences has been observed to result in gastrointestinal pain, enterocolitis and irritable colon.[8] White Chestnut would effectively address the tendency to obsessive preoccupation, yet other remedies are usually indicated in addition to heal those mental/emotional experiences which are not being mastered.[14]

DOCTRINE OF SIGNATURES: The White Chestnut tree is marked by great beauty and majesty. The branches, however, are rather brittle and easily break off in a storm, just as the bark has the tendency to crumble and fall off. This speaks of the mind's tendency to not withstand the onslaught of worrisome thoughts and be left broken in serenity and crumbling in inner steadfastness. The rosette of a set of leaves, all coming together in one point, may hint at the mind's movement of concentrating all mental powers on one point of fixation and overly adhering to it.

The flowering spike, consisting of slightly ruffled white blossoms, points upward and conveys the impression of abundance, liberation and clarity. Just by looking at these blossoms with reverence, one feels gripped by the beauty and fascination of the present moment and leaves distracting worries behind. The overall impression of the tree, when looked at from a distance, conveys serenity and peaceful grandeur.

METHOD OF PREPARATION: Individual flowers are picked and placed in a bowl of water which is left to the sun's action for several hours. The water is strained and used as medicine.

GOAL OF THERAPY: To give clarity and inner peace, reduce mental intensity and joyless, worrisome introspection; to set the mind free.

WILD OAT (BROMUS RAMOSUS)

The remedy Wild Oat belongs to the group of *Uncertainty,* as classified by Bach. The other remedies in this group are Cerato, Scleranthus, Gentian, Gorse and Hornbeam. Specifically, Wild Oat deals with lack of motivation and incentive.

MIND: In the Wild Oat state, the person is not sure as to his purpose in life and feels rather aimless, wondering about and searching for the unique calling of his life. One may try different paths or occupations but stays dissatisfied and not fully motivated, since nothing really seems to be quite right. The mind may be unsettled and absent-minded, missing that spark of motivation and incentive which stimulates and propels forward. The joyful concentration on the tasks at hand and the whole-hearted engagement in one's duties are lacking, and even play and diversion may not appeal.

This state of disinterest may actually prevent sparks of interest from developing, since active concentration and receptivity may be curtailed. A negative feedback loop is created, reinforcing aimlessness.

This lack of motivation and incentive not only applies to larger life tasks and important directions of self-realization but also occurs in regard to one's daily routine of chores and duties. These may instill boredom, lethargy and dissatisfaction.

The Wild Oat state may also come on temporarily in those pursuing their life's work. A sudden disinterest may indicate a one-sided routine with overemphasis on work and neglect of other important activities which would break up the daily pattern. Wild Oat will restore the joy of progress and instill the usual motivation.

In children, when disinterested in play or school, Wild Oat will stimulate the mind towards joyful interaction and receptivity.

In some forms of mental illness with organic dysfunction and retardation, this remedy will give maximum motivation and incentive within the physical limitations (cf. Hornbeam, Mustard).

EMOTIONS: Emotions accompanying the Wild Oat state center around frustration, joylessness, aversion, dissatisfaction, meaninglessness, boredom and futility, and feelings of not being fully awakened or activated in one's potential. There is an inner urge to growth which does not quite know how to express itself and what avenue to choose, and the result of such unanswered pressure is restlessness and frustration. Or one may have various ideas and plans and fail to integrate and ground them in reality, while a visionary longing to make important contributions to society further distracts from the small, technical details of real progress.

PHYSICAL TENDENCIES: Lethargy, a lack of appetite, and mental dullness may accompany the Wild Oat state. A depressive mood may permeate the mind and body.

In the treatment of organic mental syndromes and disorders, mental retardation, after head injuries (cf. Hornbeam, Mustard, Scleranthus), this remedy helps to spark new motivation and clarity of purpose within the given limitations.

Wild Oat will also spark interest in health matters in those unaware of the consequences of faulty living. It stimulates the intellectual understanding, lifts the desire to treat the body well, and furthers enjoyment of healthful movement. Obesity, peptic ulcer, non-insulin-dependent diabetes and drug abuse are some physical imbalances deriving largely from lack of knowledge and disinterest in taking care of the body.

DOCTRINE OF SIGNATURES: The very name of this grass reminds of unsettled activity, as one "feels one's oats" in exuberance and in preparation for adventures, and then, as one "sows one's oats" in unfocused and rather careless squandering of one's energies. The recognition of the aimlessness of such endeavor will open the mind to new horizons and instill a longing for meaning and purpose. Here, the grass will bring direction and application so that dreams and visions of fulfillment find a grounding. This wild grass actually is quite tall and delicate, gently swaying in the breeze, in the air, and seemingly barely connected with the ground. The upper portion of the stem hangs down droopily, symbolizing the lack of direction and strength of expression experienced in the Wild Oat state. Yet, the downward bow of the plant reminds of its reverence for earth, and it speaks of the person's longing to apply the self to a solid path.

"Wild" Oat will liberate the inner energies and bring the adventure of self-realization.

METHOD OF PREPARATION: The flowering ends are picked and placed in a bowl of water which is left standing in bright sunlight for several hours. The water is strained and used as medicine.

GOAL OF THERAPY: To experience fully and be aware of those challenges and possibilities uniquely suited to the self. To give renewed joy of receptivity and response, to spark interest.

WILD ROSE (ROSA CANINA)

The remedy Wild Rose is a part of Bach's group of *Not Sufficient Interest in Present Circumstances,* together with the remedies of Clematis, Honeysuckle, Olive, White Chestnut, Mustard and Chestnut Bud. Specifically, Wild Rose treats states of apathy and resignation.

MIND: In the Wild Rose state, the mind has resigned to unfavorable conditions and does not seek new opportunities for improvement. Usually, the person has made an attempt to find more wholesome or desirable options of life but has failed and given up. To protect from disappointment and continued despair, the mind chooses to resort to apathy and resignation, both of which instill a necessary tranquility and relative release from struggle.

During the initial resistance, however, Wild Rose may be indicated as well, although it is not the all-pervading state in this instance. Here, helplessness and powerlessness are present, both being characteristic of the Wild Rose state; yet, resignation has not taken hold and there is additional anger or frustration.

In other cases, the Wild Rose state does not necessarily arise out of a difficult condition that was struggled against initially. A Wild Rose tendency can be present since early childhood when a stifling environment, in combination with personality traits of shyness or uncertainty, has failed to raise the spirit of independence and adventure. These people may simply accept what comes their way, without considering options or striving for a break in the routine.

During sickness, the all-pervading Wild Rose state is portrayed in a disinterest in fighting for wellness; one gives up and may lose all incentive to live.

In mental illness, flat affect is a common occurrence and can be helped by this remedy, as in schizophrenic states, developmental disorders, psychosis, schizoid and schizotypal personality disorders. The personality disorders are less severe states than schizophrenia, with schizoid personality disorder showing more pronounced flat affect than schizotypal personality disorder. Usually, for those succumbing to these illnesses, social contact is reduced, emotional involvement low, and assertiveness yielded to passiveness.[15]

EMOTIONS: The typical Wild Rose state shows a retreat from involvement in unfavorable circumstances which could not be overcome. This withdrawal from reality helps to safeguard emotions so that the drain of despair and frustration does not take its toll. Simultaneously, however, the emotional capacity for joy and liveliness suffers as well. This stifling prevents exactly those energies from arising which the self needs to lift out of its deadlock. Outwardly, this stifled capacity for joy is visible in a disinterest in amusement and play, in a lack of hopes, wishes and dreams.

In the less complete Wild Rose state, when powerlessness is experienced with simultaneous anger and frustration, emotions may vacillate between these two extremes. If changes can be made through one's efforts, the Wild Rose state is diverted and one feels empowered again. If conditions are insurmountable, however, a Wild Rose tendency may become chronically entrenched, such as in terminal illness and disability. The remedy still helps to uplift the mind and emotions to new heights of wellness and directs the view to options of enrichment and joy within one's reach. Wild Rose liberates in the midst of hardship by changing the inner attitude from resignation and withdrawal to a new receptivity for life.

In a lifelong case of Wild Rose, although the emotional life may appear stable, there may rest hidden potential and creativity in the interior reserves of the person which this remedy helps to activate.

PHYSICAL TENDENCIES: Mental/emotional apathy permeates the physical realm as well, leading to lethargy, listlessness, lack of energy and flat affect.

In sickness, when the fighting spirit is gone and recuperation is not proceeding, or even when death is threatened due to resignation, this remedy may assist greatly.

DOCTRINE OF SIGNATURES: This abundant Wild Rose bush usually grows in the form of a hedge along the street and shields the background from view. Its branches are thick and covered with strong thorns, reminding of the canine teeth of the dog, hence its name *Rosa canina*. To draw parallels to the mind, in the initial Wild Rose state, when powerlessness and frustration are experienced, one is caught in the thorns of hardship, or by the "teeth of a dog," and one resists and does not succumb yet. Pains are raw and every movement hurts, however; and one may realize the futility of the struggle. As one ceases the struggle, the pains lessen and one may slowly retreat from life and end up swallowed up by the hedge, out of the mainstream of life and hidden from view.

The beautiful white-pink or simply white blossoms, growing out of this brambly thicket and opening their petals into the sky, speak of liberation and unfettered expression. The blossoms portray the healing quality of this remedy; they form the connection to the outside world, give and attract, and guide the view to new horizons. They give inner freedom to all, even to those who cannot quite reach the street of normal life again and have to accept a life within limiting conditions.

METHOD OF PREPARATION: Sprigs with leaves and flowers are boiled for half an hour. Subsequently, the water is strained and prepared as medicine.

GOAL OF THERAPY: To move out of dormant despair, renew incentive for life, strengthen the inner force of self-determination and liberate creative potentials.

WILLOW (SALIX VITELLINA)

The remedy Willow belongs to the group of *For Despondency or Despair*, as classified by Bach. The additional remedies in this group are Crab Apple, Oak, Star of Bethlehem, Sweet Chestnut, Elm, Pine and Larch. Specifically, Willow deals with states of resentment and bitterness regarding one's fate.

MIND: In the Willow state, one feels burdened by an unfavorable, and, as one believes, undeserved fate, and one seeks the source of such unfairness outside of the self, blaming others or even fate itself for such misfortune. One fails to perceive one's own responsibilities in such a state and does not realize how personal failures and opportunities missed due to one's own fault have caused such unhappiness. Since self-blame and regret are unbearable to the self and one refuses to deal with reality, one fixes the blame onto others and releases internal frustration and resentment towards them, even though the others may be blameless.

This unfounded resentment is differentiated from founded resentment which grows in those who truly have been hurt by another and have not been able to find justice or satisfying compensation. Unfounded resentment is based on irrational perception and on emotionally swayed interpretation of events. In extreme cases, fixed ideas, delusions and even paranoia may express the Willow dynamic. Paranoia is the most intensified blame and accusation brought towards others, as one feels persecuted and thwarted in one's destiny due to the fault of others (cf. Beech). In this state, one also projects one's strongly felt resentments onto others, believing them to be equally fixated and adverse. Founded resentment, on the other hand, stems from correct perception of events and is based on true suffering caused by another, often by someone holding the advantage of power.

This remedy is of use in all mental disorders involving resentment and blame, such as in malingering (cf. Chicory), passive aggressive personality disorder, antisocial personality disorder and in disruptive behavior disorders (cf. Holly).

EMOTIONS: Emotions accompanying unfounded resentment range from dissatisfaction and self-pity to self-righteousness, denial of reality, envy, and lack of sympathy and compassion. Wrong accusations are brought towards others without further reflection, while the own self-image is held intact and one feels offended easily when accused oneself. At the bottom of this dynamic lies the bitterness and dormant despair felt in a self not fully actualized, whose true destiny has not been fulfilled. Having missed true happiness, one also does not want others to experience such joy and advantage.

Founded resentment, on the other hand, shows genuine sadness and disappointment; despondency and despair may weigh heavily, should one be unable to rise above the limiting circumstances. Initially, one may feel tremendous anger at being mistreated but may have had to stifle such expression, either out of necessity or by choice. The locked-in outrage and sense of injustice then turns into smoldering resentment and sows bitterness, disillusionment and depression into the heart. While being in this state, one has to work very hard, with resolve and willpower, to raise the ability to forgive. The remedy Willow will make this work easier.

PHYSICAL TENDENCIES: Physical rigidity and careworn features may speak of internal bitterness and resentment. Anger, if not vented constructively and pushed within, can cause physical side effects, such as colicky pains and tension headaches, or depression on all levels of the human being. Chronically engaged-in repression of aggressive impulses, especially in the founded Willow state which is held within, can result in a variety of psychosomatic illnesses, with the heart and intestinal region being affected the most. The following psychosomatic diseases are viewed as being caused by overcompliance and suppression of aggressiveness: Hyperkinetic heart syndrome, paroxysmal supraventricular tachycardia (these two diseases being irregularities in heart activity), hypertension, hyperventilation syndrome, chronic coughs or "protest" coughs[16], constipation (cf. Chicory, Mustard), soft tissue rheumatism, rheumatoid arthritis, self-inflicted skin lesions and intermittent insomnia.[3]

DOCTRINE OF SIGNATURES: The Willow tree usually undergoes a lot of pruning, and in its cut state reminds of the losses and cutbacks in fortune experienced in the Willow state. Traditionally, Willow branches have been used for weaving of baskets and mats. The branches are very flexible and almost impossible to break. This symbolizes the power of forgiveness this remedy brings, as it helps the offended to "bow" towards the offender with a forgiving heart. Willow brings deepened steadfastness of heart and inner strength which help to stay flexible and not become rigid and burdened to the point of breaking.

Both, the branches and the catkins have a yellowish color, hence the name *vitellina,* meaning "egg yolk" in Latin. While the symbol of the egg may resonate with the healing and regenerating qualities of this tree, the yellowish shade of twigs and catkins actually speaks of bitterness or internal anger, this color being the color of the gall bladder which is traditionally seen as the seat of pent-up frustration and anger. The fuzziness of the catkins, however, hint at cozy warmth and friendship, so necessary to grow between people alienated by resentment and strife.

METHOD OF PREPARATION: Twigs with male or female catkins are boiled for half an hour. Subsequently, the water is strained and used as medicine.

GOAL OF THERAPY: To instill loving forgiveness and renew the feeling of grace. To live and let live in tolerance and gain an inner attitude of gentleness and acceptance of others.

RESCUE REMEDY

Bach also discovered a unique combination of five remedies which aim at restoring balance and calm to a person in acute emergency situations. Rescue Remedy is of great value immediately after accidents or similar moments of shock and panic when there is fainting, trembling, or other failing of normal physical functioning. This combination of remedies can prevent death if given at the right moment, and it should be the first medicine administered on arrival at the accident.

Here are the contributions of the five remedies that together give a unique synergistic effect: *Rock Rose* to counteract terror and panic; *Cherry Plum* to balance intense tension and the fear of losing mental control; *Clematis* to reduce fainting, coma; *Impatiens* to reduce tension and impatience; *Star of Bethlehem* to reduce the effects of the shock.

Rescue Remedy can also be used as a daily remedy in chronic situations of intense nervousness and tension when the vital force needs to recharge and recuperate. It helps to bring balance, calm and synchronized functioning within the levels of the human being, these being spiritual core, mind, emotions and body. After accidents, shocks, traumas or during severe illness, mental or physical, the levels move beyond a synchronized balance and can be helped to integrate anew by the repeated intake of Rescue Remedy.

CONCLUDING REMARKS

This presentation guides to the wide use of the Bach Remedies. Free of causing any side effects, they can be used generously by lay people and professionals alike. They are of use for all ages, under all circumstances of life, and for all living creation. Not only humans but animals and plants as well benefit from the remedies' healing effect after careful assessing of the problem. For humans and animals alike, should drinking or swallowing capacity be curtailed, the remedies can be applied to the lips, rubbed into the skin, vaporized, or given intravenously. Where despair is great, as in hospitals, mental institutes, prisons, or during grief, their use should not be neglected.

As deepened understanding of these unique healing gifts grows, the world will come to a full utilization and reap their liberating benefits.

NOTES

[1] Book 2, *The Psychological/Constitutional Essences of the Bach Flower Remedies,* was completed in 1993. It has been published in full by Kent Homeopathic Associates as computer software. The book is contained in: Cornelia Richardson-Boedler, *The Richardson-Boedler Bach Repertory* (San Rafael, Calif.: Kent Homeopathic Associates, 1993); and it has been included in an updated version of *Reference Works:* David Warkentin, ed., *Reference Works* (San Rafael, Calif.: Kent Homeopathic Associates, 1990).

[2] The discovery of the Bach Remedies and Bach's career are described in the biography by Nora Weeks, *The Medical Discoveries of Edward Bach, Physician* (London: C. W. Daniel, 1940).

[3] B. Luban-Plozza, W. Pöldinger, and F. Kröger, *Psychosomatic Disorders in General Practice,* trans. George Blythe from 3rd German ed. (Berlin: Springer, 1992). This work reviewed the literature concerning the known psychosomatic diseases.

[4] Factitious disorder is the voluntary production or feigning of symptoms for the sake of assuming the patient role. Malingering is the manipulative attempt to escape certain undesirable consequences, such as work or a court appearance, by feigning illness or pretending other forms of being incapacitated.

[5] In conversion disorders, the physical symptomatic expression is involuntary in contrast to factitious disorders or malingering. The patient is unaware of the underlying mental/emotional dynamic which creates inner pressure and finds an outlet on the physical plane.

[6] Luban-Plozza et al., p. 28.

[7] Luban-Plozza et al., p. 65.

[8] Luban-Plozza et al., p. 63; B. Staehelin, "Über die diagnostischen und psychotherapeutischen Möglichkeiten des einfachen Sprechstundengesprächs, dargestellt an drei Fallbeispielen mit Symptomen des Verdauungstraktes," *Praxis,* 52 (1963), 767-75.

[9] Luban-Plozza el al., p. 34; H. Huebschmann, "Psyche und Tuberkulose," in *Beiträge aus der Allgemeinen Medizin,* Vol. VIII (Stuttgart: Enke, 1952).

[10] Luban-Plozza et al., p. 30.

[11] Luban-Plozza et al., p. 41; R. H. Rosenman and M. Friedman, "The Possible Relationship of the Emotions to Clinical Coronary Heart Disease," in *Hormones and Artherosclerosis,* ed. Gregory Pincus (New York: Academic Press, 1959).

[12] Luban-Plozza et al., pp. 66-67.

[13] Luban-Plozza et al., p. 72.

[14] Explanation of terminology: "Gastralgia" refers to pain without lesions in the stomach region and right below it; "hypermotility" is excessive gastric constriction and motility; "pylorospasm" is a spasm of the lower end of the stomach where it enters the duodenum, the adjacent small intestine; and "enterocolitis" is an inflammation of the intestines and colon.

[15] Schizophrenia is defined as a major mental disorder of unknown cause, typically characterized by a separation (schism) between thought processes and emotions and accompanied by delusions, hallucinations and flat affect.

[16] Luban-Plozza et al., p. 30.

APPENDIX: BACH REMEDY REPERTORY

*T*his Bach Remedy repertory represents the distilled information of the author's Bach Remedy entries into the *Repertory of the Homoeopathic Materia Medica* by James Tyler Kent. The Bach Remedies were added in 1993 to the first part of the repertory, the section dealing with the symptoms of the mind. This expanded version of the repertory is available as part of the computerized *MacRepertory*, which was released originally by Kent Homeopathic Associates in 1987.

In addition to the Bach Remedy entries, the following repertory adds new rubrics and also gives the indications for each Bach Remedy entry, should there be several Bach Remedies listed for one particular symptom. In this way, it carries built-in materia medica of the Bach Remedies for reference.

Remedies are graded from 1 to 3 according to their indication for a specific symptom, with 3 being the highest indication.

This mark / between remedies, as in 3Agr./3Imp., suggests to take the combination of remedies for the indicated symptom.

The abbreviations of the Bach Remedies are as follows:

Agr. 　　= Agrimony (Agrimonia eupatoria)

Asp. 　　= Aspen (Populus tremula)

Beech 　= Beech (Fagus sylvatica)

Cent. 　 = Centaury (Centaurium umbellatum)

Cer. 　　= Cerato (Ceratostigma willmottiana)

Cher-P. = Cherry Plum (Prunus cerasifera)

Ch-Bd. = Chestnut Bud (Aesculus hippocastanum)

Chic. 　 = Chicory (Cichorium intybus)

Clem. 　= Clematis (Clematis vitalba)

Crb-A. 　= Crab Apple (Malus sylvestris/pumila)

Elm 　　= Elm (Ulmus procera)

Gent. 　 = Gentian (Gentiana amarella)

Gors. 　 = Gorse (Ulex europaeus)

Heath. 　= Heather (Calluna vulgaris)

Holly 　 = Holly (Ilex aquifolium)

Honey. 　= Honeysuckle (Lonicera caprifolium)

Horn. 　 = Hornbeam (Carpinus betulus)

Imp. 　　= Impatiens (Impatiens glandulifera)

Lar. 　　= Larch (Larix decidua)

Mim. 　 = Mimulus (Mimulus guttatus)

Must. 　 = Mustard (Sinapis arvensis)

Oak 　　= Oak (Quercus robur)

Oliv. 　　= Olive (Olea europaea)

Pine 　　= Pine (Pinus sylvestris)

Rd-Ch. = Red Chestnut (Aesculus carnea)

Rck-R. = Rock Rose (Helianthemum nummularium)

Rck-W. = Rock Water (Aqua petra)

Scler. = Scleranthus (Scleranthus annuus)

Star-B. = Star of Bethlehem (Ornithogalum umbellatum)

Sw-Ch. = Sweet Chestnut (Castanea sativa)

Verv. = Vervain (Verbena officinalis)

Vine = Vine (Vitis vinifera)

Waln. = Walnut (Juglans regia)

Wat-V. = Water Violet (Hottonia palustris)

Wh-Ch. = White Chestnut (Aesculus hippocastanum)

Wld-O. = Wild Oat (Bromus ramosus)

Wld-R. = Wild Rose (Rosa canina)

Will. = Willow (Salix vitellina)

REPERTORY

ABSENT-MINDED: 2Ch-Bd. 3Clem. 2Honey. Horn. 2Must. 2Oliv. Star-B. 3Wh-Ch. 2Wld-R.

depression and gloominess, from: 3Must.

drowsiness and sleepiness, from: 3Clem.

dwelling on beloved past memories, from: 3Honey.

dwelling on dream of future happiness, from: 3Clem.

exhaustion, from: Horn. 3Oliv.

grief, trauma, shock, from: 3Star-B.

inattentiveness, from: 3Ch-Bd

internal preoccupation with worrisome thoughts, from: 3Wh-Ch.

resignation, from: 3Wld-R.

ABSORBED: 3Clem. 3Honey. 2Must. 3Wh-Ch.

introspection, brooding, and gloom, from: 3Must.

persistent, worrisome thoughts, in: 3Wh-Ch.

pleasant reveries and dreams of the future, in: 3Clem.

reminiscences of past happiness, in: 3Honey.

ABSTRACTION of mind: 3Wh-Ch.

ABUSIVE: 2Cher-P. 3Holly 2Imp. 2Verv. 2Vine

anger and outrage, from: 3Holly

dictatorial and domineering, from being: 3Vine

fanaticism and fervency, from: 3Verv.

fear of losing all control, with: 3Cher-P.

impatience, from: 3Imp.

pains, with the: Cher-P.

tension, extreme, with loss of inner strength in regard to holding down abusive impulse, from: 3Cher-P. Imp. Verv.

ADVICE, seeks, from others (See Confidence): 3Cer.

AFFECTATION: 2Chic. 2Heath.

desire to be appreciated and be the center of attention, from: 3Chic.

loneliness within and need to be recognized, heard and understood, from: 3Heath.

AGITATION, internal: 3Agr. 3Cher-P. 3Holly 3Imp. 3Rd-Ch. 3Rck-R. 2Rck-W. 3Scler. 3Verv. 3Wh-Ch.

battling opposing forces within, namely dreaded impulses versus mental control, from: 3Cher-P.

fear that loved ones are in danger and one cannot assist them, from: 3Rd-Ch.

fragility of nerves, with anxiety, from: 3Rck-R.

impatience, from: 3Imp.

necessity of having to choose between two options, from: 3Scler.

overstimulation by mental impressions and ideas, with loss of overview, from: 3Scler.

persistent thoughts of deeply felt worry that evade solution, from: 3Wh-Ch.

suppression of desires, with enforced self-mastery, from: 3Rck-W.

vexation, anger and upset, from: 3Holly

willpower and inner fervent drive, excessive, due to demanding circumstances, from: 3Verv.

worry, inner restlessness and sensitivity to disquiet in one's environment, from: 3Agr.

ALOOF: 3Wat-V.

AMBITION:

absent, due to resignation and apathy: 3Wld-R.

aimless:

indecisiveness and uncertainty of attitude, from: 3Cer.

motivation, inner direction and purpose, lack of, from: 3Wld-O.

vacillating between two or several options and losing the overview, from: 3Scler.

diminished:

discouragement, from: 3Gent.

exhaustion, from: Cent. 2Horn. Oak 3Oliv.

fear of failure, from: 2Lar. 3Mim.

feeling overwhelmed, from: 3Elm

lassitude and procrastination, from: 3Horn.

self-confidence, lack of, from: 2Cer. 3Lar.

dutiful:

desire to serve others, even at own expense, from: 3Cent.

stoic perseverance in one's work, despite hardship, from: 3Oak

exaggerated:

excessive enthusiasm and inner drive, from: 3Verv.

need to lead and control, from: 2Chic. 3Vine

forceful and self-empowered attitude: 3Vine

overcare for others with expectation of gratitude and affection from others: 3Chic.

pride and desire for augmentation, from: 3Wat-V.

thwarted:

being a too willing servitor and neglecting one's destiny, from: 3Cent.

feeling underprivileged and resentful, with self-pity, from: 3Will.

AMUSEMENT:

averse to: 2Oak 2Rck-W.

negation of desires, either self-imposed or out of necessity, due to: 3Rck-W.

work-oriented attitude, due to: 3Oak

desire for: Agr.

ANARCHIST: 3Verv.

ANGER: 2Cher-P. 3Holly 2Imp. 2Verv. Vine Will.

absent persons, at: Will.

ailments after anger: 2Holly 2Will.

consoled, when: 2Chic. 2Holly

convulsion, before: Cher-P.

fanaticism, with: 3Holly/3Verv.

fear of losing all control, with: 3Cher-P./3Holly

fervency and inner tension, fueled by: 3Holly/3Verv.

former vexations, about: Will.

impatience, from: 3Holly/3Imp.

irritability, from: 3Holly 3Imp. 2Rck-R.

fragility of nerves, due to: 3Holly/3Rck-R.

selfishness and short temper, due to: 3Holly/3Imp.

jealousy, from: 3Holly

pain aggravates: Cher-P.

past events, about: Will.

perceived threat, from: 3Holly/3Rck-R.

smoldering, forming deep-seated resentment: 3Will.

stabbed, so that he could have, any one: Cher-P.

suppressed, from: 3Will.

vexation and upset, from: 3Holly

violent: 2Cher-P. 3Holly Imp. Verv. Vine

deliberate abuse of power, with: 3Holly/3Vine

unwanted loss of self-control, with: 3Cher-P./3Holly

ANGUISH: 3Agr. 3Cher-P. 2Wh-Ch. 3Sw-Ch.

faithlessness and nihilistic despair, from: 3Sw-Ch.

fear that mind will lose control and dreaded impulses will reign thought processes and conduct, with extreme tension, from: 3Cher-P.

need to control inner nervousness and feelings of inadequacy during social situation, from: 2Agr. 3Cher-P.

persistent thoughts that worry and torture the mind, from: 3Wh-Ch.

unendurable: 3Sw-Ch.

worry and internal restlessness, from: 3Agr.

ANOREXIA, mental, in hysterical girls: 2Chic. Heath.

desire to gain attention, due to unfulfilled need for affection, from: 3Chic. 2Heath.

sulkiness and self-pity, with: 3Chic.

talkativeness and need for company, with: 3Heath.

ANSWERS:

foolishly: Cer.

hastily: Cer. Ch-Bd

impulsiveness and rushing in the mind, from: 2Ch-Bd

inner insecurity, from: 2Cer.

ANTAGONISM with herself: 2Agr. 3Cher-P. 2Rck-W. 2Wh-Ch.

need to quieten inner worries and engage in diversion, from: 3Agr.

opposing forces within, one being dreaded thoughts or impulses, the other being the urgent need to keep them under control, from: 3Cher-P.

persistent unwanted thoughts that evade solution and interfere with the desire to enjoy the present moment, from: 3Wh-Ch.

urge to gain mastery over one's desires and needs, either out of necessity or self-imposed, from: 3Rck-W.

ANTICIPATION, complaints from: Cher-P. 2Lar. 3Mim. Rck-R.

envisioning a concrete situation with dread, from: 3Mim.

panic attacks and intense fear, with: 3Rck-R.

self-confidence, lack of, from: 3Lar.

tension, extreme, and fear that one is losing mental balance, may not be able to control nervousness, and fail one's job during the anticipated event, from: 3Cher-P.

ANXIETY: 3Agr. 3Asp. 3Cher-P. 3Mim. 2Pine 3Rd-Ch. 3Rck-R.

anticipating an engagement, from (See Anticipation): 3Mim.

between intervals of epilepsy: 2Cher-P. 2Rck-R.

fear of losing control over physical and mental functions, from: 3Cher-P.

terror and fright, from: 3Rck-R.

children, about his: 3Rd-Ch.

conscience, of: 3Pine

continence prolonged, from: 2Cher-P.

convulsions, before (See Anxiety; between intervals): 2Cher-P. 2Rck-R.

cruelties, after hearing of: Rck-R.

dark, in: 2Asp.

dreams, on waking from frightful: 2Rck-R.

expected of him, when anything is: 2Mim.

fear, with: 3Asp. 3Cher-P. 3Mim. 3Rd-Ch. 3Rck-R.

    fear and dread of concrete situations, from: 3Mim.

    fear of losing mental control, from: 3Cher-P.

    fear that loved ones are in danger, from: 3Rd-Ch.

    foreboding and vague fears, from: 3Asp.

    terror and extreme fright, from: 3Rck-R.

fragility of nerves, from: 3Rck-R.

friends at home, about: 3Rd-Ch.

fright, after: 3Rck-R.

future, about: Agr. 2Asp. 3Mim.

health, about: Chic. 2Crb-A. Heath. 3Mim.

    need to gain the attention one deserves and feel cared for, from: 3Chic.

    need to gain sympathetic attention, with great inner urge to share one's personal health problems, from: 3Heath.

    obsessive preoccupation with symptoms, from:3Crb-A.

    overanxiousness, with careful monitoring of symptoms, from: 3Mim.

hypochondriacal (See Anxiety; health): 2Chic. 2Crb-A. 2Heath. 3Mim.

mental exertion: 2Cher-P.

motion, from, downward: 2Rck-R.

nervousness and shyness, from: 3Mim.

night watching, from: 2Rck-R. Rd-Ch.

fear, nervousness, and worry about welfare of others, with: 3Rd-Ch.

fragility of nerves and inner tremor, with: 3Rck-R.

others, for: 3Rd-Ch.

pains, from the: Agr. 2Cher-P.

anguish, extreme, with fear of losing mental balance, from: 3Cher-P.

restlessness and attempt to hide pain and be cheerful, with: 3Agr.

pursued when walking, as if: 2Asp.

riding, while, downhill: 2Rck-R.

salvation, about: 3Pine

sedentary employment, from: 2Agr. 2Imp.

restlessness, inner disquiet, while trying to uphold calm appearance on outside, with: 3Agr.

tension and sheer need to move, with: 3Imp.

sexual desire in excess, from suppressed: 3Cher-P.

sleep, before: 2Asp. 2Mim.

concrete fears of nightmares or other discomforts: 3Mim.

fear of the unknown, of letting go: 3Asp.

sleep, loss of: 2Rck-R.

soul's welfare: 3Pine

sudden: 3Rck-R.

suicidal: 3Cher-P.

thoughts, from: 2Cher-P.

trifles, about (See Fastidious): 2Chic. 2Crb-A. Mim. Pine

worry and inner restlessness, with sensitivity to disquiet in one's environment, from: 3Agr.

ARDENT: 2Rck-W. 3Verv.

overenthusiasm and inner drive, with urge to convert others to one's viewpoint, from: 3Verv.

self-mastery and desire to inspire others with own example, from: 3Rck-W.

ARROGANCE: 3Beech 2Imp. 3Vine 3Wat-V.

attitude that one has superior judgment and has the right to criticize others, from: 3Beech

believing oneself to be capable and having the right to lead and influence others, even against their will, from: 3Vine

believing oneself to work and move more efficiently than others and having the right to urge them on, from: 3Imp.

feeling superior to others in character, endowment, or achievement, from: 3Wat-V.

ASKS for nothing: Clem. 2Wld-R.

apathy and resignation, from: 3Wld-R.

belief that only the future, not the present, holds the promise of happiness, from: 3Clem.

ATTENTION, seeks: 2Cer. 3Chic. 3Heath. 2Mim.

desire to be important to people and have them express their appreciation for her, from: 3Chic.

fear of failure or of being ridiculed, with pretended courage and outward show of confidence, from: 3Mim.

need for audience and craving to be acknowledged and listened to, from: 3Heath.

self-assurance, lack of, with need to find approval and recognition by others, from: 3Cer.

AVARICE: Chic.

AVERSION:

approached, to being: Beech 2Chic. 3Holly Wat-V. 2Will.

critical attitude and intolerance, from: 3Beech

feeling superior and not wanting to get involved, from: 3Wat-V.

resentment and bitterness, from: 3Will.

self-pity and sulkiness, from: 3Chic.

vexed and angry feelings toward someone, from: 3Holly

everything, to: 2Holly 2Wld-O.

irritability and easy annoyance, from: 3Holly

motivation and incentive, lack of, from: 3Wld-O.

husband, to: 2Will.

members of family, to: Chic. 2Holly 2Will.

men, to: 2Will.

persons, to certain: 2Holly 2Will.

religious, to the opposite sex: 2Crb-A. 2Will.

resentment against the attractive power of the opposite sex, from: 3Will.

viewing sexual issues as unclean or shameful, from: 3Crb-A.

wife, to his: 2Will.

women, to: 2Will.

BEGGING, entreating: Wld-R.

BEHAVIORAL MISTAKES, interfering in others' lives: 3Beech 3Cher-P.3Ch-Bd. 3Chic. 3Holly 3Imp. 3Verv. 3Vine 3Will.

anger, annoyance, hatred or jealousy from: 3Holly

criticism and intolerance, from: 3Beech

dominating and abusive attitude, from: 3Vine

finding excitement in rebelliousness, danger, and the negating of one's conscience, from finding: 3Cher-P./ 3Holly

impatience, from: 3Imp.

mental control, loss of, and committing unwanted dreaded acts, from: 3Cher-P.

need to meddle in others' affairs and set things right, from: 3Chic.

overenthusiasm or fanaticism, from: 3Verv.

repetitive:

failure to learn from previous mistakes, from: 3Ch-Bd

stubborn refusal to change, with: 3Ch-Bd/3Vine

resentment, bitterness and blaming others, from: 3Will.

BOREDOM: 2Agr. 2Cent. 2Clem. 2Honey. 2Horn. 2Must. 3Wld-O. 2Wld-R.

depression, gloominess and joylessness in one's activities, from: 3Must.

dwelling on:

dreams of future happiness and neglecting the present, from: 3Clem.

memories of past happiness and neglecting the present, from: 3Honey.

incentive, purpose and direction, lack of, from: 3Wld-O.

inner satisfaction, lack of, and restless need for stimulation and adventure, with: 3Agr.

lassitude and procrastination, from: 3Horn.

resignation and lack of interest in pleasurable pursuits, from: 3Wld-R.

serving others dutifully and neglecting one's own interests, from: 3Cent.

BREAK things, desire to (See Abusive): 2Cher-P. 3Holly

anger and unbridled outrage, from: 3Holly

extreme tension, emotional impact and inability to control one's behavior, although attempt has been made, from: 3Cher-P.

BROODING: 2Chic. 2Must. Oak 3Wh-Ch. 2Will.

depression and joylessness: 3Must.

harboring resentment, from: 3Will.

self-pity, from: 3Chic.

stoic attitude, bent on fulfilling one's duty, and avoiding mental diversion or recreation, from: 3Oak

worrisome thoughts of a heavy nature that evade solution, from: 3Wh-Ch.

BUSINESS:

averse to: 2Holly 3Wld-O. 2Will.

annoyance and disinclination, from: 3Holly

motivation and incentive, lack of, from: 3Wld-O.

resentment or feeling exploited, with putting blame on others, from: 3Will.

necessary: 3Agr. 3Chic. 2Oak 2Pine 2Verv. 2Vine

feel useful and still guilt feelings and self-reproach, in order to: 3Pine

find outlet for strong inner dynamic and overenthusiasm, in order to: 3Verv.

impatient urge to get "things done," from: 3Agr./3Imp. 3Verv.

adherence to strict principles and self-discipline, from: 3Verv.

inner worry and impatience about task completion, from: 3Agr./3Imp.

motivation to persevere and grind out duties, from: 3Oak

overcare for others' welfare and attention to trifles, from: 3Chic.

overcome inner disquiet and assuage worries, in order to: 3Agr.

set things right and have control over one's environment and other people's lives, in order to: 3Chic./3Vine

willing servitor, from being: 3Cent.

wish to control and accomplish task, with forceful inner attitude towards own self, from: 3Verv./3Vine

neglected:

daydreaming, from: 3Clem.

depression, lack of incentive and joylessness: 3Must.

discouragement due to obstacles, from: 3Gent.

dwelling on memories of past happiness, from: 3Honey.

exhaustion in mind and body, from: Horn. Oak 3Oliv.

exhaustion from tendency to struggle on, despite signs of fatigue: 3Oak

exhaustion, severe, with growing inability to pursue one's normal tasks: 3Oliv.

fatigue and lack of vibrancy: 3Horn.

fear of failure, from: 3Lar./3Mim.

feeling overwhelmed, from: 3Elm

feeling unappreciated and having self-pity, from: 3Chic.

guilt and self-blame, from: 3Pine

hopelessness in regard to outcome of endeavor, from: 3Gors.

inattentiveness and carelessness, from: 3Ch-Bd

indecisiveness and vacillating between options, with loss of overview from multiple internal arguments, from: 3Scler.

lassitude, fatigue and tendency to procrastination, from: 3Horn.

preoccupation with worrisome thoughts, from: 3Wh-Ch.

resignation and feelings of helplessness, from: 3Wld-R.

self-confidence, lack of, from: 3Lar. 2Cer.

sense of meaning and purpose, lack of, from: 3Wld-O.

uncertainty, lack of inner assurance, and feelings of inadequacy, from: 3Cer.

persevered in, despite set-backs and personal hardship: 3Oak

power, assuming or holding power in business and alienating others: 3Vine

willpower, excessive, necessary to attend to: 3Oak
3Verv./3Vine

determination and stoic perseverance in attending to business, from: 3Oak

need to raise one's enthusiasm and urge oneself
to attend to business, from: 3Verv./3Vine

BUSY (See Business; necessary): 2Agr.

CAPRICIOUSNESS: 3Chic. 2Heath. 2Scler. Wat-V.

feeling special and superior, and expecting special deference from others, from: 3Wat-V.

need to be noticed and find willing ears for one's problems, from: 3Heath.

need to gain attention and feel appreciated, from: 3Chic.

vacillating between ideas and wishes, moodiness, from:
3Scler.

CARES, full of: 3Agr. 2Wh-Ch.

inner restlessness and continuous worry about daily duties
or occurrences, from: 3Agr.

persistent preoccupation with thoughts of a burdensome
nature that evade solution, from: 3Wh-Ch.

CAUTIOUS: Cer. Lar. 2Mim.

anxiously: 3Mim.

indecisiveness and hesitancy, from: 3Cer.

self-confidence, lack of, and anticipation of failure, from:
3Lar.

CENSORIOUS, critical: 3Beech

CHAOTIC: 2Scler.

CHARACTER, lack of: 2Cer. 2Ch-Bd

    immaturity and impulsiveness, from: 3Ch-Bd

    indecisiveness of personality, from: 3Cer.

CHEERFUL: 3Agr.

    attempt to hide inner worries and not be a burden to others or disrupt the peace, with: 3Agr.

    headache, with: 2Agr.

    pain, with all: 2Agr.

    sadness, with: 2Agr.

    seriousness, with: 2Agr.

    thinking of death, while: 2Agr.

CHILDISH behavior: 2Cer. 3Ch-Bd

    immaturity or impulsiveness, from: 3Ch-Bd

    inner uncertainty and need to find appraisal by others, from: 3Cer.

CHILDREN:

    aversion to: 2Holly 2Will.

        irritated and vexed by them, from being: 3Holly

        resenting and blaming, with: 3Will.

    desires to beat: Cher-P. 3Holly

        anger, from: 3Holly

        tension, extreme and inability to control oneself, although attempt has been made, from: 3Cher-P.

    dislikes her own: Beech Holly 2Will.

        Criticism and intolerance, from: 3Beech

CLAIRVOYANCE: 2Clem.

COMPANY:

　　aversion to: 2Beech 3Holly Mim. Wat-V. 3Will.

　　　annoyance and irritability, from: 3Holly

　　　criticism and intolerance, from: 3Beech

　　　desires solitude to indulge her fancy: 2Clem. Honey.

　　　　　reminiscences of past happiness, due to: 3Honey.

　　　　　reveries of future happiness, due to: 3Clem.

　　　feeling superior, with indifference to others, from: 3Wat-V.

　　　resentment and bitterness, from: 3Will.

　　　shyness and fearfulness, from: 3Mim.

　　desire for: 2Agr. 2Chic. 3Heath.

　　　desire for attention and sympathy, with the urge to share one's problems and not feel isolated, from: 3Heath.

　　　need for closeness and taking care of people, from: 3Chic.

　　　seeking stimulation and release of worries through interchange with others, from: 3Agr.

COMPLAINING: 2Chic. 2Heath. 2Will.

　　feeling unappreciated and overlooked, from: 3Chic.

　　need to find sympathetic listener for one's problems and not feel isolated, from: 3Heath.

　　offenses long past: 3Will.

　　resentment and bitterness, with blaming others, from: 3Will.

CONCENTRATION:

　　aversion to: 3Horn. 2Wld-O.

　　　fatigue and mental lassitude, from: 3Horn.

　　　motivation and incentive, lack of, from: 3Wld-O.

difficult: 2Ch-Bd. 2Clem. Elm 3Horn. Must. 2Scler. Wld-O.

absent-mindedness and daydreaming, from: 3Clem.

cannot fix attention: 2Ch-Bd. 2Scler.

crazy feeling on top of head, wild feeling in head, with confusion of ideas: Scler.

dark before the eyes, becomes, on attempting to: Horn.

gloom and joylessness, from: 3Must.

having to sort through multiple impressions, losing the overview and vacillating between options, from: 3Scler.

inattentiveness and carelessness, from: 3Ch-Bd.

overwhelmed, from being: 3Elm

studying, reading, while: 2Horn.

vacant feeling, has a: 2Clem.

writing, while: 2Horn.

CONFIDENCE, want of self-confidence: 3Cer. 2Gent. 3Lar. 2Mim.

anticipation, fearful, and/or shyness, from: 3Mim.

easily discouraged attitude, with tendency to give up one's endeavors as soon as obstacles arise, from: 3Gent.

inner uncertainty, indecisiveness, and dependency on others for advice and approval of the self, from: 3Cer.

low self-esteem and lack of belief in one's capacities, from: 3Lar.

CONFUSION: Cer. 2Cher-P. 2Elm Horn. 3Scler. Wh-Ch.

concentrate the mind, on attempting to: Horn. 2Scler.

mental clarity, lack of, and mental fatigue, due to: 3Horn.

overstimulation with details and loss of overview, from: 3Scler.

identity, as to his: 2Cer.

indecisiveness and lack of intuitive or perceptive power, from: 3Cer.

injury to head, after: Elm Horn. Scler.

mind is easily overstimulated with details, prone to vacillation and lack of mental balance: 2Scler.

mind is hampered in ability to rise above situation and feel in charge: 2Elm

mind is prone to lack of clarity and fatigue: 2Horn.

intoxicated, as if: Clem.

mental exertion, from: Cher-P. Horn. 2Scler.

mental tension and extreme effort to keep mind under control, free from unwanted thoughts or impulses, from: 3Cher-P.

motion, from: 2Scler.

preoccupation with worrisome thoughts that impinge and recurrently torture the mind, from: 3Wh-Ch.

vexation, after: Holly

CONSCIENTIOUS about trifles: 2Chic. 2Crb-A. 2Pine

fussy overcare and urge to set things right, from: 3Chic.

need for cleanliness in the outside world, compensating for shame or feelings of uncleanness within, from: 3Crb-A. Pine tendency to self-reproach, with exaggerated dutiful urge to attend to each detail, from: 3Pine

religious, very: 2Pine 2Verv.

compulsive tendency, assuaging deep-seated guilt, from: 3Pine

overstrain and exaggerated willpower in regard to being conscientious, from: 3Verv.

CONSOLATION, aggravates: 3Chic. 2Holly

irritability, from: 3Holly

self-pity and sulkiness, from: 3Chic.

CONTEMPTUOUS: 2Beech 2Holly Wat-V.

critical, intolerant, and faultfinding, from being: 3Beech

hatred and antagonism, from: 3Holly

haughtiness and feeling superior, from: 2Wat-V.

of self: 2Crb-A. 2Pine

guilt and self-reproach, from: 3Pine

shame and self-loathing, from: 3Crb-A.

CONTRADICT, disposition to: 2Holly

CONTRADICTION, is intolerant of: 3Holly 2Imp. 2Vine Wat-V.

dominating attitude, from: 3Vine

feeling superior in judgment and wisdom, from: 3Wat-V.

has to restrain himself to keep from violence: Cher-P.

impatience with others, from: 3Imp.

selfishness and irritability, from: 3Holly

CONTRARY: 3Holly

COQUETTISH:

    not enough: 2Mim.

    too much so: 3Chic. 2Heath.

        desire to receive the love and attention one deserves, from: 3Chic.

        need to talk, to feel acknowledged and find sympathetic, caring audience, from: 3Heath.

COWARDICE: 3Mim.

CRUELTY (See Behavioral Mistakes): 2Cher-P. 3Holly 2Vine

    abusive, dominating attitude, from: 3Vine

    losing self-control over compelling impulses and committing dreaded, unwanted acts, from: 3Cher-P.

    malice, hatred, jealousy, from: 3Holly

CUNNING: 3Holly

CURSING: 3Holly

DEATH:

    desires: 3Cher-P. Clem. 3Sw-Ch. Wld-R.

        internal pressure, extreme and compelling suicidal impulse, from: 3Cher-P.

        longing to join deceased loved one in the beyond, from: 3Clem.

        meditates on easiest way of self-destruction: 2Cher-P.

        resignation and lack of incentive for life, from: 3Wld-R.

        unbearable anguish, loss of faith, and sense of meaninglessness of life, from: 3Sw-Ch.

    presentiment of (See Fear; death): 2Asp.

DECEITFUL: 2Holly

DEFIANT (See Behavioral Mistakes): 2Ch-Bd. 2Vine

> heedlessness, carelessness and unwillingness to learn from mistakes, from: 3Ch-Bd

> rebelliousness and wish to control one's life, from: 3Vine

DELIRIUM: 2Asp. 3Cher-P. 2Clem. 2Waln.

> angry (See Anger) (Delirium; furious): Cher-P. 2Holly

> anxious: Rck-R.

> apathetic: 2Wld-R.

> attacks people with knife: 2Cher-P.

> blames himself for his folly: Pine

> cheerful: Agr.

> erotic: 2Cher-P.

> foolish, silly: 2Cer.

> foreboding and fear of invisible forces, from: 3Asp.

> frightful: 2Rck-R.

> furious: 2Cher-P. 2Holly Imp. Verv.

>> extreme mental tension and expression of impulses that cannot be held down further despite previous desperate attempts to do so, from: 3Cher-P.

>> fervency and fanaticism, with being high-strung, from: 3Verv.

>> impatience and inner tension, from: 3Imp.

>> rage and unbridled anger, from: 3Holly

> loquacious: 2Heath. Verv.

>> need to be acknowledged and attended to, from: 3Heath.

overenthusiasm and fanatic endeavor to convert others
   to one's viewpoint, from: 3Verv.

mental balance, loss of, and unbridling of pent-up forces
   stemming from the unconscious, signaling the existence of unfulfilled needs or unresolved emotions of
   strong impact, from: 3Cher-P.

mental exertion: Cher-P.

pains, with the: Cher-P.

reality, loss of connection with, and dwelling in dreams,
   hallucinations and visions, from: 3Clem.

reproachful: 2Will.

sleepiness, with: 2Clem.

sorrowful: 2Star-B.

stability of consciousness reduced, with loss of its normal
   boundaries, opening mind to be impacted on by unconscious forces and perceived powers of the invisible
   world, in: 3Waln.

violent (See Delirium; furious): 2Cher-P. 2Holly Imp. Verv.

DELUSIONS (See Delirium): 2Asp. Cer. 3Cher-P. 2Clem.
   2Crb-A. 2Waln. 2Wh-Ch.

accused, thinks she is: 2Pine

air, that he is hovering in, like a spirit: 2Clem.

animals, frightful, of: 2Rck-R.

appreciated, that she is not: 2Chic.

argument, making an eloquent: 2Verv.

arrested, is about to be: 2Pine

asylum, that she will be sent to: 2Cher-P.

better than others, that he is: Wat-V.

business, unfit for, that he is: 2Lar.

cloud, heavy black cloud enveloped her: 2Must.

confusion, imagines others will observe her: 2Mim.

conspiracies against him, there were (See Delusions; persecuted): 2Asp. 2Will.

contaminates everything she touches: 2Crb-A.

corner, sees something coming out of: 2Asp.

crime, about to commit a: 2Cher-P.

    as if he had committed: 2Pine

criticized, that she is: Cer. Chic. Lar. 2Will.

    dependence on approval by others and lack of inner self-assurance, from: 3Cer.

    feeling incapable, with: 3Lar.

    resentment at being treated unfairly, with: 3Will.

    self-pity and feeling unappreciated, with: 3Chic.

danger, impression of (See Fear; danger): 2Rck-R.

deserted, forsaken: 2Wld-R.

despised, that she is (See Delusions; criticized): Chic. 2Will.

devil, possessed of a, is: 2Asp. 2Waln.

        fear of uncanny forces beyond one's control, with: 3Asp.

        feeling vulnerable, unstable and open to influence, with: 3Waln.

die, thought he was about to: 2Cher-P. 2Rck-R.

    intense death-anxiety and feeling threatened, with: 3Rck-R.

    threatened by suicidal impulses, from being: 3Cher-P.

diminished: Cer.

dirty, that he is: 2Crb-A.

    eating dirt: 2Crb-A.

    everything is, that: 2Crb-A.

disease, that he has every (See Anxiety; health): Chic. Heath.

    unrecognized, has an: Asp. 2Mim.

disgraced, that she is: Pine

double, of being: Cer.

dreaming when awake, imagines himself: 2Clem.

elevated in air: 2Clem.

enemy, everyone is an (See Delusions; persecuted): 2Asp. 2Will.

enlarged: Cer.

fancy, illusions of: 2Asp. Cer. 2Cher-P. 3Clem. Waln.

    compelled by images and shocking ideas: 3Cher-P.

    imaginings, born of fear of sinister forces: 3Asp.

    instability of consciousness, easily invaded by images, with loss of being grounded in reality: 3Clem./ 3Waln.

    reveries and pleasant visions: 3Clem.

    uncertainty in regard to differentiating illusions from reality, with: 3Cer.

fear of invisible, uncanny forces, presentiment of eerie dangers, and superstitions, in: 3Asp.

fixed notions and obsessions dominating consciousness, in: 3Cher-P. 2Crb-A. 2Pine 3Wh-Ch.

guilt, self-reproach, and obsessive need to release burden of conscience through repeated punishment, either self-inflicted or through authority, with: 3Pine

impulse, repeated, of shocking content, compelling to unwanted and dreaded thoughts or actions, with: 3Cher-P.

persistent distressing thought pattern, belief, or worry that evades solution and circles in the mind continually, with: 3Wh-Ch.

shame and need to be free of particular symptom that bothers and assumes unproportionate importance, with: 3Crb-A.

floating in air: 2Clem.

flying, sensation of: 2Clem.

fortune, that he was going to lose his: 2Mim.

friend has met with an accident: 3Rd-Ch.

great person, is: 2Vine 2Wat-V.

imperial, augmented attitude, with: 3Vine

pride and aloofness, with: 3Wat-V.

humility and lowliness of others, while he is great (See Delusions; great person): 2Vine 2Wat-V.

identity, errors of personal: 2Cer.

images, phantoms, sees (See Delusions; fancy): 2Asp. Cer. 2Cher-P. 2Clem. Waln.

dwells upon: 2Clem.

frightful: 2Rck-R.

pleasant: 3Clem.

injury, is about to receive: 2Mim.

insane, that she will become: 3Cher-P.

laughed at, imagines she is (See Delusions; criticized): 2Cer. Lar.

> self-confidence, lack of, and feeling inferior to others, arising from: 3Lar.

> self-distrust and concern about being appraised by others, arising from: 3Cer.

looked down upon, that she is (See Delusions; criticized; laughed at): 2Cer. Lar.

murder, thinks she is about to, her husband and child: 3Cher-P.

> that he has to, someone: 3Cher-P. 2Vine

>> compelling impulse, from: 3Cher-P.

>> urge to assume control and authority, with: 3Vine

murdered, that he would be: 2Asp. Rck-R.

> foreboding of undefined dangers, with: 3Asp.

> terror and panic attacks, with: 3Rck-R.

> conspiring to murder him, are (See Delusions; persecuted): 2Asp. 2Will.

mystery, everything around seemed a terrifying: 2Asp. Waln.

neglected his duty: 3Pine

persecuted, that he is: 2Asp. Pine Waln. 2Will.

> foreboding and perceptions of vague threats coming from others, with: 3Asp.

> guilt, underlying and unconscious wish for punishment, with: 3Pine

resenting, blaming others and transference of same emotions to perceived opponent, with: 3Will.

vulnerability and feeling unprotected from interference by unwanted, disturbing influence, with: 3Waln.

place, that he cannot pass a certain: 2Asp.

possessed, as if (See Delusion; devil): 2Asp. 2Waln.

preoccupation with recurring thought patterns of deeply felt worry, torturing and haunting the mind, in: 3Wh-Ch.

proud: 2Wat-V.

pursued, thought he was (See Delusions; persecuted): 2Asp. Pine Waln. 2Will.

rank, thinks himself a person of (See Delusions; great person): 2Vine 2Wat-V.

reproach, has neglected duty and deserves: 3Pine

repulsive fantastic imaginations: 2Cher-P.

sick, imagines himself: 2Chic. Crb-A. 2Heath. 2Mim.

    fear and concern about own self, from: 3Mim.

    need for company, for willing listeners and sympathetic attention, from: 3Heath.

    preoccupation and obsession with symptoms, with: 3Crb-A.

    self-pity and need for the attention one deserves, with: 3Chic.

  a beloved friend is sick and dying: 3Rd-Ch.

members of the family are: 3Rd-Ch.

soul, fancied body was too small for, or that it was separated from: 2Clem.

specters, ghosts, spirits, sees (See Delusions; fancy): 3Asp.
Cher-P. 2Clem. Rck-R. 2Waln.

strange, everything is: 2Asp. Cer.

strangers, friends appear as: 2Asp.

succeed, that he cannot, does everything wrong: 2Lar.

suffered, fancies he has: Chic. Heath. 2Will.

    resentment and blaming others, with: 3Will.

    self-pity and sulkiness, with: 3Chic.

    talkativeness and complaining, with: 3Heath.

superhuman control, under, is: Cher-P. Waln.

superiority: 2Wat-V.

tormented, thinks is: Sw-Ch.

transparent, seemed to be: Clem.

troubles, broods over imaginary: Must. 2Wh-Ch.

    depression and gloom, with: 3Must.

    preoccupation and persistent thought patterns, with:
3Wh-Ch.

unfortunate, that he is: Will.

vexations and offenses, of: 2Holly

visions (See Delusions; fancy): 2Clem. 2Waln.

voices, hears (See Delusions; fancy): 2Asp. Cer. 2Cher-P.
Waln.

watched, that she is being (See Delusion; persecuted): 2Asp.
Pine

weight, has no: Clem.

women are evil and will injure his soul: Asp. 2Will.

wrong:

> fancies he has done: 2Pine

> has suffered: 2Will.

DESIRES, has no more: 2Wld-R.

> more than she needs: 2Chic. Heath.

DESPAIR: 2Cher-P. 2Crb-A. 2Elm Gent. Gors. 2Lar. Must. 2Oak 2Pine 2Star-B. 3Sw-Ch. Wld-R. 2Will.

> anguish, unbearable, loss of faith, and sense of meaninglessness of life, from: 3Sw-Ch.

> criticism, from the smallest: 2Lar. 2Pine

>> feeling inferior and losing trust in one's capacities, from: 3Lar.

>> self-reproach, excessive, from: 3Pine

> depression, gloom and joylessness, from: 3Must.

> discouragement from obstacles and tendency to withdraw from struggle, with occasional despair: 3Gent.

> grief, trauma, shock, from: 3Star-B.

> guilt and self-reproach, from: 3Pine

> health, of (See Despair; recovery): 2Gent. 3Gors.

> hopelessness, from: 3Gors.

> mental tension, extreme, as compelling impulses or intense pain threaten to overtake reason, from: 3Cher-P.

> others, about: 2Rd-Ch.

> overwhelmed by tasks or emotional challenges, from being: 3Elm

> pains, with the (See Despair; anguish; mental tension): Agr. 3Cher-P. 2Sw-Ch.

restlessness and attempt to stay cheerful, with underlying despair: 3Agr.

perseverance in one's duties despite hardship and setbacks, with underlying despair: 3Oak

recovery, of: 2Gent. 3Gors.

discouragement at slow process or setbacks during healing process, from: 3Gent.

hopelessness, complete, although one goes along with new treatments to satisfy loved ones, from: 3Gors.

religious: 2Gent. 3Pine

discouragement and lack of faith in a higher power, from: 3Gent.

guilt and disquiet of conscience, with feeling unworthy before one's God, from: 3Pine

resignation in face of being unable to change one's lot, with underlying despair: 3Wld-R.

self-confidence, lack of, from: 3Lar.

shame and feelings of uncleanness, from: 3Crb-A.

unfortunate and treated unfairly, from feeling: 3Will.

DESTRUCTIVENESS (See Abusive; anger): 2Cher-P. 3Holly Imp. Verv. 2Vine

DICTATORIAL: 3Vine

DIPSOMANIA: 2Agr.

DISCIPLINE of self:

exaggerated: 2Oak 3Rck-W. 2Verv.

desire for self-mastery, due to high aspirations or out of necessity, with urge to inspire others, from: 3Rck-W.

determination to work hard and persevere despite setbacks or difficulties, from: 3Oak

necessity of raising one's willpower, inner drive and enthusiasm due to demanding task, from: 3Verv.

lack of (See Indolence): 3Ch-Bd. 2Horn. 2Wld-O.

immaturity, inattentiveness and failure to learn from mistakes, from: 3Ch-Bd.

motivation and incentive, lack of, from: 3Wld-O.

tendency to procrastination and lassitude, from: 3Horn.

DISCONTENTED: 2Agr. 2Beech 2Holly 3Wld-O. 2Will.

embitterment over one's fate, with recognition of missed opportunities and of being treated unfairly, from: 3Will.

expectancy of beauty and perfection in one's life and finding reality wanting, with expression of criticism, from: 3Beech

inner restlessness, lack of satisfaction, and need for fulfillment and adventure, from: 3Agr.

irritability; easily vexed, jealous, and upset feelings, from: 3Holly

purpose, direction and meaningful occupation, lack of, from: 3Wld-O.

DISCORDS, ailments from, between friends: Agr.

DISCOURAGED: 3Gent. 2Gors.

discouragement, lack of faith and failure to pursue tasks in face of hindrances: 3Gent.

hopelessness, with: 3Gors.

DISCRIMINATION, lack of: Ch-Bd.

DISCUSSES her symptoms with everyone: 3Heath.

DISGUST: 3Crb-A.

DISOBEDIENCE: 3Ch-Bd.

DOUBTFUL, recovery, of (See Despair; recovery): 3Gent.

DOUBTFUL, soul's welfare, of (See Despair; religious): 3Gent.
3Pine

DREAM, as if in a: 3Clem.

future, about the poetical: 2Clem.

DULLNESS: 2Clem. 3Horn. 2Must. Oak Oliv. 2Wld-O.

absent-mindedness and daydreaming, from: 3Clem.

exhaustion in mind and body, from: Horn. Oak 3Oliv.

gloominess, depression and joyless introversion, from:
3Must.

injuries of head, after: 2Horn. Must. Wld-O.

mind is prone to be less stimulated and motivated:
3Wld-O.

mind is prone to experience depression and less brightness of consciousness: 3Must.

mind is prone to have less clarity of consciousness and
reduced power of concentration, with tendency
to fatigue: 3Horn.

lassitude and fatigue, with tendency to procrastinate, from:
3Horn.

mental exertion, from: Horn. Oliv.

motivation, incentive, appeal of life, lack of, from: 3Wld-
O.

stoic, weary, one-track mind, bent on fulfilling duty at expense of recreational diversion, from: 3Oak

think long, unable to: Horn.

think or concentrate, unable to: Horn.

DWELLS on past disagreeable occurrences: 2Wh-Ch. 3Will.

recurring thoughts and disconcerting worry about past experiences, with: 3Wh-Ch.

resentment and blaming others, with: 3Will.

EAT, refuses to: 3Wld-O.

ECCENTRICITY (See Arrogance): 2Beech 2Vine 2Wat-V.

desire for realization of beauty and perfection in one's environment, with criticism, intolerance and arrogance, should these not be met, from: 3Beech

feeling superior in character and endowment, with tendency to stay aloof, from: 3Wat-V.

interest in having personal preferences met, even to the exploit or discomfort of others, from: 3Vine

ECSTASY: 2Verv.

EGOTISM (See Arrogance; Eccentricity): 2Beech 2Chic. 2Heath. 2Vine 3Wat-V.

critical and intolerant attitude toward others, while considering oneself special, from: 3Beech

leading others self-righteously, even to their disadvantage, with belief that one has higher capacities than others, from: 3Vine

overcare for others with possessiveness and expectation of being appreciated, from: 3Chic.

pride and feelings of superiority, with attitude of aloofness towards those considered less special than oneself, from: 3Wat-V.

self-centered attitude with inner need to reach out to others in order to be acknowledged and listened to, from: 3Heath.

EMBARRASSMENT, ailments after: 2Crb-A. 2Pine

guilt and self-reproach, with: 3Pine

shame at exposure of unclean aspect of self, from: 3Crb-A.

ENNUI (See Boredom): 2Clem. 2Honey. 3Wld-O.

homesickness, with: 2Honey.

ENVY: 3Holly

ESCAPE, attempts to: 2Cher-P.

ESTRANGED, family, from her: 2Will.

EXACTING, too: 2Beech Chic. Vine

dictatorial and demanding, from being: 3Vine

high standards of perfection, with tendency to judge others or their products and find fault with them, from: 3Beech

meddlesome, with urge to set things right according to one's own ideas, from being: 3Chic.

EXALTATION, politics: 2Verv.

religious: 2Verv.

EXCITEMENT: Cher-P. Heath. Holly 3Verv.

emotional, ailments from: 2Verv.

nervous: 3Verv.

religious: 2Verv.

sexual, ailments from: 2Cher-P.

talking, while: 2Heath. 2Verv.

overenthusiasm and trying to incite others, from: 3Verv.

self-centered enjoyment of having found willing listener for one's problems, from: 3Heath.

thinking of the things others have done to displease her: 2Holly

EXCLUSIVE, too (See Egotism): Beech 3Wat-V.

EXERTION, mental: 3Cher-P. 2Horn. 2Oak 2Oliv. 3Verv.

exhaustion, extreme, from prolonged mental overexertion: 3Oliv.

intense mental strain and overexertion, with threat of losing mental balance and sanity: 3Cher-P. Verv

overenthusiasm, excessive inner drive, and reinforced willpower lead to mental overexertion, threatening a nervous breakdown: Cher-P. 3Verv.

power of concentration waning due to prolonged overstudy: 3Horn.

stoic concentration on duty, with mental despondency and weariness: 3Oak

EXHAUSTION (See Wearisome).

EXHILARATION: 2Verv.

EXPANSIVE, too demonstrative: Verv.

EXTRAVAGANCE: 2Wat-V.

FANATICISM: 3Verv.

FANCIES:

absorbed in: 3Clem.

exaltation of: Cher-P. 2Clem. 2Verv.

engaging in shocking imaginations that are dreaded and yet fascinate, from: 3Cher-P.

fervency and exalted ideals that are envisioned and striven
for, from: 3Verv.

visions, reveries and dreams of beautiful or romantic
content, from: 3Clem.

frightful: 2Rck-R.

lascivious: Cher-P.

pleasant: 3Clem.

FATIGUE (See Wearisome).

FASTIDIOUS (See Conscientious): 2Chic. 2Crb-A. 2Pine

FEAR (See Anxiety; fear): 3Asp. 3Cher-P. 3Mim. 3Rd-Ch. 3Rck-R.

accidents, of: 2Mim.

agoraphobia (See Fear; phobia).

alone, of being: 2Asp. Cher-P. 3Mim. Rck-R.

dread of loneliness and its imagined discomfort or dangers, from: 3Mim.

eerie foreboding, with feeling vulnerable and lonely,
from: 3Asp.

element of terror, with: 3Rck-R.

injure himself, lest he: 3Cher-P.

alternating with mania: 3Cher-P.

animals, of: 2Mim.

approaching him, of others: 2Mim. 2Rck-R.

fear of getting hurt, either physically or emotionally, due
to sickness, fragility or emotional shyness, from:
3Mim.

tremulous nerves and easily startled state, from: 3Rck-R.

behind him, that someone is: 2Asp.

black, everything: Asp.

blood, of: Cher-P.

church or opera, when ready to go: 2Mim.

claustrophobia (See Fear; phobia).

closed places (See Fear; phobia).

cold, of taking: 2Mim.

confusion, that people would observe her: 2Mim.

contagion: 2Crb-A. 2Mim.

> fear and dread of disease, with: 3Mim.

> loathing and sense of contamination, with: 3Crb-A.

corners, to walk past certain: 2Asp.

creeping out of every corner, of something: 2Asp.

danger, impending, of: Asp. 2Mim. Rd-Ch. 2Rck-R.

> concrete fears, anticipating predictable events: 3Mim.

> fear for others: 3Rd-Ch.

> fright and inner tremor, with: 3Rck-R.

> vague fears of impending doom and sinister forces, superstitions: 3Asp.

dark: 2Asp.

death, of: 2Asp. 2Mim. 3Rck-R.

> anticipatory fears, dreading the arrival and the struggle of death, with: 3 Mim.

> fear of the unknown and foreboding, with: 3Asp.

> fright and panic attacks, with: 3Rck-R.

death, of, from pain: Cher-P.

destination, of being unable to reach his: 2Mim.

disaster, of (See Fear; danger).

disease, of impending: 3Mim.

downward motion, of: 2Rck-R.

epilepsy (See Anxiety; between intervals): 2Cher-P. 2Rck-R.

everything, constant: 2Rck-R.

evil of: 2Asp.

exertion, of: 2Mim.

fainting, of: Cher-P.

fit, of having a: 2Cher-P.

friend has met with accident, that a: 3Rd-Ch.

ghosts, of: 3Asp.

happen, something will: 3Asp.

high places (See Fear; phobia).

husband, that he would never return, that something would happen to him: 3Rd-Ch.

imaginary things: 2Asp. 2Cher-P.

   compelling imaginations of shocking, yet fascinating content, with: 3Cher-P.

   superstitions, fear of ghosts and spirits, with: 3Asp.

imbecile, that he would become: 3Cher-P.

impulses, his own: 3Cher-P.

infection, of (See Fear; contagion): 2Crb-A. 2Mim.

injured, of being (See Fear; danger): 2Mim.

insanity, of: 3Cher-P.

jumps: Rck-R.

killing, of: 3Cher-P.

knives, of: 2Cher-P.

labor, during: 2Cher-P. Rck-R.

> fear of losing control from intensity of pain and struggle, with: 3Cher-P.

> terror, fright and panic attacks, with: 3Rck-R.

losing senses: Cher-P.

medicine, of taking too much: Mim.

men of: 2Mim.

mischief, he might do, night on waking: Cher-P.

misfortune, of (See Fear; danger): 3Mim.

moral obliquity, fear of, alternating with sexual excitement: Cher-P.

murdered, of being (See Fear; danger): 2Asp. Mim. 2Rck-R.

narrow place, in (See Fear; phobia):

noise, from sudden: 2Rck-R.

observed, of her condition being: 3Mim.

opinion of others, of: 2Cer. 2Lar. 3Mim.

> fear of being appraised unfavorably, from: 3Mim.

> > self-assurance, lack of, inner indecisiveness and dependence on others for approval of self, from: 3Cer.

> > self-esteem, lack of, and distrust in one's capacities, from: 3Lar.

others and their welfare, for: 3Rd-Ch.

people, of: 2Mim.

phobia: 3Cher-P. 3Rck-R.

> fear of losing control and giving in to panic, with: 3Cher-P.

> terror and inner turmoil, with: 3Rck-R.

poverty: 3Mim.

public, appearing in, of (See Anticipation): 3Mim.

self-control, losing: 3Cher-P.

shadows, of: Asp.

sleep, before: 2Asp. 2Mim.

> concrete fears of nightmares or other discomforts: 3Mim.

> fear of the unknown, of letting go: 3Asp.

suffering, of: Mim.

suffocation, of: Rck-R.

suicide: 3Cher-P.

superstitious: 3Asp.

talking loud, as if would kill her: Mim.

thoughts, of his own: 3Cher-P. 2Wh-Ch.

> shocking impulse compelling to dreaded thoughts or actions, due to: 3Cher-P.

> worrisome thoughts that torture and cannot be released, due to: 3Wh-Ch.

touch, of: 2Rck-R.

tread lightly, must, or will injure himself: 2Mim.

tremulous: 2Rck-R.

unaccountable: 2Asp.

undertaking anything: 2Cer. 3Mim. 2Lar.

anticipatory dread and fear of failure, from: 3Mim.

inner uncertainty, lack of self-assurance and decisive power, from: 3Cer.

self-confidence, lack of, from: 3Lar.

voice, of using: Mim.

women, of: 2Mim.

work, dread of: 2Mim.

FEIGNING (See Affectation):

sick: 2Chic. Heath.

pregnancy: 2Chic. Heath.

FIGHT, wants to: 3Holly

FIRE, wants to set things on: Cher-P. 2Holly

antagonism, rebelliousness, revenge, from: 3Holly

compelling impulse that is not mastered, although known to be wrong, from: 3Cher-P.

FLATTERY, desires (See Attention): 2Chic. 2Heath.

FOOLISH behavior: 3Cer. 3Ch-Bd.

immaturity and impulsiveness of the mind, from: 3Ch-Bd.

inner uncertainty and lack of self-assurance, with inappropriate behavior, from: 3Cer.

FOREBODING: 3Asp.

FORGETFUL: 2Ch-Bd. 2Clem. 3Horn.

absent-mindedness and daydreaming, from: 3Clem.

fatigue, lassitude, and lack of power of concentration, from: 3Horn.

inattentiveness, from: 3Ch-Bd.

mental exertion, from: Horn.

FORSAKEN feeling: 3Wld-R.

FRIGHT, complaints from: 3Rck-R.

FRIGHTENED easily: 3Rck-R.

GESTURES, makes: Cer. 2Cher-P. 2Verv.

expressing internal mental force that opposes disturbing or socially unacceptable thoughts or impulses, due to: 3Cher-P.

overenthusiasm and demonstrative attempt to incite others, from: 3Verv.

ridiculous or foolish: 2Cer.

uncertainty and indecisiveness of self-expression, from: 3Cer.

violent (See Violent): 2Cher-P. 2Holly Imp. Verv. Vine

GIGGLING: 2Ch-Bd.

GLOOMY (See Sadness)(Light; desire for):

from no known cause: 3Must.

GODLESS, want of religious feeling: 2Gent. 2Sw-Ch.

faith and trust in God, lack of, from: 3Gent.

soul aspiration, loss of, and sense of meaninglessness, from: 3Sw-Ch.

GOING out, aversion to: 2Chic. 2Will.

resentment and bitterness, from: 3Will.

self-pity and not wanting to give oneself to others, from: 3Chic.

GOSSIPING: Beech 2Holly 2Will.

critical, faultfinding attitude, from: 3Beech

expressing and sharing with confidants the pent-up resentment and blame held toward an offender, from: 3Will.

jealousy of someone's advantages, fueled by: 3Holly

GRIEF: 3Star-B.

ailments, from: 2Star-B.

GRIMACES: Cher-P.

HATRED: 3Holly 2Will.

embitterment and resentment, with blaming others for one's unhappiness, from: 3Will.

response to perceived threat, with urge to fight and defend, from: 3Holly

HAUGHTY: 3Wat-V.

HEEDLESS: 2Ch-Bd.

HELPLESSNESS, feeling of: 3Wld-R.

HIGH places aggravate (See Fear; phobia): 3Cher-P. 3Rck-R.

HOMESICKNESS: 2Clem. 3Honey. 2Star-B.

ailments, from: Clem. 2Honey. Star-B.

dreaming about future and looking forward to going home, with: 3Clem.

grief and intense sadness, with: 3Star-B.

reminiscing about home life gone by and longing for past happiness, with: 3Honey.

HONOR, effects of wounded: 2Holly Wat-V.

annoyance and anger, from: 3Holly

wounded pride and augmenting oneself above offender as response, from: 3Wat-V.

HOPELESS: 3Gors.

HORRIBLE things, sad stories, affect her profoundly: 2Waln.

HURRY: 2Agr. 2Cher-P. 2Ch-Bd. 3Imp. Rck-R. 2Verv.

> anxiety and tremulous nerves, from: 3Rck-R.

> compelling impulses and compulsive thinking create inner tension and hurry, as if one seeks to escape them: 3Cher-P.

> everybody must hurry: 3Imp.

> fervency, fanaticism, or heightened willpower and speed to accomplish tasks, with urging on of oneself and others, from: 3Verv.

> impatience and inner need to move fast, from: 3Imp.

> impulsiveness and instability of mind, while not concentrating fully on the present, from: 3Ch-Bd.

> inner restlessness and worry about completion of tasks, from: 3Agr.

HYDROPHOBIA (See Fear; phobia): 3Cher-P. 3Rck-R.

HYPERACTIVE, child: 2Agr. 2Ch-Bd. 2Imp. 2Rck-R. 3Verv.

> impatience and willfulness, with inner need to move forward at a fast pace, from: 3Imp.

> inner restlessness, unfulfilled needs or discomfort, prone to be disturbed by outside influences, from: 3Agr.

> mental focus, unsettled, easily distracted, skipping from activity to activity without deepened concentration, from: 3Ch-Bd.

> overenthusiasm and excitement during play, with exaggerated speed or vehemence, from: 3Verv.

sensitivity of the nervous system, with inner tremulousness, lack of sturdy health, and nervous agitation, from: 3Rck-R.

HYSTERIA: 2Cher-P. 3Chic. 2Heath. 2Scler.

alternation of emotional and physical symptoms, with: 3Scler.

expression of self-pity and unfulfilled needs for appreciation and attention, through means other than normal verbal communication, from: 3Chic.

inner loneliness and deeply felt need for sharing and communication, expressed through heightened, exaggerated verbal flow, from: 3Heath.

lascivious: 2Cher-P.

suppression of sexual urges: 3Cher-P.

unfulfilled vital needs send compelling impulses to consciousness, threatening to be expressed at the expense of reasonable and socially acceptable conduct: 3Cher-P.

IDEAS, deficiency of: 2Clem. 3Horn. Must. 2Wld-O. Wld-R.

absent-mindedness and daydreaming, from: 3Clem.

depression, introversion and gloominess, from: 3Must.

fatigue, mental lassitude and tendency to procrastination, from: 3Horn.

motivation and incentive, lack of, from: 3Wld-O.

resignation and lack of incentive to improve one's lot, from: 3Wld-R.

IDIOCY: Horn. Wld-O.

deficiency in motivation and interest, with: 2Wld-O.

deficiency in power of concentration and lack of mental clarity, with: 2Horn.

IMBECILITY (See Idiocy): Horn. Wld-O.

IMPATIENCE: 3Imp.

IMPERTINENCE: Ch-Bd. 2Holly

    aggression, from: 3Holly

    immaturity and heedlessness, from: 3Ch-Bd.

IMPETUOUS: 3Cher-P. 3Imp. 2Verv.

    impatience and inner speed, from: 3Imp.

    overenthusiasm and fanaticism, from: 3Verv.

    pent-up inner impulses create mounting tension and inner force: 3Cher-P.

IMPERIOUS: 3Vine.

IMPOLITE (See Impertinence): Ch-Bd. 2Holly

IMPULSE:

    to set on fire (See Fire): 2Cher-P. 2Holly

    to stab his flesh with the knife he holds: 3Cher-P.

IMPULSIVE (See Impetuous): 3Cher-P. Ch-Bd. 2Imp. Verv.

    immature and unsettled mind, from: 3Ch-Bd.

INCITING others: 2Holly. 2Verv.

    inciting others into cooperation for cause considered worthy: 3Verv.

    stirring others into unkind sentiments: 3Holly

INCONSOLABLE: 2Chic. Star-B.

    deeply felt, traumatic grief, from: 3Star-B.

    self-pity and sulkiness, from: 3Chic.

INCONSTANCY: 2Agr. 2Ch-Bd. 2Chic. 2Scler. 3Wld-O.

> impulsiveness of thought and behavior, with inattentiveness and failure to learn from experience, from: 3Ch-Bd

> inability to find interesting tasks, pursuits or purposeful, deeply enriching occupation, from: 3Wld-O.

> inner restlessness, worry, lack of peace within, with feeling that important inner resources or needs are not fulfilled, from: 3Agr.

> mood swings, changeability of interests and desires, overstimulation with impressions and ideas, from: 3Scler.

> overcare or possessiveness toward others alternating with sullen retreat into self-pity, should attention and care not be returned, from: 3Chic.

INDEPENDENT: 2Wat-V.

INDIFFERENCE (See Boredom): 2Clem. 2Honey. 2Must. 2Wld-O. 3Wld-R. Wat-V.

> business affairs, to: 2Wld-O.

> complain, does not: Wld-R.

> conscience, to the dictates of: 2Ch-Bd./2Holly.

> desire, has no, no action of the will: 2Wld-R.

> everything, to: 2Wld-O. 2Wld-R.

>> apathy and lack of feeling empowered, from: 3Wld-R.

>> disinterest and lack of direction, from: 3Wld-O.

> interest in present moment, lack of, from (See Absentmindedness): 2Clem. 2Honey. 3Wld-R.

belief that future, not present, holds the key to happiness, with: 3Clem.

belief that past contained happiness that can never be repeated in this life, with: 3Honey.

burdensome hardship that one resigns oneself to, from: 3Wld-R.

introversion, depression and lack of incentive, from: 3Must.

others, to, due to feeling superior to them: 3Wat-V.

pleasure, to: 3Wld-R.

recovery, about his: 2Gors. 2Wld-R

hopelessness, due to: 3Gors.

resigning to one's sickness, from: 3Wld-R.

suffering, to: Wld-R.

INDIGNATION: 3Holly

INDOLENCE: 2Ch-Bd. 3Horn. 3Wld-O.

fatigue, lassitude, and tendency to procrastination, from: 3Horn.

inattentiveness, carelessness, no in-depth focus to tasks, from: 3Ch-Bd.

tasks neither appeal nor stimulate once engaged in: 3Wld-R.

INDUSTRIOUS: 2Agr. 2Chic. 2Imp. 2Oak 2Verv.

feels driven to work: 3Verv.

impatience and inner tension lead to fast-paced, achievement-oriented work: 3Imp.

keeping busy to assuage worry and finding outlet for inner restlessness, from: 3Agr.

overcare, exaggerated, for others and attention to trifles, from: 3Chic.

overenthusiasm and fanatic work attitude, with urging on of oneself and others, from: 3Verv.

plodding, stoic approach to work, tendency to disciplined overwork, even in face of hardship, from: 3Oak

INFANCY, complaints from:

appetite wanting: 3Wld-O.

crying, exaggerated, with urge to make needs known and have people respond: 3Verv./3Vine

frightened easily, with frequent starting: 3Rck-R.

fussiness from being pampered, with urge to be center of attention: 3Chic.

irritable, easily angered, impatient and fussy: 3Holly/3Imp.

restlessness, crying, discomfort and pain: 3Agr.

INHIBITED: 3Cer. 2Lar. 3Mim.

self-confidence, lack of, with anticipation of failure and feeling inferior to others, from: 3Lar.

shyness, timid nervousness, and fear of appraisal, from: 3Mim.

uncertainty and hesitancy of attitude, lack of decisive power, internally hampered expression of personality, from: 3Cer.

INJURE, fears to be left alone, lest he should, himself: 3Cher-P.

INSANITY: 3Cher-P. 2Sw-Ch. 2Verv.

anguish, unbearable; loss of faith, meaning and soul-joy, with nihilistic attitude: 3Sw-Ch.

compulsive impulses and ideas, stemming from unfulfilled, suppressed needs, overthrow mental balance, resulting in shocking, bizarre or antisocial behavior: 3Cher-P.

erotic: 3Cher-P.

fervency and fanaticism, with intensity of self-expression: 3Verv.

injuries to the head, from: Cher-P.

INSOLENT: 2Holly

INSPIRE, desire to inspire others by one's own example of self-mastery: 3Rck-W.

INTROSPECTION: 2Must. 3Wh-Ch.

gloominess, depression and lack of incentive to involve in present, with: 3Must.

worrisome thoughts that circle in the mind and distract from involvement in the present, from: 3Wh-Ch.

IRRESOLUTION: 3Scler. 2Cer.

timidity and hesitancy in decisions, lack of self-assurance and dependency on advice, from: 3Cer.

vacillation between two or more options, with loss of overview and dread of making the wrong choice: 3Scler.

IRRITABILITY: 2Cher-P. 3Holly 3Imp. 2Rck-R. 2Verv. 2Will.

consolation aggravates: 2Chic. 2Holly

annoyance at being interfered with, from: 3Holly

self-pity and self-centered refusal to interact with others, from: 3Chic.

contradiction, from the slightest: 2Holly

excited, when: 2Verv.

exertion, from: 2Verv.

fragility of nerves and lack of internal stamina, from: 3Rck-R.

impatience and inner need to move fast, from: 3Imp.

overexcitement, fervency, and heightened inner tension and drive, from: 3Verv.

sensitivity to disturbances in the environment, easily stirred-up and unnerved state, from: 3Holly

takes everything in bad part: Chic. 2Holly Will.

easily angered and vexed attitude, from: 3Holly

embitterment, feels treated unfairly and is offended easily, from: 3Will.

feeling unappreciated and misunderstood, from: 3Chic.

wound-up nervous system, due to having to balance internal pressures and unwanted thoughts that threaten sanity, from: 3Cher-P.

JEALOUSY: 3Holly

ailments from: 2Holly

JESTING: 2Agr. Cer. Cher-P. 2Ch-Bd.

cheer, to spread and uphold, despite internal worries: 3Agr.

impulsive, repeated jesting, with expression of internal pressures surrounding unfulfilled needs, from: 3Cher-P.

ridiculous or foolish: 2Cer. 2Ch-Bd.

immaturity of the mind, childishness, from: 3Ch-Bd.

inappropriate jokes, born of inner uncertainty, with attempt to impress others: 3Cer.

JOY:

ailments from excessive: 2Verv.

at the misfortune of others: 2Holly 2Will.

feeling unfortunate and embittered and not wishing others any happiness, from: 3Will.

revenge, jealousy, hatred, from: 3Holly.

JUMPING, impulse to jump from a height: 3Cher-P.

KILL, desire to: 2Cher-P. 3Holly.

anger or unchecked hatred, from: 3Holly

suppressed unconscious or conscious urges to kill, despite attempt to hold down intensity of impulse: 3Cher-P.

KILLED, desires to be: Cher-P.

KISSES, everyone: Cher-P.

KNEELING and praying (See Praying): 2Pine 2Verv.

LAMENTING: 2Chic. 2Will.

appreciated, because she is not: 3Chic.

unfortunate victim, from being: 3Will.

LASCIVIOUSNESS: 3Cher-P.

LAUGHING (See Jesting): 3Agr. 2Cer. 3Ch-Bd.

reprimands, at: 2Ch-Bd.

sad, when: 2Agr.

serious matters, over: 2Agr. 2Ch-Bd.

attempt to hide inner worries, from: 3Agr.

carelessness and immaturity, from: 3Ch-Bd.

silly: 2Cer. 2Ch-Bd.

impulsiveness, buoyancy, naivety, from: 3Ch-Bd.

inner insecurities, from: 3Cer.

LEARNING, difficulties during (See Concentration; Memory).

LEWDNESS: 2Cher-P.

LIGHT, desire for: 2Horn. 3Must.

> dampened spirits, with feeling of dark gloom hanging over one's head: 3Must.

> mental clarity and brightness diminished from fatigue and lassitude: 3Horn.

LOATHING: 2Crb-A. 2Holly Wld-O. Will.

> disgust toward one's own uncleanness or flaws, with tendency to see shameful or unclean aspect in one's environment as well, from: 3Crb-A.

> life: 3Sw-Ch. 2Wld-O. 3Will.

>> embitterment over one's fate, with putting blame on others, from: 3Will.

>> life does not appeal, boredom and aimlessness, no sense of destiny in regard to one's purpose and vocation: 3Wld-O.

>> life is seen as meaningless, loss of personal aspiration, nihilistic attitude: 3Sw-Ch.

> life, must restrain herself to prevent doing herself injury: 3Cher-P.

> vehemence and annoyance, with: 3Holly Will.

> work: 2Wld-O.

LONGING:

> dream of future happiness to be fulfilled, for: 3Clem.

> good opinion of others, for: 2Cent. 3Cer.

>> uncertain self-image and dependence on approval by others, from: 3Cer.

> willingness to serve and please others, from: 3Cent.

past happiness to be relived, for: 3Honey.

repose and tranquility, for: Wh-Ch.

LOOKED at, cannot bear to be: 3Chic. 2Holly Mim.

cross and upset, due to being: 3Holly.

shyness and embarrassment, due to: 3Mim.

sullen withdrawal, due to: 3Chic.

LOQUACITY: 2Agr. 2Ch-Bd. 3Heath. 2Verv.

desire for company and amusement, stemming from inner need to mix with people and find diversion and release of worries, from: 3Agr.

impulsiveness of thought and unchecked loquacity, with immaturity and childishness of the mind, from: 3Ch-Bd.

inner loneliness and need to find sympathetic understanding for one's sorrow or ailments, from: 3Heath.

overenthusiasm for a cause and attempt to convert others to one's viewpoint, from: 3Verv.

LOVE:

ailments, from disappointed: Cher-P. 2Chic. Holly Rck-W. 3Star-B.

decision, following disappointment, to forgo fulfillment of desires and be example of self-mastery, from: 3Rck-W.

love turns into hate, due to being rejected: 3Holly

sadness and deeply felt sense of loss, with: 3Star-B.

self-pity and withdrawal into hurt feelings due to being rejected: 3Chic.

suppression of sexual excitement and need, from: 3Cher-P.

love-sick, with jealousy, anger and incoherent talk: Cher-P. 2Holly.

silent grief: 3Star-B.

LUDICROUS, things seem: Agr. Cer. 2Ch-Bd.

inappropriate laughing and silliness, with: 3Ch-Bd.

need to stay cheerful and not be bogged down by serious worries, from: 3Agr.

uncertainty of judgment, with inappropriate response to situation at hand and inner lack of self-assurance, from: 3Cer.

MALICIOUS (See Hatred): 3Holly 3Will.

MANIA (See Insanity): 3Cher-P. 2Verv.

MEDDLESOME: Beech 2Chic. 2Vine

criticizing others due to their perceived imperfections: 3Beech

influencing and controlling others, from inner tendency to assume leadership: 3Vine

interfering in others' lives, with exaggerated urge to take care of them: 3Chic.

MEMORY, weakness of: 3Ch-Bd. 2Clem. 3Horn. 2Oak 2Oliv.

absent-mindedness and daydreaming on subject matter other than present theme, from: 3Clem.

fatigue, from: 3Horn. 2Oak 2Oliv.

exhaustion in mind and body and reduced ability to uphold commitments and pursue one's normal tasks: 3Oliv.

mental fatigue and reduced power of concentration: 3Horn.

persevering in duty, despite fatigue, with stoic, one-track mind: 3Oak

inattentiveness and subsequent reduced retention of subject matter, from: 3Ch-Bd.

MEN, dread of: 3Mim.

MIRTH: 3Agr.

foolish (See Foolish): 2Cer. Ch-Bd.

MISANTHROPY (See Hatred): 3Holly 3Will.

MISCHIEVOUS: 3Holly

MISTAKES :

reading, in: Horn.

speaking, in: Cer.

writing, in: Horn.

MOANING: 2Sw-Ch.

MOCKING: 2Holly

MONOMANIA (See Delusions; fixed): 3Cher-P. 2Crb-A. 2Wh-Ch.

MOOD:

agreeable: 2Agr.

alternating: 3Scler. 2Wld-O.

inconstancy of motivational interests, from: 3Wld-O.

tendency to vacillation and indecisiveness, from: 3Scler.

changeable, variable: 3Scler.

MORAL CONDUCT, mistakes in, with unwillingness to change: 3Ch-Bd./3Vine.

failure to learn from mistakes, heedlessness, from: 3Ch-Bd.

forcefulness of behavior, with disregard of others' needs, from: 3Vine.

MORAL FEELING, want of: 2Ch-Bd.

MOROSE: 2Chic. 2Horn. 3Must. 2Wld-O. 2Will.

depressive and gloomy mood, from: 3Must.

ill-tempered and resentful, from being: 3Will.

mental fatigue, lassitude and tendency to procrastination, from: 3Horn.

motivation and mental stimulation, lack of, from: 3Wld-O.

sullen retreat due to not feeling appreciated or attended to, from: 3Chic.

MORTIFICATION ailments after: 2Crb-A. Holly 2Pine Wat-V.

anger and upset feelings, from: 3Holly.

raising one's pride in defense to being offended, from: 3Wat-V.

regret, self-blame and guilt, from: 3Pine.

shame and humiliation, from: 3Crb-A.

MOTIVATION:

exaggerated: 2Rck-W. 3Verv.

fanaticism and overenthusiasm toward one's goals, with attempt to convert others, from: 3Verv.

quest for unduly harsh self-mastery and spiritual growth, with desire to inspire others, from: 3Rck-W.

lack of (See Boredom): Clem. Honey. 2Must. 3Wld-O. 2Wld-R.

MUTILATING his body: 3Cher-P.

NAKED, wants to be: 3Cher-P.

NERVOUSNESS (See Irritability; Sensitive; Timidity):

extreme: 3Cher-P. 2Imp. 2Rd-Ch. 3Rck-R. 2Verv.

fear and worry, incessant, in regard to welfare of loved ones, from: 3Rd-Ch.

fervency in one's endeavors with attempt to incite self and others to increased efforts of willpower, with mounting inner drive and nervous overexertion, from: 3Verv.

fragility of nerves, with frequent starting and underlying anxiety, from: 3Rck-R.

inner speed, tension and restlessness, tendency to sudden outbursts of impatience, from: 3Imp.

internal tension from overexerted effort to control mental balance and preserve calmness and sanity, from: 3Cher-P.

NYMPHOMANIA: Cher-P. 2Ch-Bd. Chic.

desire to gain attention and find appreciation, from: 3Chic.

impulsiveness, arising from immaturity and failure to learn from mistakes, due to: 3Ch-Bd.

sexual impulses that are carried out, though known to be inappropriate, from: 3Cher-P.

OBSTINATE: 2Ch-Bd. 2Chic. 2Verv. 3Vine

adherence to one's principles and viewpoints, with overenthusiasm and attempt to convert others, from: 3Verv.

forcefulness of opinion and behavior, with disregard for the position of others, from: 3Vine

heedlessness and failure to learn from mistakes, from: 3Ch-Bd

self-centered attitude in one's attempt to overcare for others, with obstinacy and sulkiness when not appreciated despite one's efforts: 3Chic.

OCCUPATION, ameliorates (See Business; necessary): 2Agr.

OFFENDED, easily: 3Chic. Holly 2Wat-V. 2Will.

feeling rejected and not appreciated, with self-pity, from: 3Chic.

feeling superior and expecting deference, from: 3Wat-V.

feeling treated unfairly and developing resentment, from: 3Will.

vexed and annoyed, from being: 3Holly

OVERWHELMED by tasks, duties, or emotional challenges: 3Elm

PANIC, attacks of: 3Cher-P. 3Rck-R.

fear of losing control and being subjected to attacks, with: 3Cher-P.

fright and rapid heart beat, with: 3Rck-R.

PARANOIA (See Delusions; persecuted).

PARENTING, complaints from:

anger, extreme, with great internal tension and threatened or actual abuse, although attempting to control it: 3Holly/3Cher-P.

fear and anxiety about children's safety and welfare, with nervousness: 3Rd-Ch.

impatience with children's disobedience, their emotional outbursts, and with having to adjust adult-pace to slower child-pace: 3Imp.

tension, increased and nervous overexertion from constant need to guide, control, watch and reprimand children: 3Verv./3Vine

overexertion (See Wearisome).

PERSISTS in nothing: 2Gent. 2Scler. 3Wld-O.

discouragement, lack of faith in one's work, and diminished perseverance, from: 3Gent.

disinterest and lack of motivation, from: 3Wld-O.

diversity of options and lack of decisive power, from: 3Scler.

PITIES herself: 3Chic. 2Heath. 2Will.

feeling unappreciated despite efforts made, from: 3Chic.

feeling unattended to and lonely, with need to find sympathetic listener, from: 3Heath.

feeling unfortunate and treated unfairly, from: 3Will.

PLANS, making many: 2Clem. 2Wh-Ch.

building dream castles, while neglecting the present: 3Clem.

preoccupation with plans of a worrisome and disturbing nature: 3Wh-Ch.

revengeful: 2Holly

PLAY, indisposition to play, in children: 2Ch-Bd. Clem. Gent. 3Wld-O. Wld-R.

absent-mindedness and daydreaming, from: 3Clem.

discouragement during play, due to minor obstacles, from: 3Gent.

inattentiveness and restless impulsiveness of mind, with easy distraction of focus: 3Ch-Bd.

motivation and stimulation, lack of, from: 3Wld-O.

resignation, apathy and helplessness, from: 3Wld-R.

PLEASURE, voluptuous ideas, only, in: 2Cher-P. Wld-O.

boredom and lack of motivational interests, from: 3Wld-O.

inability to free mind of compelling ideas and imaginations, from: 3Cher-P.

POWER, love of: 3Vine

POWERLESS, due to resignation: 3Wld-R.

PRAYING: 2Pine 2Verv.

guilt and desire for absolution, from: 3 Pine.

overzealous religious attitude, from: 3 Verv.

PRECOCITY: 2Wat-V.

PRESUMPTUOUS: 2Wat-V.

PRIDE: 3Wat-V.

PROSTRATION of mind: 3Horn. 2Must. 3Oak 3Oliv.

exhaustion, extreme, in mind and body, from: 3Oliv.

injuries to head, from: Horn. Must.

mind is prone to feel overshadowed or dampened: 3Must.

mind is prone to lack of clarity of consciousness: 3Horn.

introversion, depression, lack of motivation, from: 3Must.

mental fatigue, lack of power of concentration, with tendency to procrastination, from: 3Horn.

wearisome from overwork, with stoic perseverance and one-track mind, from: 3Oak

QUARRELSOME: 3Holly Will.

QUESTIONS, speaks continually in: 2Cer.

RAGE (See Anger): 3Cher-P. 3Holly 2Imp. 2Verv. Vine

　　headache, with: Cher-P.

　　kill people, tries to: 3Cher-P.

READING, averse to: 2Horn. 2Wld-O.

　　interest and motivation, lack of, from: 3Wld-O.

　　mental lassitude and lack of power of concentration, from: 3Horn.

REFUSES to take the medicine: Vine

RELIGIOUS affections: 2Pine 2Verv.

　　fanaticism: 3Verv.

　　guilt, exaggerated: 3Pine

REMINISCES with sadness about irretrievable past: 3Honey.

REMORSE: 3Pine

REPROACHES:

　　himself: 3Pine

　　others: 2Chic. 3Will.

　　　　feeling mistreated and unfortunate, due to another person's fault, from: 3Will.

　　　　feeling unappreciated despite service done, with self- pity, from: 3Chic.

REPULSIVE mood (See Loathing): 3Holly 2Will.

RESERVED: 3Wat-V.

RESIGNATION (See Indifference): Clem. Honey. 2Must. 3Wld-R.

REST, cannot, when things are not in proper place (See Conscientious): 2Agr. 2Pine

> tendency to self-reproach and heightened work ethic, from: 3Pine

> worry and restless need to accomplish tasks, from: 3Agr.

RESTLESSNESS: 3Agr. 2Cher-P. 2Ch-Bd. 3Imp. Rck-R. 2Verv.

> anxious: 2Agr. 2Cher-P. 2Rck-R.

>> fragility of nerves, starting and internal trembling, with: 3Rck-R.

>> pressure of compelling thoughts which threaten mental balance and create inner tension and agitation, from: 3Cher-P.

>> worry and internal disquiet, with need for peace in one's environment, from: 3Agr.

> conscience, of: Agr. 2Pine

>> guilt and self-reproach, from: 3Pine

>> worry about task completion, from: 3Agr.

> drives him from place to place: 2Agr. 2Imp.

> headache, during: 2Agr. 2Cher-P.

>> inner torture with attempt to stay cheerful on surface, from: 3Agr.

>> intense pain, with fear of losing sanity, from: 3Cher-P.

> inattentiveness and easy distraction of mind, from: 3Ch-Bd.

> internal speed and need to move and work fast, from: 3Imp.

> mental labor, during: 2Agr. 2Imp.

overenthusiasm and heightened tension in one's endeavors, with urge to incite oneself and others, from: 3Verv.

sitting, while: 2Agr. 2Imp.

REVERIES: 3Clem.

RIDICULE, mania to: 2Holly

ROVING about senseless, insane: 3Cher-P. 2Verv.

fervency of expression and forceful release of pent-up inner needs or impulses, from: 3Verv.

mental balance, loss of, after overexertion to suppress force of compelling internal impulses, from: 3Cher-P.

RUDENESS: 2Holly 2Vine

abusive attitude and disrespect toward others, from: 3Vine

allowing anger, vexation and annoyance to rule one's conduct, from: 3Holly

SADNESS: Beech Clem. Crb-A. Elm 2Gors. Honey. Lar. 2Must.Oak Pine 2Rck-W. 3Star-B. 2Sw-Ch. 2Wld-R. Will.

consolation aggravates: 2Chic.

continence, from: 2Rck-W.

critical attitude toward imperfect reality after loss of beautiful or beloved state, with unresolved sadness, from: 3Beech.

denial and suppression of desires, with underlying sadness and sense of loss, from: 3Rck-W.

depression and gloominess, from: 3Must.

despair, extreme, with loss of faith and meaningful aspiration, from: 3Sw-Ch.

embitterment over one's fate, with feeling unfortunate and victimized, from: 3Will.

grief, shock, trauma on emotional and cellular level, from: 3Star-B.

guilt and a burdened conscience, from: 3Pine

hopelessness, from: 3Gors.

injuries of the head, from: Must. Star-B.

> mind is prone to experience sadness and aftereffects of trauma: 3Star-B.

> mind is prone to feel less uplifted, tendency to feel gloomy: 3Must.

masturbation, from: 2Crb-A. Lar.

> self-esteem, loss of, from: 3Lar.

> shame, from: 3Crb-A.

misfortune, as if from: 2Will.

overwhelmed and subdued, from feeling: 3Elm

past happiness, loss of, with belief that it will never return, from: 3Honey.

resignation and indifference, with underlying unresolved sadness, from: 3Wld-R.

self-confidence, loss of, with feeling stifled and despondent, from: 3Lar.

sexual excitement, suppressed: Cher-P. 2Rck-W.

> forceful self-mastery, from: 3Rck-W.

>> mental imbalance and unwanted impulses, with: 3Cher-P.

shame and sense of failure, with despairing over unclean aspect of self, from: 3Crb-A.

slight, and undeserved, from: 2Will.

    stoic and heroic self-discipline despite hardship, with despondency, from: 3Oak

    unfulfilled longing, with belief that present cannot bring happiness, from: 3Clem.

    weep, cannot: 2Star-B.

SARCASM: 2Beech

SCORN: 2Beech Holly Wat-V.

    contempt and criticism, from: 3Beech

    pride and superiority, from: 3Wat-V.

    vexation and anger, from: 3Holly

SELFISHNESS: 2Chic. 2Heath. Imp. Vine Wat-V.

    assuming leadership and abusing power, with disrespect for the needs of others, from: 3Vine

    impatient urge to move and work fast, with disregard for another person's individual pace, from: 3Imp.

    inner loneliness and self-centered attitude, with overemphasis on one's personal needs and craving for attention and sympathy, from: 3Heath.

    self-centered need to overcare for and influence others, with expectation of appreciation and affection, from: 3Chic.

    superiority and pride, with aloofness toward others and expectation of deference, from: 3Wat-V.

SENSES, dullness of: 2Clem. 2Horn. 2Must.

    absent-mindedness and sleepiness, from: 3Clem.

    gloominess, introversion, depression, from: 3Must.

    mental lassitude and fatigue, with lack of strength of concentration and clarity, from: 3Horn.

SENSITIVE: 2Agr. 2Cent. 2Holly Rd-Ch. Rck-R. 3Waln

> cruelties, when hearing of: 2Waln.

> demands and needs of others, to: 3Cent. Rd-Ch.

>> desire to serve, from: 3Cent.

>>> worry and fear for the welfare of others, from: 3Rd-Ch.

> disharmony and quarrel, to: 3Agr.

> external impressions, to all: 3Waln.

>> times of emotional instability, during: 2Waln.

>> transitions of life, during: 3Waln.

> mental impressions, to: 3Waln.

> noise, to: 3Rck-R.

> pain, to unendurable: Agr. 2Cher-P.

> sensitivity of nervous system, from (See Nervousness): 2Rd-Ch. 3Rck-R.

>> fragility of nerves, with weakness, trembling, and easily aroused anxiety, from: 3Rck-R.

>> prolonged worry and fear for others, from: 3Rd-Ch.

> sensual impressions, to: 3Waln.

> vexations, to: 3Holly

SENTIMENTAL: 2Chic. Heath. 2Honey. Star-B.

> overemphasis on one's ailing, with need to find sympathy and comfort, from: 3Heath.

> reminiscences of past happiness considered lost, from: 3Honey.

> self-pity and sadness from loss of affection, from: 3Chic.

> underlying heartfelt grief, with: 3Star-B.

SERIOUS: Oak Rck-W.

> stoic, work-oriented attitude, with sense of hardship, from: 3Oak

> urge, self-imposed, or necessity to forgo pleasure and gratification of needs, from: 3Rck-W.

SERVITOR, too willing: 3Cent.

SHAMELESS: Cher-P. Ch-Bd.

> immaturity, impulsiveness, and heedlessness, from: 3Ch-Bd.

> unbridling of sexual needs, although resisted to initially, from: 3Cher-P.

SHRIEKING with the pain: Cher-P.

SITS wrapped in deep, sad thoughts, as if, and notices nothing: Must.

SLANDER, disposition to (See Hatred): 2Holly Will.

SLOWNESS of purpose: 3Wld-O.

SMILING, foolish: Cer.

SPEECH :

> childish: 2Ch-Bd.

> embarrassed: 2Cer. 2Mim.

>> shyness and timidity, from: 3Mim.

>> uncertainty and lack of decisive power, from: 3Cer.

> extravagant: Wat-V.

> foolish: 3Cer.

> hasty: Cer. 2Ch-Bd.

>> impulsiveness of mind and lack of restful concentration, from: 3Ch-Bd.

uncertainty and embarrassment, from: 3Cer.

hesitating (See Speech; embarrassed): 3Cer. 2Mim.

STARTING: 2Cher-P. 2Clem. 2Imp. 3Rck-R. 2Verv.

absent-mindedness and sleepiness, from: 3Clem.

anxious: 2Rck-R.

anxious, from downward motion: 2Rck-R.

easily: 2Clem. 3Rck-R.

fragility of nerves, with frequent shocks of anxiety and internal trembling, from: 3Rck-R.

fright, from: 3Rck-R.

irritability and mental and physical tension, from (See Nervousness): 2Cher-P. 2Imp. 2Verv.

noise, from: 2Clem. 3Rck-R.

STOIC perseverance: 3Oak

STRANGE things, impulse to do: 3Cher-P.

STRIKING (See Abusive): 2Cher-P. 3Holly Imp. Verv. Vine

STUPEFACTION (See Senses): 2Clem. 2Horn. 2Must.

SUCCEEDS, never: Gent. 2Lar. Mim.

fearful attitude, shyness and anticipation of failure, from: 3Mim.

perseverance, lack of, and discouragement, from: 3Gent.

self-confidence, lack of, and distrust in one's capacities, from: 3Lar.

SUGGESTIONS, will not receive: 2Ch-Bd. 2Vine

heedlessness and failure to learn from mistakes, from: 3Ch-Bd.

willful urge to be in control, from: 3Vine

SUICIDAL disposition: 3Cher-P. 3Sw-Ch.

> attempt to escape unbearable anguish, with loss of faith, hope, and soul peace, from: 3Sw-Ch.

> mental, emotional strain, severe, with threatened loss of mental balance, with recurring impulsive and suicidal thoughts, from: 3Cher-P.

SULKY (See Pities herself): 3Chic. 2Heath. 2Will.

SUPERSTITIOUS: 3Asp.

SURPRISES, pleasant, affections, after: 2Verv.

SUSPICIOUS: Asp. 3Holly 2Will.

> hatred, malice, with projection of own emotions onto others, from: 3Holly

> resentment, embitterment, with blaming others for one's unhappiness, from: 3Will.

> superstition, unreasonable and fearful foreboding, from: 3Asp.

SYMPATHETIC: 2Cent.

TALK:

> desires to, to some one: 3Heath.

> slow learning to: 2Cer. 3Ch-Bd.

>> immature capacity for retention, with easy distraction of mind, from: 3Ch-Bd.

>> inner uncertainty and lack of self-assurance, from: 3Cer.

TALKING, pleasure in his own talking: 2Heath.

TALKS of nothing but one subject (See Delusions; fixed) (Monomania): Cher-P. 2Heath. Wh-Ch.

> overemphasis on personal problems and urgent need to find sympathy, from: 3Heath.

TEARS things (See Abusive): 2Cher-P. 3Holly Imp. Verv. Vine

THEORIZING: Wh-Ch.

THINKING:

>aversion to (See Reading): 3Horn. 2Wld-O.

>complaints, of, aggravates: 2Crb-A. 2Wh-Ch.

>>obsession with symptoms, with despairing wish to be cleansed of them, from: 3Crb-A.

>>preoccupation with and unceasing anxious worry about symptoms, from: 3Wh-Ch.

THOUGHTS:

>disgusting thoughts with nausea: 2Crb-A.

>frightful: 2Rck-R.

>frightful, on seeing blood or a knife: 2Cher-P.

>future, of the: Clem.

>intrude and crowd around each other: Agr. 2Cher-P. Scler. 2Wh-Ch.

>>impulsive thoughts of shocking content intrude against one's wishes: 3Cher-P.

>>incessant worry and concerns, creating internal restlessness and lack of mental peace, from: 3Agr.

>>multiple impressions impinge upon the mind, with loss of overview, especially in decision-making process: 3Scler.

>>preoccupation and worry of a severe or fearful kind circle in the mind continuously, interfering with enjoyment of the present moment: 3Wh-Ch.

>sexual: 2Cher-P. Wh-Ch.

persistent (See Thoughts; intrude): Agr. 3Cher-P. 2Crb-A. 3Wh-Ch.

obsession with shameful symptom or topic and loss of proportion in regard to true importance of problem, from: 3Crb-A.

homicide: 2Cher-P.

thinks mind and body are separated: Clem.

unpleasant subjects, haunted by (See Thoughts; intrude): 2Asp. 3Cher-P. 3Wh-Ch.

foreboding, superstitions, eerie fears, from: 3Asp.

rapid, quick: 2Cher-P. Imp. 2Rck-R. Verv.

anxiety and tremulous nerves, from: 3 Rck-R.

impulsive thinking and threatened loss of mental control, from: 3Cher-P.

inner fervency and overenthusiasm, from: 3Verv.

internal impatience and hurry, from: 3Imp.

repetition, of: 2Cher-P. 2Wh-Ch.

ceaseless worry about recurring subject matter, from: 3Wh-Ch.

repeated, unwanted thought impulses, from: 3Cher-P.

tormenting (See Thoughts; intrude): 2Agr. 3Cher-P. 3Wh-Ch.

sexual: 2Cher-P.

vanishing of: 2Clem. 2Horn.

absent-mindedness and drowsiness, from: 3Clem.

mental fatigue and lack of power of concentration, from: 3Horn.

wandering: 2Ch-Bd. Clem. Honey. 2Horn.

    future, with longing, to: 3Clem.

    inattentiveness, from: 3Ch-Bd.

    mental lassitude and procrastination, from: 3Horn.

    past, with nostalgia, to: 3Honey.

THREATENING: 2Cher-P. 3Holly 2Vine.

    abusive attitude and urge to use power against others, from:3Vine

    anger or hatred, from: 3Holly

    mounting tension and fear of losing control, from: 3Cher-P.

THROWS things (See Abusive): 3Holly

TIME, fritters away his: 2Wld-O.

TIMIDITY (See Inhibited): 2Cer. 2Lar. 3Mim.

    appearing in public, about: 3Mim.

    bashful: 2Cer. 3Mim.

TORMENTS everyone with his complaints: 2Heath.

TORPOR: 2Clem.

TRANQUILITY: 2Wld-R.

TRAVEL, desire to: 2Agr. Clem. 2Wld-O.

    desire to find purpose and destiny, since unmotivated under present circumstances, from: 3Wld-O.

    inner restlessness and need for adventure, from: 3Agr.

    unfulfilled longing for love and adventure, from: 3Clem.

TRENDS, easily influenced by: 2Cer. 3Waln.

    internal instability and vulnerability, with easily impressed mind, from: 3Waln.

uncertainty of personal self-expression, lack of self-assurance, and need to find approval by others, from: 3Cer.

UNATTRACTIVE, things seem: 2Beech 2Crb-A.

critical and intolerant, based on high personal standards of perfection, from being: 3Beech

rejecting shameful aspect of self and ascribing same unattractive quality to outside world, from: 3Crb-A.

UNBEARABLE pains: 2Cher-P. Sw-Ch.

suicidal anxiety, with: 3Cher-P.

unbearable mental anguish and loss of all faith, with: 3Sw-Ch.

UNCONSCIOUSNESS: 3Clem.

UNDERTAKES:

lacks willpower to undertake anything (See Discipline; lack of): 2Ch-Bd. 2Horn. 2Wld-O.

many things, perseveres in nothing (See Persists): 2Gent. 2Scler. 3Wld-O.

nothing, lest he fail (See Fear; undertaking): 2Cer. 3Lar. 3Mim.

UNFORTUNATE, feels: 2Will.

UNFRIENDLY humor: 2Beech 3Holly 2Will.

correcting others and finding fault with them, from: 3Beech

embittered and dissatisfied, from being: 3Will.

sensitive to vexations and irritations, from being: 3Holly

USEFUL, desire to be: 2Cent. Chic.

desire to serve others in kindness, even to the detriment of one's own plans or one's health, from: 3Cent.

desire to serve, tinged with need to bind others closely to oneself and find appreciation, from: 3Chic.

VIOLENT (See Abusive): 3Cher-P. 3Holly 2Imp. 2Verv. 2Vine

pain, from: 2Cher-P.

WANDER, desires to (See Travel): 2Agr. Clem. 2Wld-O.

WANTS nothing: 2Wld-R.

WASHING always, her hands: 2Crb-A. 2Pine

guilt, self-reproach and need to be free of burden of conscience, from: 3Pine

shame about unclean aspect of self and deep-seated urge tobe cleansed of it, with fear of contamination, from: 3Crb-A.

WEARISOME: 3Cent. 2Horn. 3Oak 3Oliv.

disciplined overwork, from: 3Oak

exhaustion in mind and body, extreme, from: 3Oliv.

lassitude, from: 3Horn.

serving others at own expense, from: 3Cent.

WEARY of life: 2Horn. 2Must. 2Oliv. 3Wld-O. Will.

deeply felt exhaustion in mind and body, from: 3Oliv.

depression and sunken, gloomy mental state with joylessness, from: 3Must.

embitterment over one's fate, feels left out of the joys of lifeand seeks blame outside of self: 3Will.

fatigue and lack of vibrancy, with urge to procrastinate, from: 3Horn.

motivation, purpose, and direction, lack of, from: 3Wld-O.

WEEPING: 3Chic. 2Heath. 2Star-B.

    anger, after: 2Holly

    consolation aggravates: 2Chic.

    grief, shock, and trauma, from: 3Star-B.

    inner loneliness and need for sympathy and attention, from: 3Heath.

    offended or unappreciated, with belief that one deserves better, from feeling: 3Chic.

    pitied, if he believes he is: 2Chic.

    sad thoughts, at: 2Star-B.

    vexation, from: 2Holly

WELL, says he is when very sick: 2Agr.

WICKED disposition: 2Holly

WILD FEELING in head: Scler.

WILDNESS from vexation: 2Holly

WILL, feels as if he had two: Cher-P.

WOMEN, aversion to: 2Will.

WORK:

    aversion to mental (See Dullness): 2Clem. 3Horn. 3Wld-O.

    burdensome, yet persevered in: 3Oak

    discouragement from obstacles, during: 3Gent.

    overwhelming: 3Elm

    procrastination from lassitude, before: 3Horn.

WORRY (See Thoughts; intrude): 3Agr. Mim. 3Wh-Ch.

    anxious worry, with timid attitude and reluctance to go forward: 3Mim.

    overcareful: 2Mim.

⌘

BIBLIOGRAPHY

Sources Cited and Additional Sources

American Psychiatric Association. *Diagnostic and Statistical Manual of Mental Disorders.* 4th ed. Washington, D.C.: American Psychiatric Association, 1994.

Bach, E. *The Twelve Healers and Other Remedies.* London: C. W. Daniel, 1936.

Barnard, Julian, ed. *Collected Writings of Edward Bach.* Hereford, Eng.: Flower Remedy Programme, 1987.

Barnard, Julian and Martine. *The Healing Herbs of Edward Bach.* Hereford, Eng.: Bach Educational Programme, 1988.

Green, Stephen A. *The Psychology of Physical Illness.* Washington, D.C.: American Psychiatric Press, 1986.

Huebschmann, H. "Psyche und Tuberkulose." In *Beiträge aus der Allgemeinen Medizin.* Vol. VIII. Stuttgart: Enke, 1952.

Kent, James Tyler. *Repertory of the Homoeopathic Materia Medica.* 6th ed. 1957; rpt. New Delhi: B. Jain, 1991.

Little, Elbert L. *The Audobon Society Field Guide to North American Trees: Eastern Region.* New York: Alfred A. Knopf, 1980.

——————. *The Audobon Society Field Guide to North American Trees: Western Region.* New York: Alfred A. Knopf, 1980.

Luban-Plozza, B., W. Pöldinger, and F. Kröger. *Psychosomatic Disorders in General Practice.* Trans. George Blythe from 3rd German ed. Berlin: Springer, 1992.

Niering, William A., and Nancy C. Olmstead. *The Audobon Society Field Guide to North American Wildflowers: Eastern Region.* New York: Alfred A. Knopf, 1979.

Perry, S., A. Frances, and J. Clarkin. *A DSM-III-R Casebook of Treatment Selection.* New York: Brunner & Mazel, 1990.

Reid, William H., and Michael G. Wise. *DSM-III-R Training Guide.* New York: Brunner & Mazel, 1989.

Rosenman, R. H., _and M. Friedman. "The Possible Relationship of the Emotions to Clinical Coronary Heart Disease." In *Hormones and Artherosclerosis.* Ed. Gregory Pincus. New York: Academic Press, 1959.

Spellenberg, Richard. *The Audobon Society Field Guide to North American Wildflowers: Western Region.* New York: Alfred A. Knopf, 1979.

Staehelin, B. "Über die diagnostischen und psychotherapeutischen Möglichkeiten des einfachen Sprechstundengesprächs, dargestellt an drei Fallbeispielen mit Symptomen des Verdauungstraktes." *Praxis,* 52 (1963), 767-75.

Weeks, Nora. *The Medical Discoveries of Edward Bach, Physician.* London: C. W. Daniel, 1940.

Weeks, Nora, and Victor Bullen. *The Bach Flower Remedies: Illustrations and Preparations.* 2nd ed. Saffron Walden, Eng.: C. W. Daniel, 1990.

COMPUTER SOFTWARE

Richardson-Boedler, Cornelia. *The Richardson-Boedler Bach Repertory.* San Rafael, Calif.: Kent Homeopathic Associates, 1993.

Warkentin, David, ed. *MacRepertory*. San Rafael, Calif.: Kent Homeopathic Associates, 1987.

—————————, ed. *Reference Works*. San Rafael, Calif.: Kent Homeopathic Associates, 1990.

ADDITIONAL READING

Chancellor, Philip M. *Handbook of the Bach Flower Remedies*. 1971; rpt. New Canaan, Conn.: Keats Publishing, 1980.

Scheffer, Mechthild. *Bach Flower Therapy: Theory and Practice*. Trans. A. R. Meuss from 2nd German ed. 1984. Rochester, Vt.: Healing Arts Press, 1987.

Staehelin, B. *Haben und Sein: Ein medizinpsychologischer Vorschlag als Ergänzung zum Materialismus der heutigen Wissenschaft*. Zürich: Theologischer Verlag, 1969.

ABOUT THE AUTHOR

Dr. Cornelia Richardson-Boedler, board-certified naturopathic physician, licensed psychotherapist and forensic examiner in medicine, has completed a Doctorate in Homeopathic Medicine at the British Institute of Homoeopathy, where she is also a faculty member, tutor, Fellow, and director and instructor of Bach Flower Studies.

Born and raised in Germany, her initial academic studies were held at the University of Bonn, Germany, where she completed the "Grundstudium," comparable to a Bachelor of Arts degree, in the subjects English and Sport Science. A scholarship brought her to the United States, where she earned Bachelor of Arts degrees in the subjects Psychology, English and German. Her long-standing interest in healing broadened and led her to a Master of Arts degree in Psychology, which, among other topics, emphasized personal/ spiritual growth and the Jungian model of self-integration. Subsequently, she worked as a recreational therapist with mentally/physically handicapped children and teens. From here she widened her scope of service to Marriage, Family, and Child Therapy, until she found in homeopathic/ naturopathic medicine, as well as in the study and research of topics of standard medicine, the avenue to encompass the totality of man, thus completing her approach to healing.

She has published numerous articles, given lectures and seminars, and authored the book *Applying Bach Flower Therapy to the Healing Profession of Homeopathy,* which also contains the contents of the *Richardson-Boedler Bach Repertory.* She has also authored the treatment guide *Applying Homeopathy and Bach Flower Therapy to Psychosomatic Illness.* Currently, within the topic of homeopathic medicine, she is writing mainly on homeopathic materia medica in light of the Doctrine of Signatures, thereby assessing biological, toxicological aspects of the medicinal sources.